GUIDE TO
BREAST
CARE FOR
ONCOLOGY
NURSES

Edited by Suzanne M. Mahon, RN, DNSc, AOCN®, AGN-BC

Oncology Nursing Society
Pittsburgh, Pennsylvania

ONS Publications Department
Publisher and Director of Publications: William A. Tony, BA, CQIA
Senior Editorial Manager: Lisa M. George, BA
Assistant Editorial Manager: Amy Nicoletti, BA, JD
Acquisitions Editor: John Zaphyr, BA, MEd
Associate Staff Editors: Casey S. Kennedy, BA, Andrew Petyak, BA
Design and Production Administrator: Dany Sjoen
Editorial Assistant: Judy Holmes

Library of Congress Cataloging-in-Publication Data
Names: Mahon, Suzanne M., editor. | Oncology Nursing Society, issuing body.
Title: Guide to breast care for oncology nurses / edited by Suzanne M. Mahon.
Description: Pittsburgh, Pennsylvania : Oncology Nursing Society, [2018] |
  Includes bibliographical references and index.
Identifiers: LCCN 2017044446 (print) | LCCN 2017043118 (ebook) | ISBN
  9781635930061 (pbk.) | ISBN 9781635930115
Subjects: | MESH: Breast Neoplasms | Breast–diagnostic imaging | Cancer Care
  Facilities
Classification: LCC RC280.B8 (ebook) | LCC RC280.B8 (print) | NLM WP 870 |
  DDC 616.99/449–dc23
LC record available at https://lccn.loc.gov/2017044446

Publisher's Note

This book is published by the Oncology Nursing Society (ONS). ONS neither represents nor guarantees that the practices described herein will, if followed, ensure safe and effective patient care. The recommendations contained in this book reflect ONS's judgment regarding the state of general knowledge and practice in the field as of the date of publication. The recommendations may not be appropriate for use in all circumstances. Those who use this book should make their own determinations regarding specific safe and appropriate patient care practices, taking into account the personnel, equipment, and practices available at the hospital or other facility at which they are located. The editor and publisher cannot be held responsible for any liability incurred as a consequence from the use or application of any of the contents of this book. Figures and tables are used as examples only. They are not meant to be all-inclusive, nor do they represent endorsement of any particular institution by ONS. Mention of specific products and opinions related to those products do not indicate or imply endorsement by ONS. Websites mentioned are provided for information only; the hosts are responsible for their own content and availability. Unless otherwise indicated, dollar amounts reflect U.S. dollars.

ONS publications are originally published in English. Publishers wishing to translate ONS publications must contact ONS about licensing arrangements. ONS publications cannot be translated without obtaining written permission from ONS. (Individual tables and figures that are reprinted or adapted require additional permission from the original source.) Because translations from English may not always be accurate or precise, ONS disclaims any responsibility for inaccuracies in words or meaning that may occur as a result of the translation. Readers relying on precise information should check the original English version.

Printed in the United States of America

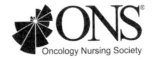

Innovation • Excellence • Advocacy

Contributors

Editor

Suzanne M. Mahon, RN, DNSc, AOCN®, AGN-BC
Professor, Internal Medicine/Division of Hematology/Oncology
Professor, Adult Nursing, School of Nursing
Saint Louis University
St. Louis, Missouri
Chapter 2. Risk Assessment

Authors

Tara S. Baney, CRNP, MS, ANP-BC, AOCNP®
Nurse Practitioner
Penn State Health
State College, Pennsylvania
Chapter 7. Chemotherapy and Biotherapy

Heidi Basinger, MS, BSN, RN, NE-BC
Director of Nursing
The James Cancer Hospital and Solove Research
    Institute
Columbus, Ohio
Chapter 1. Comprehensive Breast Centers

Elfrida Bauer, BA, RN, OCN®, CBCN®
Assistant Nurse Manager
The University of Texas MD Anderson Cancer Center
Radiation Treatment Center at Presbyterian Kaseman
    Hospital
Albuquerque, New Mexico
Chapter 6. Radiation Therapy

Susan Beikman, MSN, CRNP, AOCNP®
Nurse Practitioner
Women's Cancer Center
Magee-Womens Hospital of the University
    of Pittsburgh Medical Center
Pittsburgh, Pennsylvania
Chapter 8. Endocrine Therapy

Janet Cogswell, RN, MSN, ACNS-BC, AOCN®
Clinical Research Nurse
Memorial Sloan Kettering Cancer Center
Basking Ridge, New Jersey
Chapter 6. Radiation Therapy

**Sharon Gentry, RN, MSN, AOCN®, CBCN®, CBEC,
    ONN-CG**
Breast Nurse Navigator
Novant Health Derrick L. Davis Cancer Center
Winston-Salem, North Carolina
Chapter 10. Breast Navigation

Patricia Gordon, MSN, CRNP, NP-C
Nurse Practitioner
Women's Cancer Center
Magee-Womens Hospital of the University
    of Pittsburgh Medical Center
Pittsburgh, Pennsylvania
Chapter 8. Endocrine Therapy

Marcelle Kaplan, MS, RN, CBCN®
Oncology Nurse Consultant, Self-Employed
Merrick, New York
Chapter 9. Side Effect Management

Joanne Lester, PhD, CRNP, ANP-BC, AOCN®
Clinical Research Nurse Practitioner
The Ohio State University, Division of Surgical
    Oncology
Columbus, Ohio
*Chapter 1. Comprehensive Breast Centers; Chapter 4.
Pathology and Staging; Chapter 5. Surgical Care*

Deborah K. Mayer, PhD, ANP-BC, AOCN®, FAAN
Professor and Director of Cancer Survivorship
University of North Carolina Lineberger Comprehen-
    sive Cancer Center
Chapel Hill, North Carolina
Chapter 11. Survivorship Care

Kristen McGarry, RN, BSN, OCN®
Clinical Nurse IV
Memorial Sloan Kettering Cancer Center
Basking Ridge, New Jersey
Chapter 6. Radiation Therapy

Anna Kate Owens, MSN, RN, FNP
Nurse Practitioner
University of North Carolina Lineberger Comprehen-
    sive Cancer Center
Chapel Hill, North Carolina
Chapter 11. Survivorship Care

Marlon G. Saria, PhD, RN, AOCNS®, FAAN
Oncology Clinical Nurse Specialist
Director, Center for Quality and Outcomes Research
Pacific Neuroscience Institute and John Wayne
    Cancer Institute
Providence Saint John's Health Center
Santa Monica, California
Chapter 7. Chemotherapy and Biotherapy

Lusine Tumyan, MD
Assistant Clinical Professor
Section Chief, Women's Imaging
Department of Radiology
City of Hope
Duarte, California
Chapter 3. Breast Imaging

Mary Ann Zalewski, MSN, CRNP, AOCNP®
Nurse Practitioner
Women's Cancer Center
Magee-Womens Hospital of the University
    of Pittsburgh Medical Center
Pittsburgh, Pennsylvania
Chapter 8. Endocrine Therapy

Disclosure

Editors and authors of books and guidelines provided by the Oncology Nursing Society are expected to disclose to the readers any significant financial interest or other relationships with the manufacturer(s) of any commercial products.

A vested interest may be considered to exist if a contributor is affiliated with or has a financial interest in
commercial organizations that may have a direct or indirect interest in the subject matter. A "financial interest"
may include, but is not limited to, being a shareholder in the organization; being an employee of the commercial
organization; serving on an organization's speakers bureau; or receiving research funding from the organization.
An "affiliation" may be holding a position on an advisory board or some other role of benefit to the commercial
organization. Vested interest statements appear in the front matter for each publication.

Contributors are expected to disclose any unlabeled or investigational use of products discussed in their content. This information is acknowledged solely for the information of the readers.

The contributors provided the following disclosure and vested interest information:

Sharon Gentry, RN, MSN, AOCN®, CBCN®, CBEC, ONN-CG: Academy of Oncology Nurse and Patient Navigators,
    leadership position and honoraria; Pfizer, honoraria

Marlon G. Saria, PhD, RN, AOCNS®, FAAN: Brain Cancer Research Institute, John Wayne Cancer Institute, San
    Diego Brain Tumor Foundation, U.S. Department of the Air Force, leadership positions; CancerLife, consultant;
    ICU Medical, honoraria

Contents

Introduction

Knowledge and concepts involving the prevention, early detection, and treatment of breast cancer, as well as the long-term needs of individuals diagnosed with the disease, are continually evolving. Oncology nurses are constantly challenged to incorporate this knowledge into their care and to respond to questions about breast cancer. The importance of this role should not be underestimated. Oncology nurses guide patients at risk for and diagnosed with breast cancer through the cancer trajectory.

Epidemiology

Breast cancer is a feared disease for men and women, and with good reason. For 2017, the American Cancer Society (ACS, 2017a) estimated 252,710 new cases of invasive breast cancer and 63,410 new cases of in situ breast cancer diagnosed in women and 2,470 new cases in men. This translates to one in eight women being diagnosed with breast cancer over her lifetime. Although rates continue to decrease slowly, approximately 41,070 deaths (40,610 in women and 460 in men) were expected in 2017 (ACS, 2017a).

The 5-, 10-, and 15-year relative survival rates for all female breast cancers are 89%, 83%, and 78%, respectively (ACS, 2017a). Currently, an estimated 3.5 million women are living with a diagnosis of breast cancer (ACS, 2017a). That number is expected to rise to approximately 4.6 million women in 2026 (ACS, 2016). Female breast cancer survival rates have increased over time because of widespread mammography use leading to earlier detection and improvements in treatment (ACS, 2017b).

Trends in Diagnosis and Treatment

Approximately 61% of breast cancers are diagnosed at a localized stage, for which the five-year relative survival is 99% (ACS, 2017a). This is largely due to increased use of mammography. The Patient Protection and Affordable Care Act requires that Medicare and all new health insurance plans fully cover screening mammograms without any out-of-pocket expense for patients (ACS, 2017a). According to the most recent data available, among women aged 40 years and older, only 56% had a mammogram in the past year and 73% had one in the past two years (ACS, 2017a). Rates are lowest in women who are uninsured or underinsured. The Centers for Disease

Control and Prevention's National Breast and Cervical Cancer Early Detection Program, which was established in 1990 to improve access to breast cancer screening and diagnostic services in uninsured women, has estimated that the program only reaches about 11% of eligible women because of difficulty in recruiting women and funding shortages (Howard et al., 2015). Clearly there is room for improvement to engage more women aged 40 years and older in regular mammography.

Treatment for breast cancer can involve breast-conserving surgery such as lumpectomy or partial mastectomy and radiation therapy or mastectomy. In some women, mastectomy is the preferred option because of locally advanced stage, large or multiple tumors, or previous radiation. Recently, more patients who are eligible for breast conservation are choosing mastectomy for a variety of reasons, including reluctance to undergo radiation therapy or fear of recurrence (ACS, 2016). The most recent data available show that the number of women with early-stage disease in one breast who undergo contralateral prophylactic mastectomy has increased from 5% of total mastectomies in 1998 to 30% in 2011 (ACS, 2016). Although a bilateral mastectomy nearly eliminates the risk of developing a new breast cancer, it does not improve long-term breast cancer survival for the majority of women and is associated with potential harms. The American Society of Breast Surgeons recommends that contralateral prophylactic mastectomy be discouraged for patients with an average risk of contralateral breast cancer (Tuttle et al., 2017). Potential complications of a contralateral prophylactic mastectomy include an increased risk of bleeding, wound infection, necrosis, and embolism (Momoh et al., 2017). Women choosing a surgical approach to treat their breast cancer need honest and comprehensive information and psychosocial support so that they can make the appropriate decision for their individual situation.

Treatment for breast cancer now includes multiple chemotherapy agents, targeted therapy, radiation therapy, and hormonal manipulation. Each of these modalities continues to expand, and many research trials are currently underway. Decisions about appropriate systemic therapy, including chemotherapy, hormone therapy, and targeted therapy, are dependent on multiple factors, including the size of the tumor, the number of lymph nodes involved, the presence of estrogen or progesterone hormone receptors on cancer cells, and the amount of HER2 protein made by the cancer cells. Approximately 84% of women diagnosed with breast cancer will test positive for hormone receptors, and 14% will test positive for *HER2* gene amplification (ACS, 2016). For premenopausal women, the standard hormonal treatment is tamoxifen for at least five years. For postmenopausal women, hormonal treatment may include tamoxifen or an aromatase inhibitor for 5–10 years (ACS, 2017a). Oncology nurses are challenged to help and encourage patients to continue to take these agents for 5–10 years. Genomic tests of the tumor can help predict recurrence and are routinely used. Oncology nurses need to ensure that patients understand the meaning of these results and support them as they make decisions about systemic therapy (National Comprehensive Cancer Network®, 2017a).

Psychosocial Challenges

The body image changes that result from breast cancer surgery and related treatments serve as a constant reminder of the diagnosis. Role changes during treatment disrupt many family routines. After treatment, women need to adjust to and find a new normalcy. The psychosocial significance of the female breast in modern society compounds the ramifications of the diagnosis and associated treatment (Campbell-Enns & Woodgate, 2015). The female breast plays a significant role in nurturing and motherhood, as well as femininity and sexuality. Breast cancer threatens women's self-image and roles in her family and society. Following a diagnosis of breast cancer, women are challenged to restructure their self-image (Campbell-Enns & Woodgate, 2015).

The psychosocial ramifications for men diagnosed with breast cancer are also substantial. Only 1% of all breast cancers occur in men (ACS, 2017a). Most literature and emotional supports are geared toward women, so the unique needs of male patients are underappreciated and often ignored (Freedman & Partridge, 2017). The color pink is universally associated with breast cancer and has raised awareness about the malignancy and helped to raise money for breast cancer research (ACS, 2017a). Unfortunately, the color pink also serves as a constant and visual reminder that breast cancer is a female disease (Farrell et al., 2014). Limited research suggests that hot flashes and sexual dysfunction are very common and distressful in men (Freedman & Partridge, 2017). Optimal symptom management strategies are uncertain, and it can be difficult for men to find other male patients who can advise them on what to expect during and after breast cancer treatment.

Genetic testing has enabled the identification of individuals who have an elevated risk for developing cancer but has created a new set of psychosocial challenges (National Comprehensive Cancer Network, 2017b). Families worry about hereditary susceptibility and whether a child has inherited an increased risk for developing malignancy. Although genetic testing enables women to better understand their risks and choices available to manage the risk, it also brings about intense psychosocial reactions and ramifications. Individuals with hereditary risk live with uncertainty, including if, when, or where they will develop a malignancy, as well as the need to undergo extensive surveillance and cancer screening, making decisions about risk-reducing surgery, and dealing with the impact of the diagnosis on family relationships (Mahon, 2014).

The diagnosis of breast cancer is accompanied by many unknowns, including prognostic factors, treatment issues, and the reactions of family and friends to the diagnosis. These unknowns contribute to stress with the diagnosis. The psychological care of these patients and their families requires ongoing intervention by healthcare providers. For patients whose breast cancer cannot be cured and who will ultimately die of the disease, there is an ongoing need to recognize and implement palliative care interventions in a timely fashion.

Survivorship

The acute toxicities associated with surgery and adjuvant therapy can be significant and include hair loss, nail and skin changes, mouth sores, loss of appetite, nausea and vomiting, diarrhea, neutropenia, thrombocytopenia, and fatigue (ACS, 2016). Many research efforts are ongoing to determine how to more accurately prevent, assess, and manage these side effects. In addition to short-term side effects, many breast cancer survivors must cope with long-term consequences, including early menopause, osteoporosis, lymphedema, weight gain, cardiovascular damage, neuropathy, and cognitive changes (ACS, 2017a). Addressing the needs of this patient population through tertiary prevention practices is an ever-expanding role for nurses. Current evidence-based strategies for managing both short- and long-term toxicities and complications associated with breast cancer treatment are available on the Oncology Nursing Society's website (www.ons.org).

Research in breast cancer biology, detection, prevention, and treatment continues. Researchers are actively looking for ways to detect breast cancer as early as possible. Much effort is being made to find effective and tolerable prevention strategies. Genetic markers continue to be identified to better stratify risk. Management of the long-term complications of surgery and treatment continues to pose challenges to healthcare providers. Women need to continue to be offered clinical trials to build an evidence-based practice for the management of breast cancer.

Implications for Nurses

Many issues in breast cancer care are controversial. Patients and healthcare providers need to consider all facets and options, and patients need to make choices that are congruent and appropriate with their value systems and place in life. In some cases, no single correct answer exists.

Many resources are available to healthcare providers who care for individuals with breast cancer. Evidence-based guidelines and information are readily available from the American Cancer Society, American Society for Radiation Oncology, American Society of Clinical Oncology, National Cancer Institute, National Comprehensive Cancer Network, and Oncology Nursing Society. Oncology nurses need to be aware of these guidelines and resources and use the information to provide safe and effective clinical care.

In the age of technology, many individuals turn to the Internet for healthcare information. Some of this information is not reliable. Oncology nurses need to assess the educational needs of patients and families and provide them with accurate information in a variety of formats, including reputable, monitored websites with appropriate and current information.

For many individuals diagnosed with breast cancer, oncology nurses truly make an enormous difference in how they cope with the treatment and its associated complications. Different needs and concerns accompany each phase of the breast cancer trajectory. Nurses are challenged to provide information and care in a way that promotes health, hope, and well-being for the patients and families affected by the diagnosis of breast cancer.

References

American Cancer Society. (2016). *Cancer treatment and survivorship facts and figures 2016–2017.* Atlanta, GA: Author.

American Cancer Society. (2017a). *Breast cancer facts and figures 2017–2018.* Atlanta, GA: Author.

American Cancer Society. (2017b). *Cancer facts and figures 2017.* Atlanta, GA: Author.

Campbell-Enns, H., & Woodgate, R. (2015). The psychosocial experiences of women with breast cancer across the lifespan: A systematic review protocol. *JBI Database of Systematic Reviews and Implementation Reports, 13,* 112–121. doi:10.11124/jbisrir-2015-1795

Farrell, E., Borstelmann, N., Meyer, F., Partridge, A., Winer, E., & Ruddy, K. (2014). Male breast cancer networking and telephone support group: A model for supporting a unique population. *Psycho-Oncology, 23,* 956–958. doi:10.1002/pon.3519

Freedman, R.A., & Partridge, A.H. (2017). Emerging data and current challenges for young, old, obese, or male patients with breast cancer. *Clinical Cancer Research, 23,* 2647–2654. doi:10.1158/1078-0432.ccr-16-2552

Howard, D.H., Tangka, F.K.L., Royalty, J., Dalzell, L.P., Miller, J., O'Hara, B., ... Hall, I.J. (2015). Breast cancer screening of underserved women in the USA: Results from the National Breast and Cervical Cancer Early Detection Program, 1998–2012. *Cancer Causes and Control, 26,* 657–668. doi:10.1007/s10552-015-0553-0

Mahon, S.M. (2014). Providing care for previvors: Implications for oncology nurses. *Clinical Journal of Oncology Nursing, 18,* 21–24. doi:10.1188/14.CJON.21-24

Momoh, A.O., Cohen, W.A., Kidwell, K.M., Hamill, J.B., Qi, J., Pusic, A.L., ... Matros, E. (2017). Trade-offs associated with contralateral prophylactic mastectomy in women choosing breast reconstruction: Results of a prospective multicenter cohort. *Annals of Surgery, 266,* 158–164. doi:10.1097/sla.0000000000001840

National Comprehensive Cancer Network. (2017a). *NCCN Clinical Practice Guidelines in Oncology (NCCN Guidelines®): Breast cancer* [v.3.2017]. Retrieved from https://www.nccn.org/professionals/physician_gls/pdf/breast.pdf

National Comprehensive Cancer Network. (2017b). *NCCN Clinical Practice Guidelines in Oncology (NCCN Guidelines®): Genetic/familial high-risk assessment: Breast and ovarian* [v.1.2018]. Retrieved from https://www.nccn.org/professionals/physician_gls/pdf/genetics_screening.pdf

Tuttle, T.M., Barrio, A.V., Klimberg, V.S., Giuliano, A.E., Chavez-MacGregor, M., Buum, H.A.T., & McMasters, K.M. (2017). Guidelines for guidelines: An assessment of the American Society of Breast Surgeons contralateral prophylactic mastectomy consensus statement. *Annals of Surgical Oncology, 24,* 1–2. doi:10.1245/s10434-016-5648-7

CHAPTER 1

Comprehensive Breast Centers

Joanne Lester, PhD, CRNP, ANP-BC, AOCN®, and Heidi Basinger, MS, BSN, RN, NE-BC

Introduction

Breast cancer leads in the number of dedicated, disease-specific programs and centers in the United States. In general, dedicated cancer centers develop and translate scientific findings from the bench to patient care using laboratory discoveries to establish new treatments. This evidence-based knowledge provides state-of-the-art treatment and delivery of personalized care. Disease-focused centers use evidence-based findings and, through the experience of working with select patients, can inform treatment priorities and national research topics. Centers offer clinical trials that move science forward and most often provide the most up-to-date treatment with optimal outcomes. Breast cancer–specific centers provide public education about cancer prevention and a healthy lifestyle. Focused cancer care, resources, and research have enabled more women and men to overcome their disease than ever before in the history of cancer care.

Fundamental Components of a Comprehensive Breast Center

Radiology

Expert care begins with a comprehensive breast radiology department. Most radiology departments contain state-of-the-art equipment such as digital mammography, ultrasound, tomosynthesis, and magnetic resonance imaging (MRI). Image-guided biopsies are another important component. Some examples include core needle biopsy, ultrasound-guided core biopsy, MRI-guided core biopsy, and stereotactic image-guided biopsy.

Interprofessional Cancer Care Providers

Breast centers are staffed by a team of interprofessional cancer care providers. Departments commonly found include surgical oncology, medical oncology, and radiation oncology. In addition, breast centers employ specialists such as oncoplastic surgeons, cancer-specific pathologists, radiologists, and genetic professionals. RNs and advanced practice practitioners are typically trained to provide care to breast patients and often are certified.

Scope of Services

Upon diagnosis, through treatment, and along their cancer survivorship journey, patients receive a full scope of services from breast centers. Women and men need access to specialists who are experts in their field, as well as people who can coordinate care among services (Senter & Hatfield, 2016). In a breast center, patients will have access to the services of advanced practice nurses; RNs; professional, semiprofessional, or volunteer patient navigators; and community resources in the urban or rural setting. Specialized social workers and psychologists often are available to help patients through their journey by providing physical and psychological care.

Development of a Comprehensive Breast Center

Design Plan

Developing a new comprehensive breast center begins with a champion who starts the fundamental plan. Multiple departments are represented in a breast center, which requires coordination among administrators and oncology professionals. Developers rely on input from physicians and nurses, as well as ancillary departments. Patient advisers are interviewed, as their opinions provide critical insight into local needs. In the preparation and design of the building, developers may interview breast cancer survivors, asking them to share their experiences and what was impactful on their journeys. In this way, purposeful planning is focused on patient needs across the trajectory. Components to enhance workflow and efficiency of a freestanding comprehensive breast center are detailed in Table 1-1.

Strategic Plan

With health care and technology constantly changing, breast centers must continually evaluate and develop a strategic plan. Strategic plans may consider the need for additional services and technology, as well as continual evaluation of adequate professional staffing and ancillary service support.

Staffing

Selecting the right staffing is an important decision and necessary for the organization's success. Staffing starts with the interview process, when managers must ensure that unit expectations for staff are clear. Issues such as candidates' technical skills and expected working hours should be discussed. In addition, managers should evaluate candidates' relational expectations by asking questions about previous oncologic experiences on the job and how they might have handled a difficult or emotional situation.

Staff should expect to enter a culture of cooperation among multiple areas and departments. This culture is built on a foundation of purposeful messaging of goals and the roles of staff. Once the right staff is selected, managers should demonstrate positivity, make staff feel appreciated, and express the value of staff on an ongoing

Table 1-1. Components of a Freestanding Comprehensive Breast Center

Component	Patient Services	Patient Benefits
Boutique	Wigs, hats, jewelry, gifts, mastectomy swimsuits, mastectomy bras, lingerie, personal items, radiation creams	Privacy for wig fittings Privacy for bra fittings Volunteer staff may be survivors
Registration services	Initial check-in, separate from actual registration, patient kiosks for brief registration, financial services, initiates patients' location on electronic medical record (EMR)	Maintains privacy Timely registration Directions for financial needs Consider free parking for all services.
Radiology services	Computed tomography (CT) scan, magnetic resonance imaging (MRI), plain x-rays, bone density	Available to patients with and without cancer Easy to access on first floor Broad level of services Saves separate trip
Laboratory services	Blood draws, electrocardiograms (ECGs)	Available to patients with and without cancer, although primarily used by patients without cancer Easy to complete preadmission testing
Bistro	Food and drinks available for breakfast, lunch, and snacks Specials, outdoor grill Inside and outside tables	Convenient when fasting is required for x-rays or blood draw Variety of items Healthy food choices
Quiet area	Resembles chapel room although nonreligious	Provides quiet space Peaceful Remembrance
Dietitian	Teaching for chemotherapy-related problems Weight loss, weight gain education Healthy eating	Easy to access Helpful to improve diet Saves separate trip
Psychologist	One-to-one appointments Initial visit, follow-up Knowledgeable about breast cancer and related issues	Private Help to handle crises Available when needed Ongoing appointments Saves separate trip Easy to access
Social worker	One-to-one appointments Knowledgeable about breast cancer and community services Available to work through short-term issues Guides financial issues Guides hospital-based decision making, advance directives Development of tour of breast center for patients' children and grandchildren	Available when needed Saves separate trip Easy to access

(Continued on next page)

Table 1-1. Components of a Freestanding Comprehensive Breast Center *(Continued)*

Component	Patient Services	Patient Benefits
Chaplain	One-to-one appointments Knowledgeable about crisis management, advance directives, and end-of-life issues Knowledgeable about all types of religions Offers periodic group sessions	Available to handle crises Available when needed Saves separate trip
Genetic counselor/team	One-to-one appointments during high-risk clinic, newly diagnosed breast cancer cases, and newly metastatic breast cancer clinic Initial review of family history, genetic profile, risk profile, and relative risk Financial responsibility, sending of blood sample Genetic counseling once results received Education throughout survivorship trajectory	Easy to schedule Saves separate trip
Laboratory	Runs blood and urine specimens Courier to hospital lab for additional testing	Speedy to affirm chemotherapy Saves separate trip
Administration/clinical	Offices for administrative personnel Office supplies available Individual computers Copy, scan, fax machine Cubbies for nurse practitioners, clinical breast research personnel	Everyone in same building Continuity of providers
Conference rooms	Useful for patient classes Useful for staff meetings Useful for weekly breast conference meeting	Saves separate trip for patients as well as staff
Physical therapy/rehabilitation	Oncology-based services Lymphedema education, measurement, treatment Exercise machines/plans Available to patients with breast and gynecologic cancers and patients without cancer who have primary lymphedema	Saves separate trip Multiple services
Entire complement of oncology professionals	Oncologists, physician assistants, nurse practitioners, and RNs for newly diagnosed, newly metastatic, and high-risk cases and prevention with positive hereditary factors	Saves separate trip Provides services of all levels Research oriented Receives chemotherapy in same building
Reconstructive surgery	Oncoplastic surgeons, physician assistants, certified nurses Offer multiple services and oncoplastic procedures: tissue expander/implants Transverse rectus abdominis myocutaneous/latissimus dorsi flap Deep inferior epigastric perforator flap/free flap Nipple/areolar tattoos Teaching materials	Saves extra trip Easy access for consultation and treatment Highly skilled Wide variety of services

(Continued on next page)

Table 1-1. Components of a Freestanding Comprehensive Breast Center *(Continued)*

Component	Patient Services	Patient Benefits
Education room	Educational materials on breast cancer prevention and early detection, breast care, breast cancer, treatment of breast cancer, wellness, and overall cancer prevention and early detection	Vast array of educational materials Computers available
Surgical oncology check-in	First contact with patients as they arrive off elevators Verifies patient is in correct area Updates EMR with patient location/time Answers questions Aware of wait times	Convenient and often familiar to established patients
Surgical oncology services	Multiple clinic spaces with accompanying team rooms and physician space Nurse practitioners focus on breast cancer teaching; symptom management; postsurgical care, including drain pulls; seroma aspirations; ongoing survivor education; emotional support; referrals such as boutique, medical oncology, physical therapy, radiation oncology, and cardiology for preoperative clearance Treatment rooms for biopsy, preoperative tests (ECG), clinical research Consultation room with comfortable furniture Preoperative teaching Discharge personnel for appointments Teaching materials	Computers available Privacy Comfortable Easy to schedule appointments
Surgical suites	Available for minor surgical procedures such as skin biopsy, excision of benign breast masses, and minor oncoplastic procedures	Convenient Less expensive than hospital Same personnel as in clinic
Breast imaging services	Adjacent to surgical oncology area—separate waiting area from clinic Radiologists on site to provide same-day readings for people attending clinic Same-day biopsies Radiologists available to surgical oncology providers to examine imaging films: mammography, ultrasonography, thermography Concierge to direct patients and update EMR Educational materials	Convenient Everything done in one day
Medical oncology services	Large waiting area Soothing décor Multiple clinic spaces with accompanying team rooms and physician space Central blood draw/venous sites Consultation rooms with comfortable furniture Discharge personnel for appointments. Nurse practitioners are often providers of care.	Computers available Privacy Comfortable Easy to schedule appointments

(Continued on next page)

Table 1-1. Components of a Freestanding Comprehensive Breast Center *(Continued)*

Component	Patient Services	Patient Benefits
Chemotherapy/ infusion suites	Registration personnel to schedule continuity appointments Bed or lounge chairs One-to-one care Educational materials Certified nurses to administer drugs	Privacy Comfortable Easy to schedule appointments Convenient
Oncology pharmacy	Obtains EMR orders on specified order sheets: admix chemotherapy, IV fluids, blood product transfusions, clinical study drugs, IV antibiotics, intramuscular drugs Double pass-through hood used to admix chemotherapy	Convenience Patient education resource
Survivorship care	Review of breast cancer diagnosis, pathology, treatment (surgery, chemotherapy, radiation therapy), biologic therapy, healthy lifestyle, diet, food, weight, smoking cessation, and stress reduction Well-woman care to ensure health promotion/ risk reduction, gynecologic care, primary care provider, bone density testing, colonoscopy, dental care, safety with seat belts, and relationships	Promotes improved long-term health
Midlevel providers	Includes nurse practitioners, physician assistants, and clinical nurse specialist Provides extended care/survivorship care Offers services that busy oncologists cannot Provides continuity from practitioners to patients Leads clinics to survivorship model and transfers long-term patients from physicians' practices to nurse practitioners	Continuity of care Easy to reach with 24-hour coverage Patient education
Navigators	Often volunteers in various clinical areas Lead newly diagnosed and newly metastatic patients on their unfamiliar trajectory Depth of personal or professional experience	Patient support resource

basis. The outpatient oncology environment can be very difficult and provide emotional challenges. The emotional toll must be distanced to provide the utmost professional care, yet compassionate relief must be available at all times.

Measures of an Accredited Breast Center

National Accreditation Program for Breast Centers

The National Accreditation Program for Breast Centers (NAPBC) is the leading organization that identifies and validates the components of a full-program breast center. It is under the jurisdiction of the American College of Surgeons (ACoS). NAPBC focuses on quality performance outcomes, an interprofessional team approach, evidence-based practice, and compliance with established standards. It also provides a model to organize and manage a breast center and breast care services. NAPBC asserts that breast centers should be interprofessional, integrated, and comprehensive (ACoS, 2014).

NAPBC provides an internal and external assessment of a breast center's performance. The assessment is based on recognized standards for quality of care. Comprehensive breast centers that meet these performance measures for high-quality breast care receive national recognition and promotion from NAPBC, an established national healthcare organization.

NAPBC grants accreditation to centers that dedicate their breast program to providing the best care possible to people with breast disease and offer services across the breast cancer trajectory (see Table 1-2).

Standards of Care

NAPBC focuses on six core standards of care (ACoS, 2014):
- Center leadership
- Clinical management
- Research
- Community outreach
- Professional education
- Quality improvement

NAPBC also provides breast cancer standards of care that can be used within a breast program to ensure quality outcomes. These standards are described in the following sections.

Center Leadership

Center leadership is responsible and accountable for all breast center services. With this standard, the medical director is responsible for verification of physician board certification, establishment of essential components of medical staff, and management of codirectors or an interprofessional steering committee of the breast program.

Interprofessional Breast Conferences

Ideally, breast conferences should occur weekly. They are intended to provide consultative services for patients and education for physicians and allied health professionals. Frequency of conferences is based on annual caseload and number of case presentations; 85% of cases must be presented prospectively using a team approach (ACoS, 2014). The conference should include a comprehensive clinical summary by the provider, as well as imaging and pathology reviews for both new and previously diagnosed cases for which some phase of treatment is pending or completed. In addition, clinical trial eligibility should be considered. For patients in whom treatment has failed, a discussion of palliative care and supportive treatment is required.

Interprofessional representation must be documented at each conference with individual signatures. Required attendees include representatives from surgery, medical oncology, radiation oncology, and pathology. During the conference, participants

Table 1-2. Breast Center Component Checklist for Each Patient

Categories	Actions
Imaging	Screening mammography (digital or analog) Diagnostic mammography Ultrasound Breast MRI
Needle biopsy	Needle biopsy—palpable Image-guided, stereotactic Image-guided, ultrasound Image-guided, MRI
Pathology	Report completeness Radiology–pathology correlation Prognostic and predictive indicators Gene studies
Interprofessional conferences	Pre- and post-treatment interprofessional discussion History and physical Imaging studies Pathology
Patient navigation	Facilitate navigation of patient through system.
Genetic evaluation and management	Risk assessment Genetic counseling Genetic testing
Surgical care	Surgical correlation with imaging/concordance Preoperative planning after biopsy Breast surgery: lumpectomy or mastectomy Lymph node assessment: SLNB/AND Post-definitive surgery correlation with treatment planning
Plastic surgery consultation/treatment	Tissue expander/implants TRAM/latissimus dorsi flaps DIEP flap/free flaps
Nurses	Nurses have specialized knowledge and skills to care for patients with breast disease.
Medical oncology consultation/treatment	Discussion of appropriate treatment Hormone therapy Chemotherapy Biologics Chemoprevention
Radiation oncology consultation/treatment	Whole breast irradiation with or without boost Regional nodal irradiation Partial breast irradiation treatment or protocols Palliative radiation for bone or systemic metastasis Stereotactic radiation for isolated or limited brain metastasis
Data management	Data collection and submission

(Continued on next page)

Table 1-2. Breast Center Component Checklist for Each Patient *(Continued)*

Categories	Actions
Research	Cooperative clinical trials Research from within institution Industry-sponsored trials
Education, support, and rehabilitation	Education along the survivorship trajectory (pretreatment, during, post-treatment Psychosocial support (individual, family, support groups) Symptom management Physical therapy (e.g., lymphedema management)
Outreach and education	Community education/low income/underserved Patient education Physician/healthcare provider education: All aspects of cancer treatment, continuing education in their area of practice specific to breast cancer
Quality improvement	Continuous quality improvement through annual studies
Survivorship program	Follow-up surveillance Rehabilitation: Full complement of services to assist women and men to deal with the symptoms and long-term complications associated with treatment Health promotion/risk reduction: Group and individual education on means to promote overall health, as well as reduce modifiable risk factors associated with the development of breast cancer

AND—axillary node dissection; DIEP—deep inferior epigastric perforator; MRI—magnetic resonance imaging; SLNB—sentinel lymph node biopsy; TRAM—transverse rectus abdominis myocutaneous

Note. From *NAPBC Standards Manual, 2014 Edition* (p. 14), by American College of Surgeons, 2014. Retrieved from https://www.facs.org/~/media/files/quality%20programs/napbc/2014%20napbc%20standards%20manual.ashx. Copyright 2014 by American College of Surgeons. Adapted with permission.

will use national guidelines to validate discussion (e.g., those from the National Comprehensive Cancer Network® [NCCN®]), as well as include a visual display of pathology slides and radiology imaging and discussion of radiology–pathology correlation. Other pertinent discussion topics include clinical trial opportunities, genetic risk, and reconstructive options. The presentation should include the patient's relevant history, including physical data and family history. Conference participants will discuss the pertinent breast cancer facts, including stage of disease, patient's risk profile, surgical options, and systemic treatment such as neoadjuvant versus adjuvant chemotherapy.

Management Guidelines

The leadership team is responsible for identifying and referencing evidence-based breast care management guidelines. These guidelines are used to promote an organized approach to patient care and use of national guidelines in daily practice. Examples of guidelines include those from Adjuvant! Online (n.d.), American Society of Clinical Oncology (2016a), American Society for Radiation Oncology (ASTRO, 2017), and NCCN (2016, 2017a, 2017b), in addition to well-woman care guidelines.

Leadership also tracks the type and number of surgeries. The goal is that 50% of eligible women undergo breast-conserving surgery (ACoS, 2014), given that the tumor is localized and can attain negative margins, the procedure will result in good cosmetic outcome, and the patient can safely undergo radiation therapy. In addition, leadership is responsible for monitoring stated goals and talking with oncology teams that deviate from the treatment plan (e.g., surgeons who perform mastectomy instead of lumpectomy). Finally, management monitors physician use of American Joint Committee on Cancer staging guidelines (Amin et al., 2017), ensuring that accurate staging leads to appropriate evidence-based treatment and facilitates reliable evaluation of treatment results.

Breast Center Components

Patient Interventions and Services

From the newly diagnosed to the established patient with breast cancer, each patient seen and treated in a comprehensive breast center is offered a wide range of evidence-based interventions and services (ACoS, 2014). The checklist in Table 1-2 summarizes component categories and actions.

Patient Navigation

Breast center management identifies patient navigators, including their qualifications and roles, and indicates the number of patient navigators who are to provide navigation from prediagnosis through all phases of the cancer experience. (See Chapter 10 for more details on breast navigation.)

Diagnostic Imaging

Screening and diagnostic mammography must be performed at Mammography Quality Standards Act–certified facilities. Management should adopt nationally recognized mammography screening guidelines (American Cancer Society, n.d.; National Cancer Institute, 2016; NCCN, 2016). Centers performing advanced diagnostic imaging services must meet the regulations of the Medicare Improvements for Patients and Providers Act with appropriate in-house capabilities or referrals. The American College of Radiology (ACR) guidelines provide information on mammographic screening (ACR, 2013), diagnostic imaging, and breast MRI (ACR, 2016).

Ultrasonography

Various procedures can be performed at certified facilities. Diagnostic ultrasound and ultrasound-guided needle biopsy are performed at ACR ultrasound–accredited facilities. ACR accrediting includes the facility, radiologists, procedures, equipment, quality control, quality assurance, accuracy of needle placement, and image quality (ACR Accreditation, n.d.-a). The American Society of Breast Surgeons' (n.d.) Breast Ultrasound Certification Program ensures that surgeons meet criteria in clinical experience, training, and quality assurance.

Radiation Oncology Services

Breast centers should provide radiation oncology treatment services for all patients, whether on-site or as a referral to a community hospital. Multiple accreditation groups are associated with radiation oncology, including ACR's Radiation Oncology Practice Accreditation (ACR Accreditation, n.d.-b), and the American Society for Radiation Oncology's (n.d.) ASTRO Accreditation Program for Excellence.

These groups help ensure that minimal quality assurance practices are met. Quality assurance practices include verification that patient identification is confirmed by two independent methods prior to each radiation encounter; verification of daily, monthly, and annual radiation treatment machine quality assurance procedures; verification of independent check of dose calculation for every new or changed treatment prior to starting treatment; and verification that patient-specific quality assurance is done prior to initiation of intensity-modulated radiation therapy. As a standard of care, NAPBC requires that radiation therapy is administered within one year (365 days) of diagnosis for women younger than age 70 receiving breast-conserving surgery (ACoS, 2014).

Biopsies

An important component of breast centers is performing biopsies. Sentinel lymph node biopsy should be performed on early-stage breast cancer when possible and appropriate for neoadjuvant treatment (ACoS, 2014; NCCN, 2017a; see Chapter 5 for more details). Pathologists should use guidelines from the College of American Pathologists (CAP, n.d.) for pathologic evaluation of breast specimens. At least 90% of all charts should have evidence of CAP guidelines (ACoS, 2014). Estrogen and progesterone receptors and HER2 need to be evaluated on only one specimen (core biopsy vs. surgical specimen) unless clinical evidence exists to repeat them. In addition, studies performed at outside institutions must be reported as an addendum on the pathology report, whether repeated or not. If studies were performed at an outside institution, pathologists at the breast center must review the study and repeat if necessary. Imaging studies should be correlated with the pathology reports when possible. A synoptic format should be used for breast cancer pathology reports.

Needle biopsy should be the initial biopsy approach versus open biopsy (ACoS, 2014; NCCN, 2017a). The physician performing the biopsy must communicate a radiographic presentation to the pathologist. The ACR Stereotactic Breast Biopsy Accreditation Program reviews staff qualifications, equipment, quality control, quality assurance, accuracy of needle placement, imaging quality, and handling of biopsy specimens.

Medical Oncology Services

Medical oncology encompasses the systemic treatment of breast cancer, including treatments such as chemotherapy, biologic therapy, hormonal therapy, and chemoprevention.

Breast cancer quality measures are endorsed by National Quality Measures for Breast Centers (2016). These measures validate that combination chemotherapy is considered or administered within four months (120 days) from the date of diagnosis for women younger than age 70 with stage IC, II, or III hormone receptor–negative disease. Antiestrogen or aromatase inhibitors are considered or administered within one year (365 days) of diagnosis for women younger than age 70 with stage II or III hormone receptor–positive disease. The American Society of Clinical Oncology (2016b) has also developed an oncologist-led, practice-based quality improvement program—the Quality Oncology Practice Initiative (QOPI®)—recommended by NAPBC (ACoS, 2014).

Nursing

A necessary component of any breast center is nursing. Nursing care is provided by RNs with specialized knowledge and skills in breast disease. Nursing assessment and interventions are guided by evidence-based practice and symptom management.

Breast oncology nurses are integral members of the oncology breast team to achieve optimal outcomes. Integral to this outcome are certified staff nurses in breast centers.

Advanced practice nurses (APNs) provide a different level of care in a breast-dedicated center. Each team comprises an oncologist (e.g., medical, surgical, radiation), APN, and RN. This union provides continuity of care and a direct point of contact for each patient. The APN is responsible for advanced assessment, symptom management, and documentation of the care plan.

Support and Rehabilitation Services

Support and rehabilitation services are provided by, or referred to, people with specialized knowledge of breast disease. Included in these services are mental health specialists who address patient needs throughout the breast cancer continuum. In addition, support services help patients and families cope with day-to-day needs. On-site personnel include social workers who specialize in the care of patients with cancer and have knowledge about community services. Local agencies are available in patients' communities and therefore are easier for patients to access. Multiple resources are available online, allowing patients access to information from the comfort of their own home.

The goals of supportive care and rehabilitation include the following:
- Assistance to patients and family members with adjustment to breast cancer diagnosis and treatment
- Lymphedema management and risk reduction practices
- Integrative medicine (e.g., yoga, tai chi, exercise)
- Psychosocial distress screening and support
- Nutrition counseling
- Palliative care
- Support groups
- Transportation services
- Complementary services (e.g., music or art therapy, relaxation, massage)

Genetic Evaluation and Management

Genetic evaluation and management of breast and ovarian cancer must be available on site or by referral to a credentialed genetic professional (see Chapter 2). Institutions without these professionals may utilize a nationwide network of genetic experts available by telephone or online, including the DNA Direct Genomic Medicine Network (www.dnadirect.com/dnaweb/products/genomic-medicine-network.html) and InformedDNA (https://informeddna.com).

Educational Resources

Breast centers should provide culturally and educationally appropriate resources. A process should be in place to provide materials in multiple formats (print, electronic, etc.). Resources should be reviewed and updated annually. Centers should have a full spectrum of resources regarding breast disease, treatment options, symptom management, and survivorship needs.

Reconstructive Surgery

Breast centers are required to offer all people considering or undergoing breast surgery (e.g., mastectomy) a preoperative referral to a plastic surgery team. Ideally, all people who are considering a mastectomy or lumpectomy should be referred, as reconstructive options may be available for both types of surgeries. Medical records should include documentation that the person saw a plastic surgeon and did not desire reconstruction or was not physically appropriate (e.g., morbidly obese).

Reconstructive surgery can be immediate or delayed, performed with a mastectomy, and unilateral or bilateral. The low chance of contralateral disease should be documented. If a patient chooses lumpectomy versus mastectomy, documentation of data supporting the equivalence of lumpectomy plus radiation to mastectomy should be included. This process enables informed decision making and educates patients that reconstruction does not interfere with ongoing surveillance of cancer (Rainsbury & Willett, 2012).

Survivorship Care

Comprehensive breast cancer survivorship care (see Chapter 11) is a necessary component for any breast center. Patients should be provided with a survivorship care plan within six months of completing active treatment (e.g., surgery, chemotherapy, radiation therapy), but no longer than one year from diagnosis. Survivorship plans should include genetics/family history, support services provided or referred, psychologist referral, rehabilitation plan, nutritional services, vocational therapy, and contact information for all team members.

Follow-up care should include possible late and long-term side effects of treatment and symptoms; possible sexual dysfunction effects, symptoms, and management; possible psychological effects and potential need for support; referral services for insurance, employment, and financial issues; contraindicated medications for the future, including hormone replacement therapy and specific antidepressants (if on hormonal therapy); and over-the-counter estrogenic products.

Finally, a treatment summary should be completed, detailing tumor characteristics, site, stage, grade, prognostic factors, and details of active treatment (NCCN, 2017b).

Research

Research in breast centers promotes advancements in prevention, early diagnosis, and treatment. Breast centers should make available clinical trial information, eligibility, and possible participation.

Fewer than 5% of patients with breast cancer nationally are accrued to clinical trials (Breastcancer.org, 2017), including National Cancer Institute–sponsored programs, the Community Clinical Oncology Program, cooperative groups, and the Alliance for Clinical Trials in Oncology. Other research includes university-related research and pharmaceutical-sponsored research. The research team comprises principal investigators, study coordinators, and data managers, as well as institutional research board support.

Community Outreach

Effective community outreach can increase breast cancer awareness for patients and families with and without a diagnosis of breast cancer.

Professional and Breast Center Staff Education

To increase the knowledge of breast center staff, professional and staff education should be conducted regularly. Educational activities can be held at the breast center and should include continuing medical and nursing education. Professional and staff education helps maintain competence and validates what staff are doing with patients and families. Multiple venues to obtain this information should be available for all team members. Options include educational activities such as breast cancer–related lecture series; local, state, regional, or national breast cancer meetings or workshops; breast cancer–related video conferences; breast cancer–related web-based training modules; journals of continuing medical and nursing education; and web conferences.

Quality Improvement

A commitment to quality improvement ensures that breast services, care, and patient outcomes are continuously evaluated and reviewed. Monthly, quarterly, and annual review of quality outcomes should be conducted. These reviews should measure quality, correct deficiencies, enhance patient outcomes, and represent interprofessional effort and responsibility. Quality improvement studies include process, scope of issue, reason why the issue is addressed, and available data. Quality improvement studies define the following: the issue of concern, the area requiring investigation or improvement, contributing factors, initiatives and interventions needed for resolution, and an opportunity for change.

Several organizations offer center-specific quality improvement programs, including the National Consortium of Breast Centers' National Quality Measures for Breast Centers (2016), the American Society of Clinical Oncology's (2016b) QOPI, and the American Society of Plastic Surgeons' (n.d.) Tracking Operations and Outcomes for Plastic Surgeons.

Accreditation Review

Centers that receive program accreditation must comply with NAPBC standards and undergo a review every three years. To apply for accreditation, breast centers must provide electronic records for review prior to arrival, including the following:
• Survey application record
• Roster of breast steering committee
• Copy of year's meeting minutes from steering committee

- Breast conference schedule/calendar for full year

Centers should also supply deidentified access to breast cancer cases diagnosed within the past year. These cases should include the following:
- Medical record number
- Age of patient
- Histology
- Date of diagnosis
- Definitive surgical resection for stage I, II, or III breast cancers
- Charts, graphs, and reports demonstrating participation in national quality breast care improvement initiative

On site, cancer centers must provide 20 medical records as identified by the surveyor to be assessed for breast conservation, sentinel lymph node biopsy, breast cancer staging, pathology reports, core needle biopsy, radiation oncology, medical oncology, and reconstructive surgery. In addition, cancer centers must make available 10 medical records for benign disease and 5 records reflecting diagnoses of atypical lobular hyperplasia or atypical ductal hyperplasia. Annual reports of radiation oncology quality assurance and annual reports from support and rehabilitation leaders must be provided. Other records that must be submitted include samples of educational resources and clinical trial materials provided to patients and examples of prevention, education, and early detection programs held within the last year.

Cancer centers also must demonstrate the system used for participation in breast cancer national quality improvement initiatives. Examples include attendance at weekly interprofessional meetings and review of attendance records or grids. Centers also must provide annual performance rates to demonstrate use of core needle biopsy for diagnosis (e.g., versus open biopsy), the breast conservation rate in stage 0, I, or II disease, and administration of radiation therapy within one year of diagnosis in women younger than 70 years of age.

Accredited breast programs are found in academic settings, treatment centers, hospital-based breast centers, and private practice.

Women who need qualified breast care and healthcare providers can search for NAPBC-accredited breast centers by geographical location and zip code at www.facs .org/search/accredited-breast-centers. To earn NAPBC accreditation, a center must have the items listed in Table 1-2.

Summary

The development and completion of a comprehensive breast center is a long process led by champions for the cause and astute managers. These projects often must compete with other institutional needs and priorities and may be overlooked for more important ones. A breast center begins with imaging and surgical oncology and expands with various components of a comprehensive program, one by one. It must start somewhere in order to grow into something larger.

Continual review and compliance with interprofessional national standards is a critical step in providing the best possible care to women and men, as well as their families, who are affected by a diagnosis of breast cancer.

These services should encompass the entire breast cancer trajectory from screening and genetic services for asymptomatic women through diagnosis, treatment, survivorship, and palliative care.

References

ACR Accreditation. (n.d.-a). Modalities. Retrieved from http://www.acraccreditation.org/modalities

ACR Accreditation. (n.d.-b). Radiation oncology. Retrieved from http://www.acraccreditation.org/modalities/radiation-oncology-practice

Adjuvant! Online. (n.d.). Welcome to Adjuvant! Online. Retrieved from https://adjuvantonline.com

American Cancer Society. (n.d.). Breast cancer screening guidelines. Retrieved from https://www.cancer.org/health-care-professionals/american-cancer-society-prevention-early-detection-guidelines/breast-cancer-screening-guidelines.html

American College of Radiology. (2013). *ACR practice parameter for the performance of screening and diagnostic mammography.* Retrieved from https://www.acr.org/-/media/ACR/Files/Practice-Parameters/Screen-Diag-Mammo.pdf

American College of Radiology. (2016). *ACR practice parameter for the performance of magnetic resonance imaging-guided breast interventional procedures.* https://www.acr.org/-/media/ACR/Files/Practice-Parameters/mr-guided-breast.pdf?la=en

American College of Surgeons. (2014). *NAPBC standards manual, 2014 edition.* Retrieved from https://www.facs.org/quality-programs/napbc/standards

American Society for Radiation Oncology. (n.d.). ASTRO Accreditation Program for Excellence. Retrieved from https://www.astro.org/Daily-Practice/Accreditation/Accreditation

American Society for Radiation Oncology. (2017). *Clinical practice statements: Breast cancer.* Retrieved from https://www.astro.org/Clinical-Practice-Statements.aspx

American Society of Breast Surgeons. (n.d.). Breast ultrasound certification. Retrieved from https://www.breastsurgeons.org/certification/breast_ultrasound_certification.php

American Society of Clinical Oncology. (2016a). *Breast cancer.* Retrieved from http://www.asco.org/practice-guidelines/quality-guidelines/guidelines/breast-cancer

American Society of Clinical Oncology. (2016b). Quality Oncology Practice Initiative (QOPI®). Retrieved from http://www.instituteforquality.org/quality-oncology-practice-initiative-qopi

American Society of Plastic Surgeons. (n.d.). Tracking Operations and Outcomes for Plastic Surgeons (TOPS). Retrieved from https://www.plasticsurgery.org/for-medical-professionals/quality-and-registries/tracking-operations-and-outcomes-for-plastic-surgeons

Amin, M.B., Edge, S., Greene, F., Byrd, D.R., Brookland, R.K., Washington, M.K., … Meyer, L.R. (Eds.). (2017). *AJCC cancer staging manual* (8th ed.). New York, NY: Springer.

Breastcancer.org. (2017). Clinical trials. Retrieved from http://www.breastcancer.org/treatment/clinical_trials

College of American Pathologists. (n.d.). CAP guidelines. Retrieved from http://www.cap.org/web/home/protocols-and-guidelines/cap-guidelines?_adf.ctrl-state=2zbolg9tp_4&_afrLoop=3154458158 57561#!%40%40%3F_afrLoop%3D315445815857561%26_adf.ctrl-state%3De4k00y05p_9

National Cancer Institute. (2016, December 7). Mammograms. Retrieved from http://www.cancer.gov/types/breast/mammograms-fact-sheet

National Comprehensive Cancer Network. (2016). *NCCN Clinical Practice Guidelines in Oncology (NCCN Guidelines®): Genetic/familial high-risk assessment: Breast and ovarian* [v.2.2017]. Retrieved from https://www.nccn.org/professionals/physician_gls/pdf/genetics_screening.pdf

National Comprehensive Cancer Network. (2017a). *NCCN Clinical Practice Guidelines in Oncology (NCCN Guidelines®): Breast cancer* [v.2.2017]. Retrieved from https://www.nccn.org/professionals/physician_gls/pdf/breast.pdf

National Comprehensive Cancer Network. (2017b). *NCCN Clinical Practice Guidelines in Oncology (NCCN Guidelines®): Survivorship* [v.2.2017]. Retrieved from https://www.nccn.org/professionals/physician_gls/pdf/survivorship.pdf

National Quality Measures for Breast Centers. (2016). Becoming a Certified Quality Breast Center of Excellence™. Retrieved from http://www2.nqmbc.org/pdfs/NQMBC_brochure_2016.pdf

Rainsbury, D., & Willett, A. (Eds.). (2012). *Oncoplastic breast reconstruction: Guidelines for best practice.* Retrieved from http://associationofbreastsurgery.org.uk/media/1424/oncoplastic-breast-reconstruction-guidelines-for-best-practice.pdf

Senter, L., & Hatfield, R. (2016). Nurse practitioners and genetic counselors: Collaborative roles in a complex system. *Nurse Practitioner, 41*(7), 43–49. doi:10.1097/01.NPR.0000470355.00838.a2

CHAPTER 2

Risk Assessment

Suzanne M. Mahon, RN, DNSc, AOCN®, AGN-BC

Introduction

Understanding breast cancer risk is a challenge both for women to comprehend and for healthcare professionals to communicate in understandable terms. All women are at risk for developing breast cancer, given the overall incidence of breast cancer; however, women with multiple risk factors are at higher risk. A risk factor is a trait or characteristic that is associated with a statistically significant increased likelihood of developing a disease. The presence of a risk factor does not absolutely mean that a person will develop breast cancer, nor does the absence of a risk factor make a person immune to developing breast cancer. Basic elements of a breast cancer risk assessment generally include a review of medical history, a history of exposures to carcinogens in daily living, and a detailed family history. Clinicians consider these elements when making recommendations for breast cancer prevention and early detection. This chapter will review the principles of risk assessment, risk factors for developing breast cancer, the genetic testing process, and evidence-based breast cancer prevention and detection measures.

Breast Cancer Incidence and Risk Assessment

An estimated 252,710 women are diagnosed with invasive breast cancer annually (American Cancer Society [ACS], 2017a). Additionally, an estimated 63,410 women are diagnosed with in situ breast cancer each year. Breast cancer is the most common cancer diagnosed in women, accounting for 30% of cancer diagnoses in women. The median age for developing breast cancer is 62, but women of all ages are affected (see Figure 2-1). An estimated 2,470 men are diagnosed with breast cancer annually. Breast cancer incidence rates have remained basically stable since 2004. An estimated 40,610 women and 460 men die annually from breast cancer. It is the second most common cause of cancer deaths in women, accounting for 14% of all cancer deaths in women. The breast cancer death rates declined by 38% from 1989 to 2014 (ACS, 2017a).

Breast cancer risk assessment is the critical initial step in helping individuals to better comprehend the ramifications of the disease and to take appropriate steps to prevent it or detect it early, when it is most treatable. Risk assessment guides refer-

Figure 2-1. Percentages of New Cases by Age Group

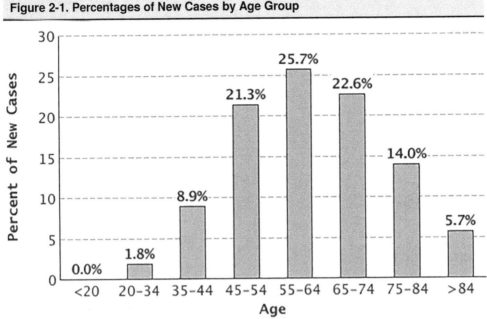

Female breast cancer is most common in middle-aged and older women. Although rare, men can develop breast cancer as well. The number of new cases of female breast cancer was 125.0 per 100,000 women per year based on 2009–2013 cases.

Note. From "Cancer Stat Facts: Female Breast Cancer," by National Cancer Institute Surveillance, Epidemiology, and End Results Program, n.d. Retrieved from http://seer.cancer.gov/statfacts/html/breast.html.

rals to genetic counseling for some and ultimately the selection of screening recommendations for all. It also provides an opportunity for nurses to teach patients about primary prevention measures to prevent, delay, or reduce the risk of developing cancer.

Definitions of Types of Risk

Absolute Risk

Absolute risk is a measure of the occurrence of cancer, by either incidence (new cases) or mortality (deaths), in an identified population. Absolute risk is helpful when patients need to understand what the chances are for all individuals in a population of developing a specific disease. It can be expressed either as the number of cases for a specified denominator (for example, 125 cases of breast cancer per 100,000 women annually) or as a cumulative risk up to a specified age (for example, one in eight women will develop breast cancer if they live to age 85) (ACS, 2017a). The one-in-eight figure describes the average risk of breast cancer in Caucasian American women, and its calculation considers other causes of death over the life span. This figure will possibly overestimate breast cancer risk for some people with no risk factors and will greatly underestimate the risk for people with several risk factors or those with a genetic mutation.

Relative Risk

Relative risk refers to a comparison of the incidence or number of deaths among those with a specific risk factor compared to those without the risk factor. Relative risk is helpful for comparing risk of developing breast cancer between individuals who have a risk factor and those who do not. If the risk for a woman with no known risk factors is 1.0, one can evaluate those with risk factors in relation to this figure (see Table 2-1). When using relative risk, it is important to specify the anchor, or the comparison. Relative risk factors cannot be added together. Women with multiple risk factors, especially those with higher relative risk figures, should consider that information carefully when making decisions about breast cancer prevention and detection measures.

Table 2-1. Relative Risk Factors for Developing Breast Cancer

Risk Factor	Comparison	Relative Risk
Early menarche (before age 12)	Menarche after age 15	1.1–2.1
Late menopause (after age 55)	Menopause age 45 or younger	1.5–2.3
First live birth after age 30	First live birth before age 25	1.9
Nulliparous	First live birth before age 25	3.0
Recent hormonal contraceptive use	No contraceptive use	1.1–2.0
Biopsy-proven proliferative disease	No proliferative disease	1.9–2.5
Biopsy-proven proliferative disease with atypical hyperplasia	No proliferative disease	4.4–5.3
Alcohol intake (two or more drinks per day)	No or minimal alcohol intake	1.2
Obesity/increased body mass (in 80th percentile or higher at age 55)	Body mass in 20th percentile or less at age 55	1.2–2.6
First-degree relative with postmenopausal breast cancer	No first-degree relative with postmenopausal breast cancer	1.8
First-degree relative with premenopausal breast cancer	No first-degree relative with premenopausal breast cancer	3.3
Past history of invasive breast cancer	No past history of invasive breast cancer	6.8–8.2
Current hormone replacement therapy use with estrogen and progesterone for at least five years	No history of hormone replacement therapy use	1.3–1.8
BRCA1 and *BRCA2* or other inherited gene mutation	No inherited gene mutation	5–30
High breast density	Average breast density	3–5

Note. Based on information from American Cancer Society, 2015; National Comprehensive Cancer Network, 2017a; Yang et al., 2011.

From "Risk Factors for Breast Cancer" (p. 9), by S.M. Mahon in S.M. Mahon (Ed.), *Site-Specific Cancer Series: Breast Cancer* (2nd ed.), 2011, Pittsburgh, PA: Oncology Nursing Society. Copyright 2011 by Oncology Nursing Society. Adapted with permission.

Rationale for Breast Cancer Risk Assessment

From a scientific perspective, the identification of risk factors contributes to the understanding of breast cancer biology. When identified, such risk factors may be altered to decrease the number of new cases or deaths from cancer.

Risk assessment guides public policy for the allocation of funding for screening, especially for cancer sites in which reasonable screening tests exist, incidence is substantial, and for which screening directly affects the morbidity and mortality associated with the disease.

Risk assessment also guides screening and prevention recommendations. Women of average risk can follow the guidelines for the general population. Women with increased risk may benefit from modification of the guidelines. For example, women with a lifetime risk of breast cancer of 20%–25% or greater may benefit from the addition of breast magnetic resonance imaging (MRI) starting at age 30 (ACS, 2015).

Communicating Breast Cancer Risk Assessment

When nurses discuss risk factors with patients, they need to carefully articulate the type of risk (absolute or relative) and the physiologic basis of the risk factor, if known. To communicate effectively, nurses need to understand the pathophysiologic basis of each risk factor for breast cancer.

Breast cancer risk assessment should be documented and include the patient's past medical history and personal history factors that may increase the risk of developing cancer. Family history of malignancy is also an important part of the assessment. Modifiable risk factors are amenable to cancer prevention measures and adoption of a healthier lifestyle. Many risk factors for breast cancer are nonmodifiable. Risk models are available that combine various risk factors to estimate the risk of developing breast cancer (see Table 2-2).

Risk assessment models are based on assumptions and epidemiologic studies, which may be weak or deficient and limit the accuracy of the model. If these assumptions and studies are weak or deficient, the resulting assessment can be inaccurate or inappropriate. No model completely and accurately explains an individual's risk for developing breast cancer (Schonberg et al., 2016).

Risk Factors for Breast Cancer

The most consistently documented uncontrollable risk factor for the development of breast cancer is increasing age (ACS, 2015). Most cases occur after age 45 (see Figure 2-1). Age is a nonmodifiable risk factor.

Endogenous hormonal factors also play a role in breast cancer risk. Female hormone levels fluctuate throughout life and are associated with changes in the breast tissue. Prolonged exposure to ovarian hormones, especially estrogen, increases breast cancer risk and is associated with estrogen receptor–positive breast cancer (National Comprehensive Cancer Network® [NCCN®], 2017a). Risk increases in women who have early menarche (before age 12), a later menopause (after age 55), later first pregnancy (age 30 or later), and in nulliparous women (NCCN, 2017a). Pregnancy

Table 2-2. Models for Predicting the Lifetime Risk of Developing Breast Cancer

Model	Indications	Strengths	Limitations
Gail model Also known as Breast Cancer Risk Assessment Tool (BCRAT) (Costantino et al., 1999; Schonberg et al., 2016)	Estimates breast cancer risk in the next five years and over a lifetime Most effectively used in women with a limited to moderate family history of breast cancer Often used to determine whether the patient should be enrolled in a chemoprevention trial or treatment	Readily available to use on computers and handheld devices Freely available at www.cancer.gov /bcrisktool Considers previous biopsies Considers previous pregnancies Considers menstrual history	Does not consider personal or family history of ovarian cancer Does not consider the age at which other relatives were diagnosed (the model does not take into account the impact of early-onset breast cancer in the family) Does not consider paternal side of family with a diagnosis of breast or ovarian cancer Does not consider second-degree relatives with a diagnosis of breast or ovarian cancer Has not been used extensively with many ethnic minorities and may have limited usefulness
Claus model (Claus et al., 1991, 1994)	Provides age-specific estimates for the risk of developing breast cancer Most effectively used in women with a significant family history of breast cancer	Considers the age at diagnosis of breast cancer Considers both maternal and paternal family history Calculates risk in 10-year increments, which is helpful to younger women or when trying to keep risk in perspective	Does not consider ethnicity Does not consider ovarian cancer history Might significantly underestimate risk in people with a *BRCA1* or *BRCA2* mutation
Pedigree Assessment Tool (PAT) (Hoskins et al., 2006)	Identifies women at increased risk for hereditary breast cancer and whether to offer genetic testing Best used with women being seen in primary care settings with multiple family members diagnosed with breast cancer	Simple point scoring system based on family history with points weighted according to features associated with *BRCA1* or *BRCA2* mutations	May over-refer some women for genetic counseling

(Continued on next page)

Table 2-2. Models for Predicting the Lifetime Risk of Developing Breast Cancer *(Continued)*

Model	Indications	Strengths	Limitations
IBIS Breast Cancer Risk Evaluation Tool (Tyrer Cuzick Model) (Tyrer et al., 2004)	Identifies women who might benefit from modified screening recommendations or genetic assessment	Freely available at www.ems-trials.org /riskevaluator Considers multiple risk factors including age, height, weight, parity, maternal and paternal family history of breast and ovarian cancer, and benign breast disease	May overestimate risk in women with multiple risk factors

Note. From "Risk Factors for Breast Cancer" (pp. 22–23), by S.M. Mahon in S.M. Mahon (Ed.), *Site-Specific Cancer Series: Breast Cancer* (2nd ed.), 2011, Pittsburgh, PA: Oncology Nursing Society. Copyright 2011 by Oncology Nursing Society. Adapted with permission.

interrupts the exposure of breast cells to circulating estrogen. It also lowers the total number of menstrual cycles a woman has in her lifetime (ACS, 2015). Endogenous hormonal factors are largely nonmodifiable.

Use of exogenous hormonal agents, on the other hand, is a largely modifiable risk factor. Hormone replacement therapies (especially those that are estrogen based) increase the risk of breast cancer. Current or recent users of combined hormone replacement therapy for five years or longer have an increased risk of breast cancer (Marjoribanks, Farquhar, Roberts, Lethaby, & Lee, 2017). Risk is also greater for women who start hormone therapy soon after the onset of menopause compared to those who begin use later (ACS, 2015).

Hormonal contraceptives that contain both estrogen and progesterone can slightly increase the risk for breast cancer, especially among women who have used them for 10 or more years (Beaber et al., 2014). Current and recent (less than 10 years since last use) users have a slightly increased risk compared with women who have never used hormonal contraceptives (Yang et al., 2011). Infertility treatment may increase the risk of developing breast cancer, although the exact risk is not clear. Long-term prospective studies are needed to better characterize this risk (Brinton et al., 2014).

Previous history of breast cancer is another risk factor. Women who had breast cancer in the past have a higher risk of developing breast cancer again. Overall, these women are 1.5 times more likely to develop a new breast cancer. For women with breast cancer diagnosed before age 40, the risk of a second breast cancer is 4.5 times higher (ACS, 2015). The new primary breast cancer can develop in the same breast as the first cancer or in the opposite breast (NCCN, 2017a). This is a nonmodifiable risk factor.

Another nonmodifiable risk factor is ionizing radiation exposure. Women who have received radiation therapy to the chest, neck, and axilla area (called the mantle radiation field) have a higher risk of developing breast cancer. This increased risk has been particularly noted in women who received treatment to these areas for Hodgkin lymphoma before the age of 30 (NCCN, 2017a).

Proliferative lesions (often referred to as ductal and lobular hyperplasia) without atypia are associated with a 1.5–2 times higher risk compared to people who do not have one of these lesions (ACS, 2015). Proliferative lesions (including ductal and lobular hyperplasia) with atypia are associated with four to five times higher risk compared to those who do not have one of these lesions (ACS, 2015; Hartmann et al., 2014). This is a nonmodifiable risk factor.

Obesity is a modifiable risk factor that increases the risk of breast cancer in postmenopausal women. Women with a body mass index (BMI) of 31.1 kg/m^2 or higher have a 2.5 times greater risk of developing breast cancer than those with a BMI of 22.6 kg/m^2 or lower (Emaus et al., 2014). Adipose tissue (especially in postmenopausal women) produces a small amount of estrogen. Having more fat tissue can increase estrogen levels and therefore increase the chance that breast cancer will develop (ACS, 2015). A large meta-analysis of women who did not use hormone replacement therapy suggests that for each 11 pounds gained during adulthood, the risk of postmenopausal breast cancer increases by 11% (Emaus et al., 2014).

Alcohol consumption, another modifiable risk factor, increases the risk of breast cancer by about 7%–10% for each drink of alcohol consumed daily on a regular basis. The risk increases with the amount of alcohol consumed (ACS, 2015). Alcohol is associated with higher levels of estrogen (Chen, Rosner, Hankinson, Colditz, & Willett, 2011). Alcohol may also lower levels of some essential nutrients that protect against cell damage, such as folate (a type of B vitamin), vitamin A, and vitamin C (NCCN, 2017a).

Family history is also a risk factor. Women with a family history of breast cancer are at increased risk for developing breast cancer. Nurses need to be able to identify families with possible hereditary predisposition for developing cancer and refer them for comprehensive genetic assessment (see Figure 2-2).

Figure 2-2. Key Indicators of Hereditary Risk for Developing Cancer

- Several relatives have developed breast and/or ovarian cancer. In general, the pedigree will show two or more first-degree relatives on the same side of the family who have developed the same or related cancers.
- Cancers are diagnosed at an age that is younger than seen in the general population (breast cancer before age 50).
- A pattern of autosomal dominant transmission is evident. Usually the cancer is seen in more than one generation, and there is evidence of vertical transmission.
- Unique tumor site combinations may be present, especially families with breast, ovarian, pancreatic, melanoma, and prostate cancers.
- An excess of multifocal or bilateral breast cancers may exist.
- An excess of multiple primary tumors may be seen. After successful treatment of one cancer, individuals from these families might go on to develop a completely new cancer, such as ovarian cancer after breast cancer.
- The family is of Ashkenazi Jewish background with a history of one or more breast cancers.
- Family history includes triple-negative breast cancer diagnosed before the age of 60.
- A history of male breast cancer exists in the family.
- There is a confirmed genetic mutation associated with breast cancer.

Note. Based on information from American Cancer Society, 2015; National Comprehensive Cancer Network, 2017c; Weitzel et al., 2011.

From "Risk Factors for Breast Cancer" (p. 16), by S.M. Mahon in S.M. Mahon (Ed.), *Site-Specific Cancer Series: Breast Cancer* (2nd ed.), 2011, Pittsburgh, PA: Oncology Nursing Society. Copyright 2011 by Oncology Nursing Society. Reprinted with permission.

Genetic Risk for Developing Breast Cancer

Approximately 10% of all cases of breast cancer are related to a hereditary predisposition (ACS, 2015). This predisposition usually results from the inheritance of a single germ-line mutation, which is usually autosomal dominant. Given the high incidence of breast cancer, even a seemingly small incidence of 10% potentially translates into a large number of affected patients.

The first step in identifying these families is to take a detailed family history and construct a pedigree that includes both maternal and paternal relatives (see Figure 2-3). First-degree relatives include parents, siblings, and children and share 50% of genetic material. Second-degree relatives include grandparents, aunts, and uncles. Second-degree relatives have 25% of their genes in common. The pedigree should also include nieces and nephews because these younger family members can provide information about childhood cancers, which also has implications for the genetic risk assessment. Third-degree relatives (cousins, great-aunts and great-uncles, and great-grandparents) can be included as well, although the accuracy of reports on these relatives is not always high. These relatives share 12.5% of the same genes. The pedigree

Figure 2-3. Three-Generation Pedigree of a Family at Risk for Developing Breast Cancer

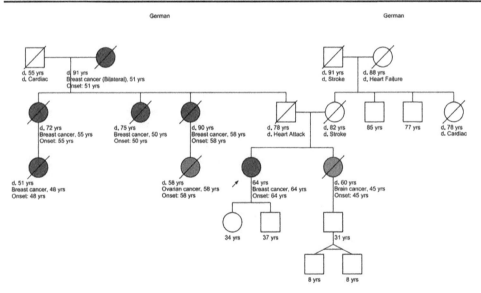

The pedigree provides an organized way to document the risk factors related to family history, such as whether a relative is alive or dead, age at death if applicable, significant medical diagnoses, or a diagnosis of cancer. Space can be provided to describe in detail the specific type of cancer, age at diagnosis, and other characteristics, such as whether a breast cancer was premenopausal or bilateral. This is a typical pedigree constructed with the purpose of visually portraying hereditary risk of developing breast and/or ovarian cancer. The arrow indicates the proband, or the member initiating inquiry about risk. Circles represent women, and squares represent men. Three generations are recorded. Current age or age at death is listed. A slash indicates a deceased family member. Cancer diagnoses and age at diagnosis are listed. This pedigree also illustrates how a male can pass the mutation on to a female because the mutation is on an autosome, not a sex chromosome. First-degree relatives have a 50% risk of having a mutation.

is used to calculate the risk of developing a cancer and the risk of having a mutation for an individual based on the number of relatives diagnosed with a malignancy, as well as how close genetically the relatives are related.

Taking a family history in the primary care setting may take 15–30 minutes depending on the size of the family and the level of reported detail. Pursuing pathology reports to confirm diagnoses takes additional time. Interpreting that information can take even longer (Mahon, 2013a). Nurses should ask patients about specific relatives and their health individually rather than asking a more general question such as, "Have any of your relatives been diagnosed with cancer?"

Pedigree assessment includes documentation of ethnicity because this is a consideration when deciding whether testing may be appropriate, and this information may alter testing strategies. For example, 1 in 40 Ashkenazi people carry one of three mutations: 185delAG and 5382insC for *BRCA1* and 6174delT for *BRCA2* (Finkelman et al., 2012). This results from a phenomenon referred to as the *founder effect*, which occurs when a population has descended from a relatively small number of people and results in the loss of genetic variation and often an increased number of deleterious mutations.

Interpreting pedigrees is further complicated by the concept of *penetrance*, which is the likelihood that a genetic change will be expressed. Not everyone with a mutation will go on to develop the cancer or cancers. For example, mutations in *BRCA1* and *BRCA2* are about 87% penetrant, meaning that approximately 87% of the women with the mutation will go on to develop breast cancer by age 70 (Petrucelli, Daly, & Pal, 2016). Sometimes a family will have members who have the mutation but, for whatever reason, have not gone on to develop the cancer. This makes evaluation of family histories challenging.

Pedigrees document potential genetic risk and can be used to teach patients and families basic genetic concepts. Reliability of patient information should be considered when obtaining and communicating the risk assessment. Reports suggest that personal recall of a family history of malignancy may be inaccurate as much as 11% of the time for first-degree relatives and even more frequently for second- and third-degree relatives (Bennett, 2010). This limits the accuracy of the risk assessment and may result in the selection of the wrong genetic test or the unnecessary use of financial resources for genetic testing that is not likely to yield informative results.

In many cases, patients may be unsure of the accuracy of the information, and ideally, healthcare providers should use pathology reports, medical records, and death certificates to confirm information about cancers. Once such records are collected, the family history often appears very different, and this ultimately may change recommendations regarding testing. Family members can find this process extremely stressful. Nurses need to educate patients on the importance of this activity and encourage them to collect the data. Figure 2-4 describes limitations of pedigree assessment.

A variety of models are available to calculate the risk of having a *BRCA1* or *BRCA2* mutation. These calculations typically provide a range of risk calculations because different models are based on different risk factors. Typically, the genetics professional provides a range of risk for having a mutation. Few models exist for calculating the risk of less common, lower penetrance genes associated with hereditary breast cancer (see Table 2-3).

When the genetics professional offers genetic testing, it is important to provide the rationale for why it is being offered. The decision to offer testing may be based on a clinical checklist, an extensive family history as reflected in a pedigree, and a high

---

Figure 2-4. Limitations and Challenges of Pedigree Assessment

---

- Most hereditary cancer syndromes have incomplete penetrance. Most families have carriers of the mutation who have lived to older ages without developing cancer.
- Family histories often are incomplete or inaccurate. Families may have inaccurate information, or family dynamics may lead to incomplete information because family members are unable or unwilling to communicate with each other.
- Sometimes family members who have the mutation may have died early from other causes such as accidents, infections, or other unexpected deaths.
- There may be false paternity. This creates challenges when counseling family members about the pedigree. The same conflicts arise if an individual learns he or she is adopted. Adoptees may have difficulty obtaining family records.
- There may be a phenocopy in the family. This means that a person develops a sporadic cancer that is the same as the cancer for which the family has hereditary risk. For example, two sisters are diagnosed with breast cancer in their mid-40s. One tests positive for a mutation, and one does not. The sister who tests negative is a phenocopy, meaning that on paper assessment, she appears to have genetic risk because she has early-onset breast cancer, but genetically, she did not inherit the mutation; rather, she developed a sporadic cancer.
- Medical records are sometimes destroyed or impossible to obtain, so an accurate pedigree cannot be constructed.
- The family may be very small or, in the case of assessing breast and ovarian cancer risk, have only a small number of female relatives. A statistical 50% chance of developing hereditary cancers may not be evident.
- Sometimes women who are mutation carriers may have already had prophylactic surgery, especially an oophorectomy, which might mask their risk or may have prevented them from developing the cancer.

Note. From "Risk Factors for Breast Cancer" (p. 17), by S.M. Mahon in S.M. Mahon (Ed.), *Site-Specific Cancer Series: Breast Cancer* (2nd ed.), 2011, Pittsburgh, PA: Oncology Nursing Society. Copyright 2011 by Oncology Nursing Society. Reprinted with permission.

probability of having a mutation. Using risk models can be confusing if the range of risk is large. At this point, clinical judgment remains a key component in estimating an individual's risk for having a mutation or hereditary risk (Weitzel, Blazer, MacDonald, Culver, & Offit, 2011).

Genetic Testing Process

Genetic testing may best be carried out by an individual who is credentialed in genetics. Some insurance companies now require that individuals be seen by a credentialed genetics professional for coverage of genetic testing costs.

Genetic credentials include certified genetic counselors credentialed by the American Board of Genetic Counseling or American Board of Medical Genetics and Genomics; American College of Medical Genetics and Genomics physician/PhD board-certified in medical genetics; and advanced genetics nursing–board certified (AGN-BC) credentialed through the American Nurses Credentialing Center.

Many professional groups advocate that genetic testing should only be ordered by credentialed genetics professionals. This includes NCCN, the American College of Medical Genetics and Genomics, the American College of Surgeons, and the National Society of Genetic Counselors (American College of Surgeons Commission on Cancer, 2015; Hampel, Bennett, Buchanan, Pearlman, & Wiesner, 2015; NCCN, 2017c). The American Society of Clinical Oncology emphasizes that patients should have access to extensive pre- and post-testing counseling but does not specify who should

Table 2-3. Models That Predict the Risk of Having a Mutation Associated With Hereditary Breast Cancer

Model	Indications	Strengths	Limitations
BRCAPRO Model (Katki, 2007)	Calculates the chance of having a *BRCA1* or *BRCA2* mutation in women with or without breast cancer	Considers the age of onset of breast cancer in family Considers both first- and second-degree relatives Considers breast and ovarian cancer history Considers oophorectomy history Considers Ashkenazi Jewish ancestry	Limited data in some minority groups May overestimate risk in women with bilateral breast cancer Requires a computer program and extensive data entry
BOADICEA Model (Antoniou et al., 2004)	Calculates the chance of having a *BRCA1* or *BRCA2* mutation in women with or without breast or ovarian cancer	Considers exact age at breast and ovarian cancer diagnosis Considers Ashkenazi Jewish ancestry Includes all first- and second-degree relatives with and without cancer	Limited data in minority groups Requires a computer program and extensive data entry
Manchester Model (Evans et al., 2004)	Estimates the risk of carrying a *BRCA1* or *BRCA2* mutation	May be useful in identifying women who have *BRCA2* mutations Targets non-Jewish women with a family history of breast and/or ovarian cancer	May be less useful in identifying women who have *BRCA1* mutations
Tyrer Cuzick (Tyrer et al., 2004)	Estimates the risk of carrying a *BRCA1* or *BRCA2* mutation	Also calculates lifetime risk of developing breast cancer	Proband must not have a diagnosis of breast cancer. Requires a computer program and some data entry

provide that counseling—only that the provider should have a knowledge of genetics (Robson et al., 2015).

However, limitations exist when genetic testing is provided outside of formal counseling by a credentialed genetics professional (Mahon, 2013c). For instance, the wrong genetic test could be ordered, and genetic test results can be misinterpreted. Inappropriate or inadequate genetic counseling results in psychosocial distress or other negative outcomes, and care is not coordinated for the rest of the family.

Hereditary Breast Cancer Syndromes

Historically, genetic testing for hereditary breast cancer was limited to the *BRCA1* and *BRCA2* genes, which was done by Sanger sequencing in which short pieces of DNA are separated by capillary electrophoresis into fragments of DNA and then analyzed by detecting the final fluorescent sequences of base pairs on each fragment. Testing for these genes became commercially available in 1998 (Matloff & Brierley, 2010).

Since 2013, testing for other genes associated with hereditary breast cancer has become commercially available. This is largely due to next-generation sequencing, or NGS (Mahon, 2013b). NGS panels analyze less common high- and intermediate-penetrance genes associated with cancer susceptibility (NCCN, 2017c).

NGS is accomplished by sequencing massive numbers of DNA sequences in a single reaction, which is often referred to as *massive parallel sequencing* and requires only one sample (blood or saliva). Benefits of NGS include lower cost than multiple, individual tests; detection of deletions, translocations, insertions, and copy number alterations; and usefulness in clinically confusing presentations when an obvious syndrome is unclear, thereby increasing the possibility of detecting a mutation and identifying a hereditary cancer syndrome (NCCN, 2017c).

Common genetic syndromes associated with breast cancer are shown in Table 2-4. Most hereditary cancer syndromes are autosomal dominant so they can be passed from either the maternal or paternal side, and each offspring of an affected person has a 50% chance of also inheriting the mutation. Management depends on the specific gene and considers family and personal history. Knowledge about risks associated with each gene, as well as recommendations, is constantly evolving. People with hereditary risk should be instructed to inquire about updated risks and management every 12–18 months.

Table 2-4. Autosomal Common Hereditary Breast Cancer Syndromes

Syndrome/Gene Location	Associated Cancers	Management Considerations
Hereditary breast and ovarian cancer syndrome • BRCA1 at 17q21 • BRCA2 at 13q21 • Affects 1 in 800–2,500 people	Female breast (55%–90%) Ovarian/fallopian tube/primary peritoneal (25%–55%) Prostate Male breast Pancreatic Melanoma Risk of second breast cancer can be as high as 65%.	**Screening for women:** • Breast self-awareness • Professional breast examination • Mammography and breast MRI at a younger age • Ovarian screening to include transvaginal ultrasound and pelvic examination • Full body dermatologic examination • Consider pancreatic cancer screening. **Screening for men:** • Breast self-awareness • Professional breast examination • Consider baseline mammogram with repeat imaging if there is gynecomastia or parenchymal/glandular breast density. • Prostate cancer screening with PSA testing and digital rectal examination beginning at about age 40 • Full body dermatologic examination • Consider pancreatic cancer screening. **Prevention for women:** • Consider chemoprevention with an agent such as tamoxifen. • Prophylactic mastectomies • Prophylactic bilateral salpingo-oophorectomy

(Continued on next page)

Table 2-4. Autosomal Common Hereditary Breast Cancer Syndromes *(Continued)*

Syndrome/Gene Location	Associated Cancers	Management Considerations
Li-Fraumeni syndrome • *TP53* at 17p13.1 • Very rare—an estimated 400 nonrelated families	Female breast Soft tissue sarcoma Osteosarcoma Brain tumors (benign and malignant) Hematologic malignancies Adrenocortical carcinoma Overall risk for cancer: nearly 100% in females, 73% in males	**Screening for women:** • Breast self-awareness • Professional breast examination • Mammography and breast MRI at a younger age • Ovarian screening to include transvaginal ultrasound and pelvic examination **Screening for men and women:** • Colonoscopy at an earlier and more frequent interval than in the general population • Annual dermatologic examination • Annual neurologic examination • Annual physical examination with attention to any new vague, unexplained symptoms • Exercise caution regarding exposure to ionizing radiation. **Prevention for women:** • Consider chemoprevention with an agent such as tamoxifen. • Consider prophylactic mastectomies and oophorectomies.
Cowden syndrome • *PTEN* at 10q23 • Affects 1 in 200,000–250,000 people	Female breast (25%–50%) Thyroid (10%) Endometrial (10%) Colon Renal Melanoma Skin manifestations, including multiple trichilemmomas, oral fibromas, and acral, palmar, and plantar keratoses	**Screening for women:** • Breast self-awareness • Professional breast examination • Mammography and breast MRI at a younger age • Ovarian screening to include transvaginal ultrasound with endometrial biopsy and pelvic examination **Screening for men and women:** • Full body dermatologic examination • Colonoscopy at a younger age and more frequent interval than in the general population • Annual thyroid ultrasound beginning at age 20 • Consider routine renal ultrasound starting at about age 20 **Prevention for women:** • Consider chemoprevention with an agent such as tamoxifen. • Prophylactic mastectomies • Prophylactic total hysterectomy with bilateral salpingo-oophorectomy
Ataxia telangiectasia • *ATM* at 11q22.3 • Affects 1 in 30,000–100,000 people	Female breast Colon Pancreatic	**Screening for women:** • Breast self-awareness • Professional breast examination • Mammography and breast MRI at a younger age **Screening for men and women:** • Colonoscopy at a younger age and more frequent interval than in the general population • Consider pancreatic screening. • Exercise caution regarding exposure to ionizing radiation. **Prevention for women:** • Consider chemoprevention with an agent such as tamoxifen. • Consider prophylactic mastectomies.

(Continued on next page)

Table 2-4. Autosomal Common Hereditary Breast Cancer Syndromes *(Continued)*

Syndrome/Gene Location	Associated Cancers	Management Considerations
Peutz-Jeghers syndrome • *STK11* at 19p13.3 • Affects 1 in 120,000 people	Female breast (30%–60%) Ovarian tumors (25%) Colorectal (35%–40%) Pancreatic (10%–35%) Gastric (30%) Lung (15%) Small intestine (15%) Cervical (10%) Endometrial (10%) Testicular tumors (10%) Characterized by melanocytic macules on the lips, perioral, and buccal regions Multiple gastrointestinal polyps including hamartomas	**Screening for women:** • Breast self-awareness • Professional breast examination • Mammography and breast MRI at a younger age • Ovarian screening to include transvaginal ultrasound with endometrial biopsy and pelvic examination **Screening for men and women:** • Full body dermatologic examination • Colonoscopy, upper endoscopy, and small bowel visualization at a younger age and more frequent interval than in the general population • Consider pancreatic screening. • Annual physical examination with attention to any new vague, unexplained symptoms **Prevention for women:** • Consider chemoprevention with an agent such as tamoxifen. • Consider prophylactic mastectomies. • Consider prophylactic bilateral salpingo-oophorectomy with or without a hysterectomy.
CDH1 • 16q22.1	Female breast (40%–55%) Diffuse gastric cancer (40%–85%) Colon	**Screening for women:** • Breast self-awareness • Professional breast examination • Mammography and breast MRI at a younger age **Screening for men and women:** • Routine endoscopy starting in teenage years with biopsies • Colonoscopy at a younger age and more frequent interval than the general population **Prevention for women:** • Consider chemoprevention with an agent such as tamoxifen. • Consider prophylactic mastectomies. **Prevention for men and women:** Strongly consider prophylactic gastrectomy.
CHEK2 • 22q12.1	Female breast Male breast Colon, prostate Thyroid Endometrial (serous) Ovarian	**Screening for women:** • Breast self-awareness • Professional breast examination • Mammography and breast MRI at a younger age • Ovarian and endometrial screening to include transvaginal ultrasound, possible endometrial biopsy and pelvic examination **Screening for men:** • Breast self-awareness • Professional breast examination • Consider baseline mammogram with repeat imaging if there is gynecomastia or parenchymal/glandular breast density

(Continued on next page)

Table 2-4. Autosomal Common Hereditary Breast Cancer Syndromes *(Continued)*

Syndrome/Gene Location	Associated Cancers	Management Considerations
CHEK2 (cont.)		• Prostate cancer screening with PSA testing and digital rectal examination beginning at about age 40 **Screening for men and women:** • Annual thyroid examination, which might include ultrasound • Colonoscopy at a younger age and more frequent interval than the general population • Colonoscopy at a younger age and more frequent interval than the general population **Prevention for women:** • Consider chemoprevention with an agent such as tamoxifen. • Prophylactic mastectomies • Prophylactic bilateral salpingo-oophorectomy
PALB2 • 16p12.2	Female breast (25%–60%) Male breast Pancreatic Ovarian	**Screening for women:** • Breast self-awareness • Professional breast examination • Mammography and breast MRI at a younger age • Ovarian screening to include transvaginal ultrasound and pelvic examination • Consider pancreatic cancer screening. **Screening for men:** • Breast self-awareness • Professional breast examination • Consider baseline mammogram with repeat imaging if there is gynecomastia or parenchymal/glandular breast density. • Consider pancreatic cancer screening. **Prevention for women:** • Consider chemoprevention with an agent such as tamoxifen. • Consider prophylactic mastectomies. • Consider prophylactic bilateral salpingo-oophorectomy.
FANCC • 9q22.3	Female breast	**Screening for women:** • Breast self-awareness • Professional breast examination • Mammography and breast MRI at a younger age **Prevention for women** • Consider chemoprevention with an agent such as tamoxifen. • Consider prophylactic mastectomies.
XRCC2 • 7q36.1	Female breast Pancreatic	**Screening for women:** • Breast self-awareness • Professional breast examination • Mammography and breast MRI at a younger age • Consider pancreatic cancer screening. **Prevention for women:** • Consider chemoprevention with an agent such as tamoxifen. • Consider prophylactic mastectomies.

(Continued on next page)

Table 2-4. Autosomal Common Hereditary Breast Cancer Syndromes *(Continued)*

Syndrome/Gene Location	Associated Cancers	Management Considerations
BARD1 • 2q35	Female breast Ovarian	**Screening for women:** • Breast self-awareness • Professional breast examination • Mammography and breast MRI at a younger age • Ovarian screening to include transvaginal ultrasound and pelvic examination **Prevention for women:** • Consider chemoprevention with an agent such as tamoxifen. • Consider prophylactic mastectomies. • Consider prophylactic bilateral salpingo-oophorectomy.
NN • 8q21	Female breast Ovarian Prostate	**Screening for women:** • Breast self-awareness • Professional breast examination • Mammography and breast MRI at a younger age • Ovarian screening to include transvaginal ultrasound and pelvic examination **Prevention for women:** • Consider chemoprevention with an agent such as tamoxifen. • Consider prophylactic mastectomies. • Consider prophylactic bilateral salpingo-oophorectomy.
RAD51C • 17q22 *RAD51D* • 17q11	Female breast Ovarian	**Screening for women:** • Breast self-awareness • Professional breast examination • Mammography and breast MRI at a younger age • Ovarian screening to include transvaginal ultrasound and pelvic examination **Prevention for women:** • Consider chemoprevention with an agent such as tamoxifen. • Consider prophylactic mastectomies. • Consider bilateral prophylactic salpingo-oophorectomy.
BRIP1 • 17q22.2	Female breast Ovarian	**Screening for women:** • Breast self-awareness • Professional breast examination • Mammography and breast MRI at a younger age • Ovarian screening to include transvaginal ultrasound and pelvic examination **Prevention for women:** • Consider chemoprevention with an agent such as tamoxifen. • Consider prophylactic mastectomies. • Consider bilateral prophylactic salpingo-oophorectomy.

MRI—magnetic resonance imaging; PSA—prostate-specific antigen

Note. Based on information from Hampel et al., 2015; Mahon, 2014a, 2014b, 2016; National Comprehensive Cancer Network, 2017c; Petrucelli et al., 2016; Walsh et al., 2011; Weitzel et al., 2011.

Components of Genetic Counseling

Pretest Counseling

Pretest counseling includes multiple steps and can take approximately 90 minutes to ensure that all concerns are adequately addressed (Mahon, 2013a; Weitzel et al., 2011). The genetics professional performs the following steps:

- Introduces self to the patient and family and discusses the purpose of the visit and the agenda
- Assesses if the patient and family have concerns, motivations, or expectations regarding genetic testing
- Constructs a three-generation pedigree that includes maternal and paternal sides with current ages or age at death, diagnoses of cancer, cause of death, and ethnicity
- Assesses other risk factors based on lifestyle and past medical history
- Assesses current screening practices and dates and outcomes of most recent screening tests
- Assesses family dynamics regarding sharing information and support, as well as other support systems, and how the patient and family have managed other stressful situations in the past
- Performs targeted physical examination to identify features associated with hereditary cancer syndromes as appropriate, such as head circumference or presence of dermatologic lesions
- Provides calculations regarding risk of developing cancer in the context of absolute and relative risk and the risk of having a mutation
- Describes any factors that limit the accuracy of the risk assessment or make it difficult to interpret
- Discusses basic principles of cancer genetics in understandable terms using the pedigree to augment teaching
- Identifies the best candidate in whom to initiate testing and explains why that person is best
- Discusses that the alternative to genetic testing is not testing and manages the patient based on risk assessment
- Discusses the possible risk of discrimination and the impact of genetic test results on life insurance, disability insurance, or long-term care insurance
- Provides the rationale for the testing strategy and why a specific test or panel of tests is being ordered
- Discusses how the specimen will be collected (usually blood or saliva), the test's turnaround time, costs of testing, insurance coverage, and preauthorization for the genetic test
- Discusses the possible outcomes of testing, including positive, negative, and variant of unknown significance, as well as possible management strategies for each outcome, including prophylactic surgery, chemoprevention, or aggressive surveillance (see Table 2-5)
- Discusses potential psychological risks and responses to genetic testing results and decisions
- Discusses the responsibility of communicating genetic information to at-risk family members and healthcare providers

Ordering genetic testing may occur at the end of the pretest session or in a separate appointment. Additional steps in the pretest session include completion of test req-

Table 2-5. Classification of Variants

Classification	Definition	Clinical Implications
Negative (polymorphism)	Very strong evidence that the genetic change is not associated with increased susceptibility for developing a disease; such changes may be detected during genetic testing but are not routinely reported.	At-risk family members should not be offered targeted testing. Medical management (e.g., screening, prevention measures) is based on personal and family history, not genetic testing.
Pathogenic mutation	Sufficient evidence that the genetic change is capable of causing increased risk for developing a disease	Affects medical management (e.g., screening, prevention measures); can offer targeted testing to at-risk family members
Variant (likely benign)	Strong evidence that the genetic change is not associated with increased susceptibility for developing a disease	At-risk family members should not be offered targeted testing. Medical management (e.g., screening, prevention measures) is based on personal and family history, not genetic testing.
Variant (likely pathogenic)	Strong evidence that the genetic change is capable of causing increased risk for developing a disease; more evidence is needed to classify as a pathogenic mutation.	Affects medical management, particularly screening recommendations. Prevention measures may be offered, depending on what is known about the variant. Targeted testing can be offered to at-risk family members to help them clarify the risk.
Variant of unknown significance	Genetic changes with limited and conflicting evidence regarding whether the genetic change is associated with an increased risk for developing a disease	Targeted testing of family members to collect cosegregation data may help to clarify the meaning of the variant in the context of a laboratory-supported reclassification study. Medical management (e.g., screening, prevention measures) is based on personal and family history, not genetic testing.

Note. Based on information from Couzin-Frankel, 2014; Eggington et al., 2014; Rehm et al., 2013; Sijmons et al., 2013.

From "Management of Patients With a Genetic Variant of Unknown Significance," by S.M. Mahon, 2015, *Oncology Nursing Forum, 42,* p. 317. Copyright 2015 by Oncology Nursing Society. Reprinted with permission.

uisition form and necessary documentation, including pedigree and clinical notes; review and acknowledgment of informed consent document; collection of the specimen; and discussion of how genetic test results will be disclosed.

Post-Test Counseling

Post-test counseling includes disclosure of results and can take up to an hour depending on family dynamics, results, and emotional response to the results. Post-test counseling consists of the genetics professional performing the following steps:
- Discusses and interprets what the test results mean for the patient and other family members, including a discussion of the benefits and limitations of testing
- Discusses personalized recommendations for cancer prevention and early detection based on genetic testing results, personal risk factors, and family history

- Identifies at-risk family members who also would benefit from genetic testing or modification of screening and prevention interventions
- Provides and discusses strategies for informing other family members about test results and offers coordination of care for relatives who live in a different geographic area
- Identifies clinical trials appropriate for the patient and at-risk family members
- Provides psychosocial support as needed
- Provides the individual and family with written recommendations summarizing the pre- and post-test counseling sessions, including a copy of the pedigree, genetic testing results, and risk calculations as appropriate

Benefits of Genetic Testing

Cancer susceptibility genetic testing has the potential to identify whether a person is at increased risk for a specific cancer or cancers associated with a hereditary cancer syndrome. Individuals with known genetic predisposition can develop a plan for cancer screening and prevention consistent with their values and needs. Individuals who test negative for a known mutation in their family often can experience decreased anxiety, as their risk for developing malignancy is that of the general population, and their children will not inherit the risk. They can engage in population-based screening recommendations. Ultimately, this saves healthcare financial resources as well.

Risks of Genetic Testing

Psychological distress, both short and long term, may result from genetic testing (Mahon, 2014c). Parents may be distressed and worry about risks that have been passed to their children. Patients may be confused and overwhelmed by the many recommendations for management, especially if the result is indeterminate or positive. Individuals who test negative for a known familial mutation may feel guilty because they did not inherit the risk but other siblings did.

Loss of privacy is another potential risk. Friends and employers may learn of a genetic mutation if the individual needs to take time off for necessary prevention measures. Another privacy concern is that family members who did not want to know their genetic status may learn about it indirectly. For example, a parent has a sister with a known mutation. The parent refuses testing. The offspring of the parent opts to test and is found to have the familial mutation. The parent is an obligate carrier and now realizes he or she carries the mutation despite not wanting to know.

Discrimination by employers and insurers also can be an issue. Federal legislation prohibits group health insurers and employers from discriminating against people based on their genetic risk. This legislation is the Genetic Information Nondiscrimination Act of 2008, commonly referred to as GINA (U.S. Department of Health and Human Services, 2009). A genetic mutation might make it more difficult to obtain life, disability, or long-term care insurance. This risk should be discussed in the pre-test counseling session in the event the patient wants to purchase more of this type of insurance prior to testing.

Individuals who test negative for a known familial mutation may develop a false sense of security about their risks for developing cancer. They still have the population risk for developing malignancy and need to follow population-based guidelines for prevention and early detection. Their risk for developing cancer is not zero.

Limitations of Genetic Testing

Genetic tests cannot predict when, where, or if an individual will be diagnosed with cancer. One of the challenges in the communication of genetic risk information and genetic test results is that probabilities and uncertainties surround genetic information. Not all mutations are detectable. Families with substantial family histories who test negative for mutations even with NGS may still have increased risk. A negative result is only truly negative if there is a known mutation in the family. Otherwise, a negative result is noninformative and only means that the individual tested negative for known mutations on whatever genes were tested (Mahon, 2015).

For many genetic mutations, the clinical significance is not completely clear, or there is not a clear plan for management.

Primary Prevention of Breast Cancer

Definitions of Prevention

Primary prevention measures are the direct steps to prevent or delay breast cancer from developing. *Secondary prevention* is the implementation of screening or early detection measures to detect cancer in the asymptomatic phase, when treatment is most likely to be effective and the least toxic. *Tertiary prevention* includes measures to screen for second malignancies in cancer survivors, as well as the management and prevention of long-term complications due to cancer therapies.

Lifestyle Factors

Breast-feeding for at least one year may slightly reduce the risk of developing breast cancer, especially triple-negative cancers (ACS, 2015). This may be because breast-feeding stops menstruation, thereby reducing the lifetime number of menstrual cycles, and because breast-feeding induces protective structural changes in the breast.

Women who engage in regular physical activity have a 10%–25% lower risk of breast cancer, especially for postmenopausal women (ACS, 2015). ACS recommends at least 150 minutes of moderate-intensity or 75 minutes of vigorous-intensity activity each week spread out over the week (ACS, 2017b).

Women who eat a diet high in fruits and vegetables may reduce their risk of hormone receptor–negative breast cancer (ACS, 2015). ACS recommends at least two and a half cups of fresh fruits and vegetables daily, which leads to higher levels of protective carotenoids (ACS, 2017b).

Chemoprevention

Two medications (tamoxifen and raloxifene) have received U.S. Food and Drug Administration approval for the prevention of breast cancer in women with an increased risk for developing breast cancer (at least 20%–25%) (ACS, 2015).

These medications are known as selective estrogen receptor modulators because they block estrogen in some tissues of the body but have an estrogen-like effect in others. A meta-analysis of more than 83,000 high-risk women from nine breast cancer prevention trials found that taking a selective estrogen receptor modulator reduced estrogen receptor–positive breast cancer risk by 38% over 10 years (Cuzick et al., 2013). Tamoxifen is approved for both pre- and postmenopausal women, and raloxifene is approved for postmenopausal women. Rare but significant side effects include embolus and endometrial cancer. Currently, aromatase inhibitors are in clinical trials with postmenopausal women to prevent breast cancer. These agents are associated with an increased risk for developing osteoporosis. Women who opt to take a chemoprevention agent should do so only after a risk assessment validates that their risk is increased and they have had a discussion of the potential risks and benefits of taking a chemoprevention agent. They need to be monitored closely for side effects. Data are conflicting on when to start chemoprevention; it depends on the family history and how long to use the agent (usually 5–10 years) (Cuzick et al., 2013).

Prophylactic Surgery

Prophylactic surgery generally is reserved for women who have a documented mutation associated with increased risk for developing breast cancer and should only be done after careful evaluation of the potential risks and benefits, especially given the variable penetrance of many genetic mutations. Not every woman with a mutation will go on to develop breast cancer (Weitzel et al., 2011). A prophylactic mastectomy will reduce the risk of developing breast cancer by 90%–95% (NCCN, 2017c). A prophylactic oophorectomy, especially before the age of 50, may reduce the risk of developing breast cancer by up to 50% (NCCN, 2017c).

Patient Education Regarding Early Detection

Women should receive information about the strengths and limitations of screening tools, including information about the recommended time interval for each. Nurses should be aware of barriers to the early detection of breast cancer and take steps to remove the barriers (see Figure 2-5).

Women should be informed that screening is for asymptomatic women. Symptomatic women need to be referred directly for a diagnostic evaluation. Signs and symptoms of breast cancer that warrant immediate evaluation should be discussed (see Figure 2-6). Education also includes discussion and reminders of ways to prevent breast cancer, especially lifestyle factors. Patients must be made aware that if their family history changes or a change occurs in another risk factor, screening recommendations may be modified. Risk assessments should be updated annually. Women should be instructed that once they have been provided information about risk and screening options, they need to make the decision about what options they would like to pursue.

Nurses need to be able to instruct patients on the possible outcomes and the accuracy of screening tests.

- A true-positive (TP) test result is one that correctly identifies cancer in a person who has a diagnosis of cancer.

Figure 2-5. Barriers to Engaging in Breast Cancer Screening

System Barriers
• Conflicting recommendations create confusion about recommendations.
• Facilities may be geographically inaccessible or have inconvenient hours.
• Healthcare providers may be confused about the variety of recommendations from different agencies.
• Healthcare providers may not focus on wellness.
• Healthcare providers may not recommend screening.
• Risk assessment may not be conducted or may not be accurate to recommend appropriate screening.

Patient Barriers
• The woman underestimates the magnitude of her risk.
• The woman does not understand the potential benefits of screening.
• The woman lacks insurance or ability to pay for screening.
• The woman cannot access transportation to get to screening.
• The woman has other complications that prevent access to screening, including lack of screening availability during off working hours or difficulty obtaining child care.
• Mammography or breast examination might be considered embarrassing.
• Mammography or a breast examination might be culturally unacceptable.
• The woman may have language barriers.
• The woman may not have spousal, partner, or social support to complete screening.

Note. Based on information from American Cancer Society, 2015; Centers for Disease Control and Prevention, 2017; Nadalin et al., 2016.

From "Prevention and Detection" (p. 41), by S.M. Mahon in S.M. Mahon (Ed.), *Site-Specific Cancer Series: Breast Cancer* (2nd ed.), 2011, Pittsburgh, PA: Oncology Nursing Society. Copyright 2011 by Oncology Nursing Society. Adapted with permission.

• A true-negative (TN) test result is a normal or negative screen for cancer in an individual who is subsequently found not to have cancer within a defined period after the last test.
• A false-negative (FN) test result is one that fails to identify cancer in an individual who actually has cancer.
• A false-positive (FP) test result is an abnormal test for cancer screening in an individual who does not have cancer. A high FP test rate can result in unnecessary follow-up testing and anxiety in people who have a positive screen.

The sensitivity of a screening test is its ability to detect those individuals with cancer. It is calculated by taking the number of TPs and dividing it by the total number of cancer cases (TP + FN). The specificity of a test is its ability to identify those individuals who do not have cancer. It is calculated by dividing the number of TNs by the sum of the TN and FP cases.

Figure 2-6. Signs and Symptoms of Breast Cancer

• A mass or lump in the breast or axilla, which may or may not be painful
• Swelling or thickening in all or part of the breast
• Skin irritation or change in color, redness, or scaliness of the skin
• Dimpling or indentation of the breast skin
• Nipple inversion in a previously everted nipple
• Nipple eversion in a previous inverted nipple
• Change in the direction a nipple points
• Nipple discharge other than breast milk
• Any persistent change in the breast

Note. Based on information from American Cancer Society, 2015; National Comprehensive Cancer Network, 2017a.

Access in Special Populations

Disparities among racial groups exist in utilization of screening mammography (ACS, 2015). These disparities stem from many factors, including misconceptions or a lack of knowledge, low income status, unemployment, and lack of insurance. Overall, in 2013, 69% of women aged 45 and older had undergone a mammogram in the past two years (ACS, 2015). The rates by race/ethnicity were 69% of non-Hispanic White women, 60% of non-Hispanic African American women, 69% of Asian American women, 61% of Native American and Alaska Native women, and 64% of Hispanic women. Lower utilization (54%) was seen in women with a high school or less education. Lack of insurance is another major barrier; only 39% of women without insurance aged 45 and older had undergone a mammogram in the past two years (ACS, 2015).

Disparities in mammography screening for people with disabilities are related to physical and sociologic barriers. Many mammography facilities are ill-equipped to service people using a wheelchair. Women with disabilities are living longer, and preventive measures should be available for health maintenance.

Women who are uninsured or underinsured may not know how to access free and low-cost screening mammograms. Congress passed the Breast and Cervical Cancer Mortality Prevention Act of 1990, which resulted in the National Breast and Cervical Cancer Early Detection Program, or the NBCCEDP (Centers for Disease Control and Prevention, 2017). The program provides low-income, uninsured, and underserved women access to breast and cervical cancer screening and diagnostic services. An estimated 10% of U.S. women of screening age are eligible to receive NBCCEDP breast cancer screening services (Centers for Disease Control and Prevention, 2017). Federal guidelines establish an eligibility baseline to direct services to uninsured and underinsured women who are at or below 250% of federal poverty level and aged 21–64 for cervical cancer screening or aged 40–64 for breast cancer screening. Services include clinical breast examinations, mammograms, Pap tests, diagnostic testing for women with abnormal screening outcomes, surgical consultation, and referrals to treatment. Since 1991, the NBCCEDP has served more than 4.8 million women, provided more than 12 million screening examinations, and diagnosed 67,959 breast cancers. At age 65, women become eligible for Medicare, which provides coverage for breast cancer screening, including mammography.

Recommendations for Early Detection of Breast Cancer

Early detection and screening measures are referred to as secondary prevention measures. Recommendations for early detection are based on the risk assessment. The ultimate goal of risk assessment is a decrease in cancer morbidity and mortality. Risk assessment also provides the foundation for shared decision making and informed consent so that individuals can make appropriate decisions about genetic testing, cancer screening, and cancer prevention maneuvers (Jimbo et al., 2013). Average-risk women can follow population-based recommendations for the early detection of breast cancer (see Table 2-6). Women at increased risk may benefit from a modification of these guidelines (NCCN, 2017c).

Breast Self-Awareness

Breast self-awareness is sometimes referred to as breast self-examination (BSE). BSE has been routinely recommended in the past by physicians, nurses, and profes-

Table 2-6. Recommendations for the Early Detection of Breast Cancer

Organization	Breast Self-Examination	Clinical Breast Examination	Mammography	Breast MRI
American Cancer Society (2015)	Not recommended Women should be instructed on changes that should be evaluated promptly.	Not recommended	Begin at age 45, with opportunity to begin annual screening between ages 40 and 44. Interval: Annually for women aged 45–54, with option to continue annual screening or transition to biennial screening at age 55 Women should continue screening mammography as long as their overall health is good and they have a life expectancy of 10 years or more.	Women at high lifetime risk Those with known BRCA1 or BRCA2 or other genetic susceptibility mutations Had radiation therapy to the chest when they were 10–30 years of age Have a lifetime risk of breast cancer of 15%–20%, according to risk assessment tools that are based mainly on family history Have a personal history of breast cancer, ductal carcinoma in situ, lobular carcinoma in situ, atypical ductal hyperplasia, or atypical lobular hyperplasia
American College of Obstetricians and Gynecologists (2011)	Consider for high-risk patients. Breast self-awareness is recommended for all women.	Age 20–39: every 1–3 years Age 40 and older: annually	Begin at age 40 and perform annually. No recommendation as to when to stop screening mammography.	Not recommended for screening women at average risk of developing breast cancer. Women who are estimated to have a lifetime risk of breast cancer of 20% or greater, based on risk models that rely largely on family history, but who are either untested or tested negative for BRCA mutations can be offered enhanced screening, which might include breast MRI. Women who test positive for BRCA1 and BRCA2 mutations should be offered enhanced screening and education about risk reduction methods.

(Continued on next page)

Table 2-6. Recommendations for the Early Detection of Breast Cancer *(Continued)*

Organization	Breast Self-Examination	Clinical Breast Examination	Mammography	Breast MRI
Canadian Task Force on Preventive Health Care (2011)	Not recommended	Not recommended	For women aged 40–49 years, recommended to not routinely screen with mammography. Begin at age 50 and perform every 2–3 years until age 75.	Not recommended
National Comprehensive Cancer Network (2017b)	Breast awareness is encouraged for asymptomatic women beginning at age 25.	Age 20–39: every 1–3 years Age 40 and older: annually	Begin at age 40 and perform annually. No recommendation as to when to stop screening mammography.	Women with a lifetime risk of breast cancer of greater than 20% can consider breast MRI to start 10 years before the youngest diagnosis of breast cancer in the family but not before age 30.
U.S. Preventive Services Task Force (Siu, 2016)	Not recommended	Not recommended	The decision to start at age 40 should be an individualized one. Recommended to start at age 50 and perform every 2 years for women aged 50–74. No recommendation as to when to stop screening mammography.	Not recommended

MRI—magnetic resonance imaging

Note. From "Prevention and Detection" (p. 43), by S.M. Mahon in S.M. Mahon (Ed.), *Site-Specific Cancer Series: Breast Cancer* (2nd ed.), 2011, Pittsburgh, PA: Oncology Nursing Society. Copyright 2011 by Oncology Nursing Society. Adapted with permission.

sional organizations as an adjunct tool to facilitate the early detection of breast cancer (ACS, 2015). Very few studies have been done to substantiate its effectiveness (i.e., decrease in mortality) or associated financial and emotional costs. The underlying rationale has been that women who perform BSE find lumps earlier than women who do not perform BSE and that the lumps are smaller and more easily treated, thereby decreasing mortality. The current focus is on breast self-awareness and emphasizes that women may choose to practice it if they desire. The goal is to detect changes in the breast and includes both observing the breasts for changes and palpating the breast for lumps or other changes in breast tissue.

Clinical Breast Examination

Historically, screening for breast cancer has included a recommendation for a clinical examination (ACS, 2015). The premise for this recommendation is that some breast cancers may not be detected on mammography but on clinical examination (NCCN, 2017b). A clinical breast examination includes inspection of the breast, as well as palpation. Many professional groups have moved away from recommending a clinical examination in women of average risk because research suggests that a clinical breast examination in conjunction with mammography has been shown to detect only a small proportion of breast cancer tumors and increases the probability of FPs (ACS, 2015).

Screening Mammography

The goal of screening mammography is to detect breast cancer when it is still too small to be felt by a healthcare provider or the patient. During mammography, the technologist will position the patient and image each breast separately. Each breast is carefully positioned on a special plate and then gently compressed with a paddle (often made of clear Plexiglas® or other plastic). This compression flattens the breast so that the maximum amount of tissue can be imaged and examined. Correct positioning of the breast during mammography is extremely important. If the entire breast is not in the field or if something is blocking the field, the diagnosis can be compromised. It is also easier to apply proper compression when the breast is positioned correctly. Breast compression may cause some discomfort, but it only lasts for a brief time during the mammography procedure. Patients should feel firm pressure from the compression but no significant pain. Regular mammography in women older than the age of 40 reduces the risk of dying of breast cancer by 20% (ACS, 2015).

Screening Magnetic Resonance Imaging

Women at increased risk for developing breast cancer (lifetime risk greater than 20%–25%) might benefit from screening breast MRI (ACS, 2015; NCCN, 2017b). MRI uses magnetic fields and dedicated breast MRI equipment with biopsy capability to create detailed, cross-sectional images of the breast following the IV injection of contrast material (usually gadolinium-DTPA). MRI is an adjunct rather than a replacement for mammography (NCCN, 2017b). Insurance coverage can be variable and usually requires justification of risk and benefit.

Nursing Implications

Education

Healthcare professionals need continual updates on risk assessment models and strategies, as well as current guidelines for cancer prevention and early detection. Genetics professionals need continual updates on new genes associated with increased cancer risk and management strategies for those at increased risk. Resources for healthcare providers to stay updated are shown in Table 2-7.

Table 2-7. Selected Resources on Breast Cancer Genetics, Prevention, and Early Detection

Resource	Contents
American Cancer Society Breast Cancer Facts and Figures www.cancer.org	Detailed statistics about breast cancer risk, epidemiology, and screening recommendations
Facing Our Risk of Cancer Empowered (FORCE) www.facingourrisk.org	Organization that provides support and education for women and families affected by hereditary risk for developing breast cancer
GeneReviews® www.ncbi.nlm.nih.gov/books/NBK1116	Searchable database of common human genes with detailed information about the epidemiology, testing strategies, and management recommendations for specific mutations
National Comprehensive Cancer Network www.nccn.org	Evidence-based guidelines on breast cancer risk assessment and reduction, breast cancer screening, and hereditary risk for developing breast cancer
National Guideline Clearinghouse www.guideline.gov	Comprehensive list of guidelines from multiple professional organizations; allows for search and comparison of guidelines
National Society of Genetic Counselors www.nsgc.org	Searchable database to locate genetics professionals by geographic region

Administration

If the institution cannot provide a specific service, such as access to a genetics professional, arrangements need to be made to contract for such services. If the institution provides screening services, it needs to have a careful protocol for informing patients of results and arranging for prompt diagnostic workup for those with abnormal screens.

Clinical Practice

The implementation of cancer prevention and early detection is based on an accurate risk assessment (see Figure 2-7). Nurses in all areas of oncology practice can instruct patients and families on the importance of understanding their risk and engaging in cancer prevention and early detection maneuvers. Advanced practice nurses can order screening and diagnostic evaluations as appropriate, and advanced practice nurses with additional training and credentialing can perform genetic risk assessments, order genetic tests, and provide recommendations for prevention and early detection based on the risk assessment and genetic testing results.

Research

More research is needed to find the best ways to communicate risk to patients and families and to engage patients in recommended screening and prevention measures. In addition, more research is needed to better understand how patients make deci-

Figure 2-7. Summary of Breast Cancer Risk Assessment Procedures

Address Psychosocial Concerns
- Assess for any psychosocial concerns that may limit the patient's ability to understand or engage in breast cancer prevention and early detection.
- Assess beliefs about the causes of cancer.
- Assess motivations for seeking cancer risk assessment.
- Assess experiences with cancer and feelings, perceptions, concerns, or fears related to those experiences.
- Consider cultural, religious, and socioeconomic background.
- Provide an opportunity for the patient to describe any fears and concerns.
- Assess for depression, anxiety, or other signs that might suggest difficulty adjusting to the information. Refer the patient for further services when indicated.
- Assess if the patient has the financial resources or insurance to pay for screening and if there are patient barriers to accessing screening. If barriers are identified, the patient should be referred to the appropriate social services and programs.

Gather Information for the Risk Assessment
- Gather family history, which includes at least three generations, age at onset of cancer, and diagnoses. Confirm diagnoses with reports whenever possible.
- Assess reproductive risk factors:
  - Age at menarche
  - Age at first pregnancy and number of pregnancies
  - Hormonal contraceptive use
  - Hormone replacement therapy use
  - Age at menopause
- Assess past history of breast biopsies (confirm with pathology report).
- Assess lifestyle risk factors:
  - Alcohol use
  - Exercise patterns
  - Dietary patterns
  - Height and weight to assess for obesity

Construct the Risk Assessment
- Select a model to predict risk for the individual patient.
- When appropriate, select a model to predict the patient's risk of carrying a mutation.

Communicate the Risk Assessment
- Discuss the patient's absolute risk of developing breast cancer.
- Discuss the patient's relative risk of developing breast cancer.
- Families with suspected hereditary risk should be referred to a genetics professional who will communicate:
  - The risk of carrying a mutation in families with a suspected hereditary predisposition
  - Basic concepts of genetics and inheritance
  - Options for genetic testing
- Discuss the strengths and limitations of cancer risk assessment.
- Discuss the options available for risk management:
  - Specific recommendations for prevention, including lifestyle changes
  - Specific recommendations for screening, including data on the accuracy and limitations of the recommended screening strategies, including mammography
- Inform the patient regarding signs and symptoms of cancer.
- Provide culturally appropriate written materials when possible.
- Explain how the screening results will be communicated to the patient. Follow the office visit with a written letter summarizing the recommendations made in the office.
- Provide guidance on discussing the risk assessment with family members, especially in the case of a hereditary predisposition.

(Continued on next page)

Figure 2-7. Summary of Breast Cancer Risk Assessment Procedures *(Continued)*

Long-Term Follow-Up
• Engage the patient in regular follow-up, with reminders if needed.
• Assess whether the patient is practicing the recommended prevention and early detection strategies.
• Update the family history and risk assessment. Revise recommendations as indicated.
• Assist patients with a hereditary risk in contacting and informing other family members who also may have a hereditary risk.

Note. From "Risk Factors for Breast Cancer" (p. 28), by S.M. Mahon in S.M. Mahon (Ed.), *Site-Specific Cancer Series: Breast Cancer* (2nd ed.), 2011, Pittsburgh, PA: Oncology Nursing Society. Copyright 2011 by Oncology Nursing Society. Adapted with permission.

sions about genetic testing and how to facilitate positive outcomes. Nurses can serve as a resource to the media to explain information for the public on new research and findings on breast cancer risk factors, as well as concepts related to cancer prevention and early detection.

Summary

Risk factor assessment forms the foundation for providing appropriate recommendations for breast cancer prevention and early detection. Oncology nurses should provide education to all women about the epidemiology of breast cancer and the rationale for a comprehensive breast cancer risk assessment. Whenever possible, efforts should be made to encourage individuals to reduce their risk for developing breast cancer, including the adoption of a healthy lifestyle. Women and men with a suspected or known predisposition for developing breast cancer should undergo evaluation with a genetics professional to determine if genetic testing is appropriate and to interpret genetic testing results. These individuals often require more aggressive screening and prevention efforts and often at an earlier age than recommended for those in the general population. Nurses should educate women on recommended screening measures, including the strengths and limitations of the recommended measures. When properly implemented, breast cancer screening measures can be a powerful tool in reducing the morbidity and mortality associated with breast cancer.

References

American Cancer Society. (2015). *Breast cancer facts and figures 2015–2016*. Atlanta, GA: Author.

American Cancer Society. (2017a). *Cancer facts and figures 2017*. Atlanta, GA: Author.

American Cancer Society. (2017b). *Cancer prevention and early detection facts and figures 2017–2018*. Atlanta, GA: Author.

American College of Obstetricians and Gynecologists. (2011). Practice Bulletin No. 122: Breast cancer screening. *Obstetrics and Gynecology, 118,* 372–382. doi:10.1097/AOG.0b013e31822c98e5

American College of Surgeons Commission on Cancer. (2015). *Cancer program standards: Ensuring patient-centered care* (2016 ed.). Retrieved from https://www.facs.org/quality-programs/cancer/coc/standards

Antoniou, A.C., Pharoah, P.P.D., Smith, P., & Easton, D.F. (2004). The BOADICEA model of genetic susceptibility to breast and ovarian cancer. *British Journal of Cancer, 91,* 1580–1590. doi:10.1038/sj.bjc.6602175

Beaber, E.F., Malone, K.E., Tang, M.-T.C., Barlow, W.E., Porter, P.L., Daling, J.R., & Li, C.I. (2014). Oral contraceptives and breast cancer risk overall and by molecular subtype among young women. *Cancer Epidemiology, Biomarkers and Prevention, 23,* 755–764. doi:10.1158/1055-9965.EPI-13-0944

Bennett, R.L. (2010). *The practical guide to the genetic family history* (2nd ed.). Hoboken, NJ: Wiley-Blackwell.

Brinton, L.A., Scoccia, B., Moghissi, K.S., Westhoff, C.L., Niwa, S., Ruggieri, D., ... Lamb, E.J. (2014). Long-term relationship of ovulation-stimulating drugs to breast cancer risk. *Cancer Epidemiology, Biomarkers and Prevention, 23,* 584–593. doi:10.1158/1055-9965.EPI-13-0996

Canadian Task Force on Preventive Health Care. (2011). Recommendations on screening for breast cancer in average-risk women aged 40–74 years. *Canadian Medical Association Journal, 183,* 1991–2001. doi:10.1503/cmaj.110334

Centers for Disease Control and Prevention. (2017). National Breast and Cervical Cancer Early Detection Program (NBCCEDP). Retrieved from http://www.cdc.gov/cancer/nbccedp/about.htm

Chen, W.Y., Rosner, B., Hankinson, S.E., Colditz, G.A., & Willett, W.C. (2011). Moderate alcohol consumption during adult life, drinking patterns, and breast cancer risk. *JAMA, 306,* 1884–1890. doi:10.1001/jama.2011.1590

Claus, E.B., Risch, N., & Thompson, W.D. (1991). Genetic analysis of breast cancer in the Cancer and Steroid Hormone Study. *American Journal of Human Genetics, 48,* 232–242. Retrieved from http://www.ncbi.nlm.nih.gov/pmc/articles/PMC1683001

Claus, E.B., Risch, N., & Thompson, W.D. (1994). Autosomal dominant inheritance of early-onset breast cancer. Implications for risk prediction. *Cancer, 73,* 643–651. doi:10.1002/1097-0142(19940201)73:3<643::AID-CNCR2820730323>3.0.CO;2-5

Costantino, J.P., Gail, M.H., Pee, D., Anderson, S., Redmond, C.K., Benichou, J., & Wieand, H.S. (1999). Validation studies for models projecting the risk of invasive and total breast cancer incidence. *Journal of the National Cancer Institute, 91,* 1541–1548. doi:10.1093/jnci/91.18.1541

Couzin-Frankel, J. (2014). Unknown significance. *Science, 346,* 1167–1170.

Cuzick, J., Sestak, I., Bonanni, B., Costantino, J.P., Cummings, S., DeCensi, A., ... Wickerham, D.L. (2013). Selective oestrogen receptor modulators in prevention of breast cancer: An updated meta-analysis of individual participant data. *Lancet, 381,* 1827–1834. doi:10.1016/S0140-6736(13)60140-3

Eggington, J.M., Bowles, K.R., Moyes, K., Manley, S., Esterling, L., Sizemore, S., ... Wenstrup, R.J. (2014). A comprehensive laboratory-based program for classification of variants of uncertain significance in hereditary cancer genes. *Clinical Genetics, 86,* 229–237. doi:10.1111/cge.12315

Emaus, M.J., van Gils, C.H., Bakker, M.F., Bisschop, C.N.S., Monninkhof, E.M., Bueno-de-Mesquita, H.B., ... May, A.M. (2014). Weight change in middle adulthood and breast cancer risk in the EPIC-PANACEA study. *International Journal of Cancer, 135,* 2887–2899. doi:10.1002/ijc.28926

Evans, D.G.R., Eccles, D.M., Rahman, N., Young, K., Bulman, M., Amir, E., ... Lalloo, F. (2004). A new scoring system for the chances of identifying a *BRCA1/2* mutation outperforms existing models including BRCAPRO. *Journal of Medical Genetics, 41,* 474–480. doi:10.1136/jmg.2003.017996

Finkelman, B.S., Rubinstein, W.S., Friedman, S., Friebel, T.M., Dubitsky, S., Schonberger, N.S., ... Rebbeck, T.R. (2012). Breast and ovarian cancer risk and risk reduction in Jewish *BRCA1/2* mutation carriers. *Journal of Clinical Oncology, 30,* 1321–1328. doi:10.1200/JCO.2011.37.8133

Hampel, H., Bennett, R.L., Buchanan, A., Pearlman, R., & Wiesner, G.L. (2015). A practice guideline from the American College of Medical Genetics and Genomics and the National Society of Genetic Counselors: Referral indications for cancer predisposition assessment. *Genetics in Medicine, 17,* 70–87. doi:10.1038/gim.2014.147

Hartmann, L.C., Radisky, D.C., Frost, M.H., Santen, R.J., Vierkant, R.A., Benetti, L.L., ... Degnim, A.C. (2014). Understanding the premalignant potential of atypical hyperplasia through its natural history: A longitudinal cohort study. *Cancer Prevention Research, 7,* 211–217. doi:10.1158/1940-6207.CAPR-13-0222

Hoskins, K.F., Zwaagstra, A., & Ranz, M. (2006). Validation of a tool for identifying women at high risk for hereditary breast cancer in population-based screening. *Cancer, 107,* 1769–1776. doi:10.1002/cncr.22202

Jimbo, M., Rana, G.K., Hawley, S., Holmes-Rovner, M., Kelly-Blake, K., Nease, D.E., Jr., & Ruffin, M.T. (2013). What is lacking in current decision aids on cancer screening? *CA: A Cancer Journal for Clinicians, 63,* 193–214. doi:10.3322/caac.21180

Katki, H.A. (2007). Incorporating medical interventions into carrier probability estimation for genetic counseling. *BMC Medical Genetics, 8,* 13. doi:10.1186/1471-2350-8-13

Mahon, S.M. (2013a). Allocation of work activities in a comprehensive cancer genetics program. *Clinical Journal of Oncology Nursing, 17,* 397–404. doi:10.1188/13.CJON.397-404

Mahon, S.M. (2013b). Next-generation DNA sequencing: Implications for oncology care. *Oncology Nursing Forum, 40,* 437–439. doi:10.1188/13.ONF.437-439

Mahon, S.M. (2013c). Ordering the correct genetic test: Implications for oncology and primary care healthcare professionals. *Clinical Journal of Oncology Nursing, 17,* 128–131. doi:10.1188/13.CJON.128-131

Mahon, S.M. (2014a). Breast cancer risk associated with *CHEK2* mutations. *Oncology Nursing Forum, 41,* 692–694. doi:10.1188/14.ONF.692-694

Mahon, S.M. (2014b). Cancer risks for men with *BRCA1/2* mutations. *Oncology Nursing Forum, 41,* 99–101. doi:10.1188/14.ONF.99-101

Mahon, S.M. (2014c). Providing care for previvors: Implications for oncology nurses. *Clinical Journal of Oncology Nursing, 18,* 21–24. doi:10.1188/14.CJON.21-24

Mahon, S.M. (2015). Management of patients with a genetic variant of unknown significance. *Oncology Nursing Forum, 42,* 316–318. doi:10.1188/15.ONF.316-318

Mahon, S.M. (2016). Management of individuals with a mutation in the ataxia telangiectasia mutated gene. *Oncology Nursing Forum, 43,* 114–117. doi:10.1188/16.ONF.114-117

Marjoribanks, J., Farquhar, C., Roberts, H., Lethaby, A., & Lee, J. (2017). Long-term hormone therapy for perimenopausal and postmenopausal women. *Cochrane Database of Systematic Reviews, 2017*(1). doi:10.1002/14651858.CD004143.pub5

Matloff, E.T., & Brierley, K.L. (2010). The double-helix derailed: The story of the *BRCA* patent. *Lancet, 376,* 314–315. doi:10.1016/S0140-6736(10)61150-6

Nadalin, V., Maher, J., Lessels, C., Chiarelli, A., & Kreiger, N. (2016). Breast screening knowledge and barriers among under/never screened women. *Public Health, 133,* 63–66. doi:10.1016/j.puhe.2015.11.028

National Comprehensive Cancer Network. (2017a). *NCCN Clinical Practice Guidelines in Oncology (NCCN Guidelines®): Breast cancer risk reduction* [v.1.2016]. Retrieved from https://www.nccn.org/professionals/physician_gls/pdf/breast_risk.pdf

National Comprehensive Cancer Network. (2017b). *NCCN Clinical Practice Guidelines in Oncology (NCCN Guidelines®): Breast cancer screening and diagnosis* [v.1.2017]. Retrieved from http://www.nccn.org/professionals/physician_gls/pdf/breast-screening.pdf

National Comprehensive Cancer Network. (2017c). *NCCN Clinical Practice Guidelines in Oncology (NCCN Guidelines®): Genetic/familial high-risk assessment: Breast and ovarian* [v.2.2017]. Retrieved from https://www.nccn.org/professionals/physician_gls/pdf/genetics_screening.pdf

Petrucelli, N., Daly, M.B., & Pal, T. (2016). *BRCA1*- and *BRCA2*-associated hereditary breast and ovarian cancer. In R.A. Pagon, M.P. Adam, H.H. Ardinger, S.E. Wallace, A. Amemiya, L.J.H. Bean, ... K. Stephens (Eds.), *GeneReviews®*. Retrieved from https://www.ncbi.nlm.nih.gov/books/NBK1247

Rehm, H.L., Bale, S.J., Bayrak-Toydemir, P., Berg, J.S., Brown, K.K., Deignan, J.L., ... Lyon, E. (2013). ACMG clinical laboratory standards for next-generation sequencing. *Genetics in Medicine, 15,* 733–747. doi:10.1038/gim.2013.92

Robson, M.E., Bradbury, A.R., Arun, B., Domchek, S.M., Ford, J.M., Hampel, H.L., ... Lindor, N.M. (2015). American Society of Clinical Oncology policy statement update: Genetic and genomic testing for cancer susceptibility. *Journal of Clinical Oncology, 33,* 3660–3667. doi:10.1200/JCO.2015.63.0996

Schonberg, M.A., Li, V.W., Eliassen, A.H., Davis, R.B., LaCroix, A.Z., McCarthy, E.P., ... Ngo, L.H. (2016). Performance of the Breast Cancer Risk Assessment Tool among women aged 75 years and older. *Journal of the National Cancer Institute, 108*(3). doi:10.1093/jnci/djv348

Sijmons, R.H., Greenblatt, M.S., & Genuardi, M. (2013). Gene variants of unknown clinical significance in Lynch syndrome: An introduction for clinicians. *Familial Cancer, 12,* 181–187. doi:10.1007/s10689-013-9629-8

Siu, A.L. (2016). Screening for breast cancer: U.S. Preventive Services Task Force recommendation statement. *Annals of Internal Medicine, 164,* 279–296. doi:10.7326/M15-2886

Tyrer, J., Duffy, S.W., & Cuzick, J. (2004). A breast cancer prediction model incorporating familial and personal risk factors. *Statistics in Medicine, 23,* 1111–1130. doi:10.1002/sim.1668

U.S. Department of Health and Human Services. (2009). "GINA": The Genetic Information Nondiscrimination Act of 2008; Information for researchers and health care professionals. Retrieved from http://www.genome.gov/Pages/PolicyEthics/GeneticDiscrimination/GINAInfoDoc.pdf

Walsh, T., Casadei, S., Lee, M.K., Pennil, C.C., Nord, A.S., Thornton, A.M., ... Swisher, E.M. (2011). Mutations in 12 genes for inherited ovarian, fallopian tube, and peritoneal carcinoma identified by massively parallel sequencing. *Proceedings of the National Academy of Sciences, 108,* 18032–18037. doi:10.1073/pnas.1115052108

Weitzel, J.N., Blazer, K.R., MacDonald, D.J., Culver, J.O., & Offit, K. (2011). Genetics, genomics, and cancer risk assessment. *CA: A Cancer Journal for Clinicians, 61,* 327–359. doi:10.3322/caac.20128

Yang, X.R., Chang-Claude, J., Goode, E.L., Couch, F.J., Nevanlinna, H., Milne, R.L., ... Garcia-Closas, M. (2011). Associations of breast cancer risk factors with tumor subtypes: A pooled analysis from the Breast Cancer Association Consortium Studies. *Journal of the National Cancer Institute, 103,* 250–263. doi:10.1093/jnci/djq526

CHAPTER 3

Breast Imaging

Lusine Tumyan, MD

Introduction

Breast imaging is a critical tool in breast care. Breast imaging tools include mammography, ultrasound, and breast magnetic resonance imaging (MRI). These modalities can be used for both screening and diagnostic examinations. Improvements in breast imaging have led to the earlier detection of breast cancers and less-invasive biopsy techniques. Oncology nurses need to understand the capabilities of various breast imaging modalities to provide optimal patient education and support.

Mammography

Screening Mammography

Mammogram screening is the examination of an asymptomatic woman in an attempt to detect abnormal lesions of the breast when they are small, not palpable, and confined to the breast. Overall sensitivity of screening mammography ranges from 73% to 88%, with specificity ranging from 83% to 94% (Ikeda, 2011).

Screening mammograms include two standard projections per breast, craniocaudal (CC) and mediolateral oblique (MLO). In a CC mammogram (see Figure 3-1), an x-ray beam is directed from the superior aspect of the breast to the inferior aspect of the breast. The entire breast parenchyma is depicted, including the pectoralis muscle and retromammary space. The nipple should be in profile. In the MLO view (see Figure 3-2), the x-ray beam is directed from the superior-medial aspect of the breast to the inferior-lateral aspect of breast at an angle of 30°–60°. An optimal MLO view should include nipple in profile, concave pectoralis muscle, an open intramammary fold, and fat visualized posterior to all fibroglandular tissue.

Diagnostic Mammography

Diagnostic mammography is an examination used to evaluate a patient with a breast mass or other symptoms, an abnormal or questionable screening mammogram, or special cases such as a history of breast cancer with breast-conserving sur-

Figure 3-1. Craniocaudal (CC) Mammographic View

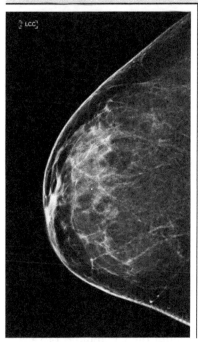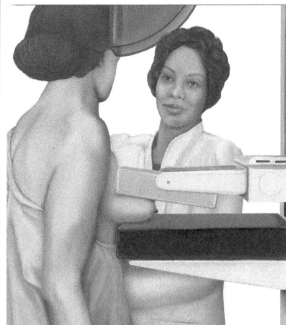

X-ray beam directed from the superior to the inferior of breast

Note. Figures courtesy of National Cancer Institute. Illustration created by Alan Hoofring. Retrieved from https://visualsonline.cancer.gov/details.cfm?imageid=9405 and https://visualsonline.cancer.gov/details.cfm?imageid=4361.

gery. Diagnostic mammography includes additional mammographic views tailored to the problem. Some of the common views include the true lateral view, spot compression view, spot compression magnification view, rolled views, and exaggerated CC view.

A true lateral view is a 90° lateral view of the breast. In the mediolateral view, the x-ray beam is directed from medial to lateral breast. In the lateromedial view, the x-ray beam is directed from lateral to medial breast (see Figure 3-3). A mediolateral view is useful in determining the exact location of an abnormality. A mediolateral view is best for evaluating a central or lateral breast abnormality, whereas a lateromedial view is best for evaluating a medial breast abnormality.

The spot compression view (see Figure 3-4) provides an examination of a smaller area of breast tissue with a small compression paddle. This view provides greater effective pressure, resulting in better tissue separation and better visualization of the breast tissue, as well as improved resolution because of reduction of thickness.

The spot compression magnification view (see Figure 3-5) focuses on a smaller area of the breast by using a magnification device and allows visualization of microcalcifications. Rolled views provide a view of the breast rotated medially or laterally around the axis of the nipple. Changing tissue distribution allows determination of whether a true lesion is present or if a pseudolesion was created by overlapping fibroglandular tissue. Rolled views can also be used to determine the location of the lesion based on its migration compared to the standard view.

Figure 3-2. Mediolateral Oblique (MLO) Mammographic View

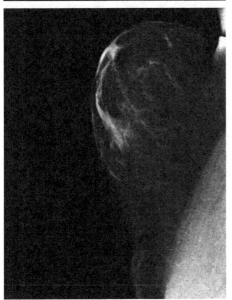

X-ray beam directed from the superior-medial to the inferior-lateral aspect of breast at a 30°–60° angle

Note. Figure courtesy of National Cancer Institute. Retrieved from https://visualsonline.cancer.gov/details .cfm?imageid=9410.

Figure 3-3. 90° Mediolateral View of Breast

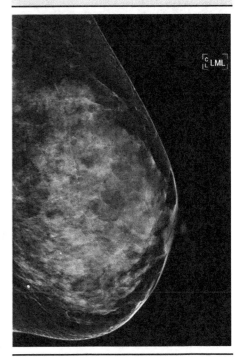

Note. Figure courtesy of City of Hope. Used with permission.

An exaggerated CC view can be obtained as an exaggerated lateral CC view with more inclusion of the lateral breast or an exaggerated medial CC view with more inclusion of the medial breast. This view is ideal for depicting lateral or medial lesions located in the far posterior breast.

Breast Lesions

Breast masses are space-occupying lesions in three dimensions, seen on two different mammographic projections with complete or partially convex outward borders (see Figure 3-6). Masses are characterized based on shape, margin, and density (D'Orsi, Sickles, Mendelson, & Morris, 2013).

The shape of a breast lesion can take several forms:
- Oval—elliptical shape that may include two or three undulations
- Round—spherical or circular shape
- Irregular—neither oval nor round
  Margins can range from sharply defined to indistinct, as follows:
- Circumscribed—sharply demarcated margin with abrupt transition between mass and tissue; at least 75% of margin well defined
- Obscured—margins (greater than 25%) hidden by superimposed fibroglandular tissue

---

Figure 3-4. Craniocaudal Views of Breast Mass

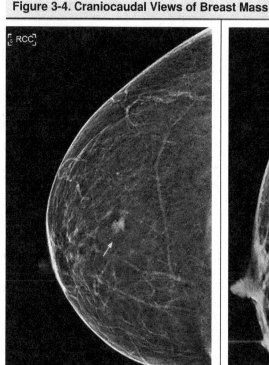 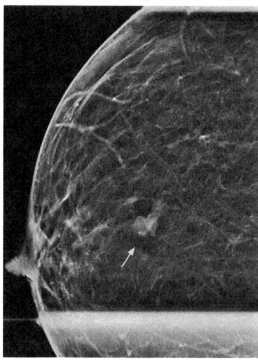

Left: Standard right craniocaudal view (CC) with mass in central right breast (arrow)
Right: Spot compression craniocaudal view (sCC) demonstrates mass in central breast with better defined lobulated boarders (arrow).

Note. Figures courtesy of City of Hope. Used with permission.

- Microlobulated—short cycle undulations
- Indistinct—no clear demarcation of the margin or any portion of the margin from surrounding tissue
- Spiculated—lines radiating from the mass
  The density of a lesion can range based on the composition of fat and tissue, as follows:
- High density—mass is denser or whiter than the expected volume of fibroglandular tissue
- Equal density—mass is the same density as the expected volume of fibroglandular tissue
- Low density—mass is lighter than the expected volume of fibroglandular tissue
- Fat-containing—mass density is the same as the fat density; almost always represents a benign mass

Calcifications

Calcifications may form in breast cancer as a result of central necrosis or secretions by malignant cells and may be the only sign of malignancy on mammogram (Ikeda,

Figure 3-5. Mediolateral Views of Breast

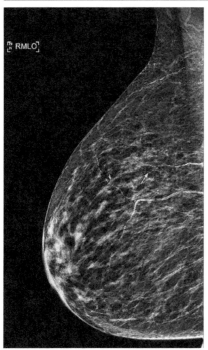
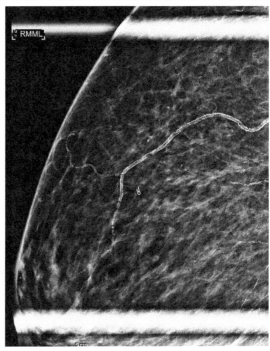

Left: Right mediolateral oblique view (MLO)—cluster of calcifications in upper breast (arrow)
Right: Magnification mediolateral view (MML)—magnification view demonstrates cluster of pleomorphic calcifications (arrow)

Note. Figures courtesy of City of Hope. Used with permission.

2011). They are characterized based on distribution and calcification type, either typically benign or typically suspicious (D'Orsi et al., 2013).

Typically benign calcifications (see Figure 3-7) can be found in various types and forms:

- Skin—lucent-centered calcification most commonly seen along the inframammary fold, parasternally, overlying the axilla and around the areola
- Vascular—parallel track or linear tubal calcifications associated with blood vessels
- Coarse or "popcorn-like"—large (larger than 2–3 mm in diameter) and usually produced by a degenerating fibroadenoma
- Large rod-like—calcifications associated with ductal ectasia form solid or discontinuous smooth linear rods, most of which are 0.5 mm or larger in diameter; generally bilateral
- Round—multiple round calcifications are frequently formed in acini or lobules
- Rim—calcium deposits on the surface of a sphere, such as an oil cyst
- Dystrophic—irregular shape calcifications often with lucent centers in an irradiated breast or following trauma or surgery
- Milk of calcium—calcifications in cysts that layer on mediolateral view and appear amorphous on CC view

Figure 3-6. Mammographic Projections of Breast Lesions

Shape	Margins
Oval elliptical shape that may include two or three undulations	**Circumscribed** 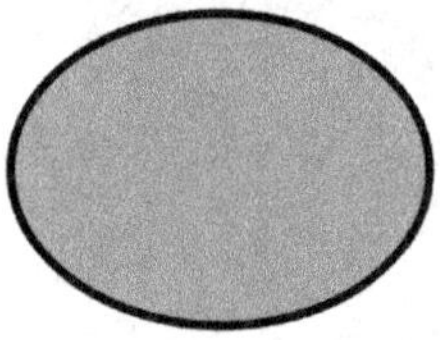 sharply demarcated margin with abrupt transition between mass and tissue
Round spherical or circular shape	**Obscured** 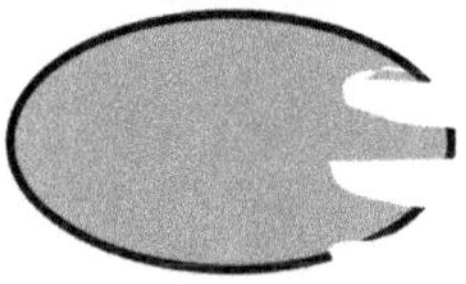 margins (> 25%) are hidden by superimposed fibroglandular tissue
Irregular 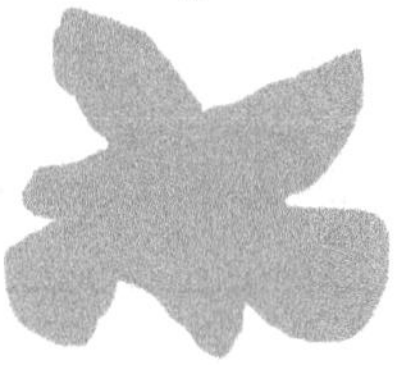 neither oval nor round	**Microlobulated** 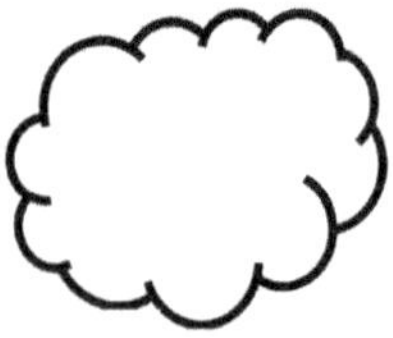 short cycle undulations
	Indistinct 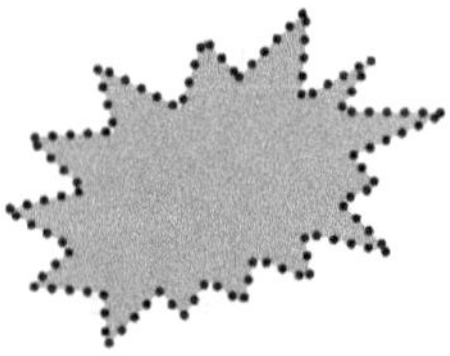 no clear demarcation of the margin
	Spiculated 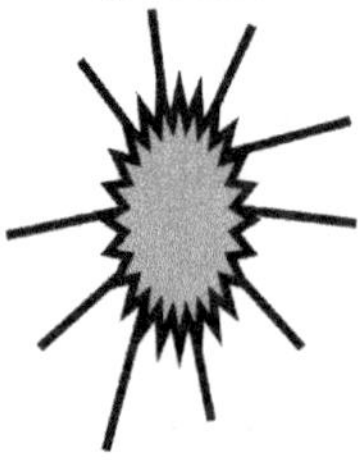 lines radiating from the mass

Figure 3-7. Typically Benign Calcifications

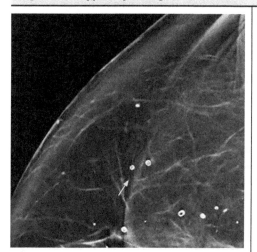

Skin calcifications with lucent centers

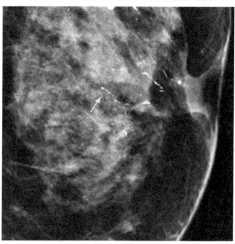

Large rod-like calcifications associated with ductal ectasia

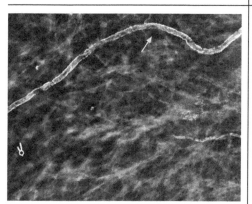

Vascular calcifications—parallel track associated with blood vessels

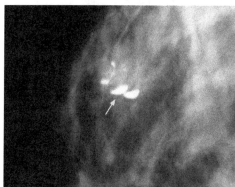

Milk of calcium—calcifications layering in cysts

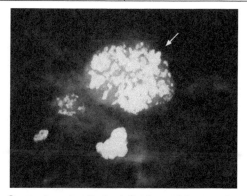

Coarse "popcorn-like" calcifications of degenerating fibroadenoma

Note. Figures courtesy of City of Hope. Used with permission.

- Suture—calcifications deposited on suture material, typically linear or tubular
  Typically suspicious calcifications (see Figure 3-8) also present as varying types:
- Coarse heterogeneous—irregular calcifications that tend to cluster but are smaller than dystrophic calcifications
- Fine pleomorphic—irregular calcifications that vary in size and shape and are usually less than 0.5 mm in diameter
- Amorphous—small or hazy calcifications where the shape cannot be characterized

Distribution

Distribution is the arrangement of calcifications in the breast (see Figure 3-9) and can range from diffuse to segmental, as follows:
- Diffuse—calcifications distributed randomly throughout the breast. Diffuse punctate and amorphous calcifications, especially if they are bilateral, are generally benign.

Figure 3-8. Typically Suspicious Calcifications

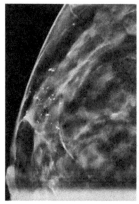

Coarse heterogeneous calcifications—irregular shapes

Fine pleomorphic calcifications—irregular calcifications that vary in size and shape

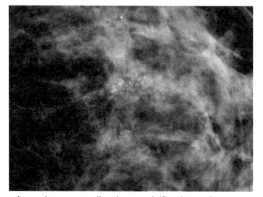

Amorphous—small or hazy calcifications where the shape is difficult to determine

---

Note. Figures courtesy of City of Hope. Used with permission.

- Regional—calcifications that occupy a large portion of breast tissue (larger than 2 cm in greatest dimension) and do not conform to ductal distribution. Malignancy is less likely with regional calcifications. However, complete characterization of regional calcifications must take into account the morphology as well as distribution.
- Grouped—few calcifications occupy a small portion of breast tissue. Both malignant and benign calcifications can have grouped distribution.
- Linear—calcifications in linear array, suggestive of ductal distribution. In general, calcifications with linear distribution are considered with suspicion.
- Segmental—triangular or cone-shaped calcifications with the apex toward the nipple, suggestive of enhancement within or around ducts. Segmental distribution in general is also considered with suspicion.

Asymmetries

Asymmetries (see Figure 3-10) are fibroglandular tissue areas that do not occupy three-dimensional space and are characterized based on appearance on one mammographic view or two mammographic views, as follows:
- Asymmetry—area of fibroglandular tissue visible on only one mammographic view

---

Figure 3-9. Distribution of Calcifications

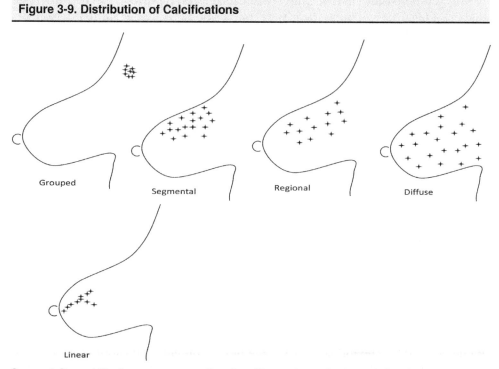

Grouped: Few calcifications occupy a small portion of breast tissue. **Segmental:** Calcifications are triangular or cone-shaped with apex toward the nipple and are suggestive of enhancement within or around ducts. **Regional:** Calcifications occupy a large portion of breast tissue (> 2 cm in greatest dimension) and do not conform to duct distribution. **Diffuse:** Calcifications are distributed randomly throughout the breast. **Linear:** Calcifications occur in a linear array, suggestive of ductal distribution.

- Focal asymmetry—fibroglandular tissue visible on two mammographic projections
- Global asymmetry—large amount of fibroglandular tissue over at least one quadrant of breast visible on two mammographic projections
- Developing asymmetry—focal asymmetry that is new or larger compared to previous examination. About 15% of developing asymmetries are found to be malignant (D'Orsi et al., 2013).

Architectural Distortion

Architectural distortion is distortion of the breast parenchyma with no visible mass (D'Orsi et al., 2013). Thin lines or spiculations are seen radiating from a point with focal retraction or distortion of the anterior or posterior edge of the parenchyma.

Breast Magnetic Resonance Imaging

Invasive breast tumors are generally associated with neovascularity, or formation of new vascular networks, with an abnormal leaky endothelium leading to rapid uptake (rapid wash-in) of contrast agent during initial phase MRI and rapid decline of contrast enhancement (rapid washout) during delayed phase MRI.

MRI is very sensitive in detecting breast cancer, with reported sensitivity of greater than 90% regardless of breast density or composition (Warren et al., 2005). Note that breast density has an inverse effect on sensitivity of mammogram. Sensitivity decreases with background enhancement, but more research is necessary to fully understand this effect (Telegrafo, Rella, Ianora, Angelelli, & Moschetta, 2016). Enhancement is also present in many benign conditions; therefore, specificity of breast MRI varies from 35% to 95% (Ikeda, 2011). Both morphology and kinetics are important in differentiating benign from malignant lesions.

Screening Magnetic Resonance Imaging

Screening MRI is an examination of asymptomatic patients with increased risk of breast carcinoma (typically 20% or higher lifetime risk) (D'Orsi et al., 2013). Studies have found sensitivity for MRI to be 71%–100% and specificity to be 81%–99% (Saslow et al., 2007). Because of increased false-positive rates and overall cost, breast MRI is not recommended for routine screening in average-risk patients at this time. Abbreviated MRI protocols have been proposed for screening average-risk patients, but more research is necessary to determine the effectiveness.

Diagnostic Magnetic Resonance Imaging

Diagnostic MRI is an examination of symptomatic patients (American College of Radiology, 2014). The following are some of the common indications for diagnostic MRI. In patients with a new breast malignancy, MRI is important for screening of the ipsilateral and contralateral breasts for occult malignancy, as well as for determining the extent of disease for surgical planning. In patients with positive margins following lumpectomy, MRI is crucial in surgical planning and determining the presence of residual carcinoma. For patients receiving neoadjuvant chemotherapy, MRI

Figure 3-10. Examples of Asymmetry

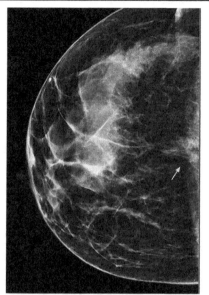

A. Focal asymmetry on CC view (arrow)

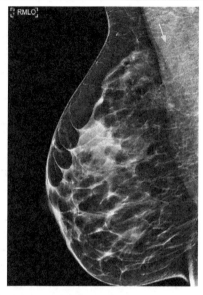

B. Focal asymmetry on MLO view (arrow)

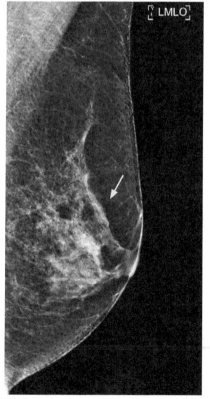

C. Global asymmetry on MLO view (arrows)

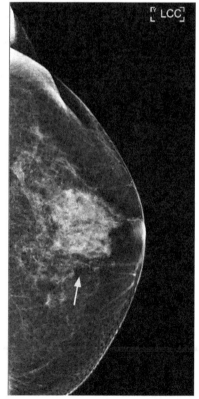

D. Global asymmetry on CC view (arrows)

(Continued on next page)

Figure 3-10. Examples of Asymmetry *(Continued)*

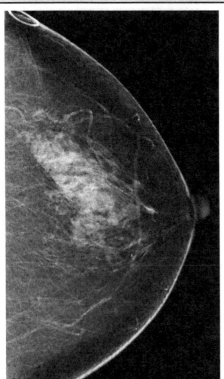

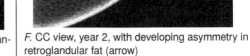

E. CC view, year 1, with no asymmetry in retroglandular fat

F. CC view, year 2, with developing asymmetry in retroglandular fat (arrow)

CC—craniocaudal; MLO—mediolateral oblique

Note. Figures courtesy of City of Hope. Used with permission.

is used for determining response to treatment and surgical planning. MRI is also used for additional evaluation of clinical or imaging findings. In patients with metastatic carcinoma for which the primary is not known but is suspected to be of breast origin, diagnostic MRI is especially useful. It also is used in the case of suspected cancer recurrence in patients with mastectomy and tissue or implant reconstruction. Implant-specific MRI is the most sensitive modality for evaluating implants and thus also is used to evaluate implant integrity.

Breast Magnetic Resonance Imaging Findings and Reporting

Equivalent to breast density on mammogram, breast MRI records the amount of *fibroglandular tissue* in relation to fat, which is assessed and reported. Fibroglandular tissue is assessed (see Figure 3-11) on fat-saturated T1-weighted imaging or non–fat-saturated T1-weighted imaging and described as one of the following:
• Almost entirely fatty—majority of the breast is composed of fat with interspersed fibroglandular tissue

Figure 3-11. Examples of Magnetic Resonance Imaging Results

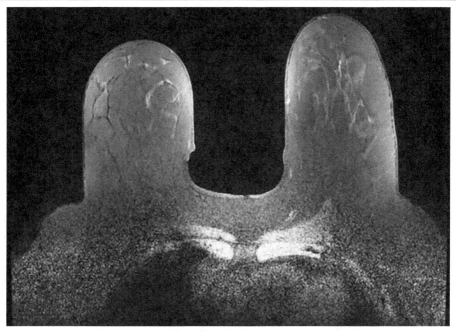

Predominantly fatty background parenchyma (T1 precontrast)

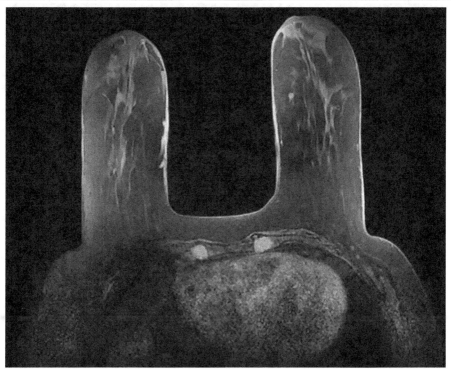

Fatty with scattered fibroglandular elements background parenchyma (T1 precontrast)

(Continued on next page)

Figure 3-11. Examples of Magnetic Resonance Imaging Results *(Continued)*

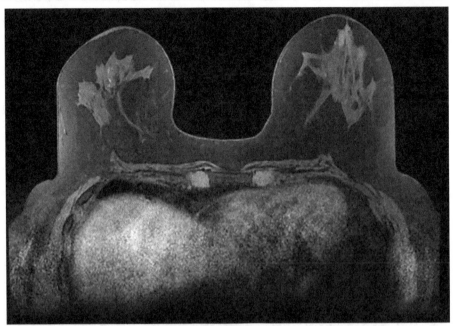

Heterogeneously dense background parenchyma (T1 precontrast)

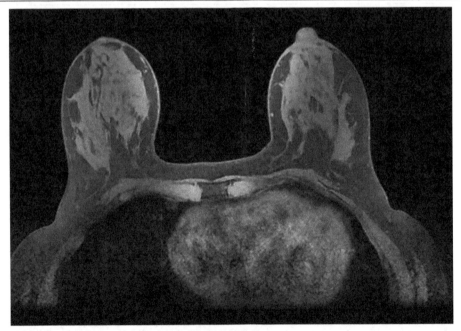

Extremely dense background parenchyma (T1 precontrast)

Note. Figures courtesy of City of Hope. Used with permission.

- Scattered fibroglandular tissue—most of the breast is composed of fat with interspersed fibroglandular tissue that is more than the almost entirely fatty category but less than the heterogeneous category
- Heterogeneous fibroglandular tissue—most of the breast is composed of fibroglandular tissue with interspersed fatty tissue
- Extreme fibroglandular tissue—majority of the breast is composed of fibroglandular tissue with very little interspersed fat

Background parenchyma enhancement (see Figure 3-12) is the enhancement of parenchyma excluding mass lesions. It is characterized by the percentage of glandular tissue enhanced, as follows (Morris, 2007):

- Minimal—less than 25%
- Mild—25%–50%
- Moderate—50%–75%
- Marked—greater than 75%

A *mass* (see Figures 3-13 and 3-14) is a lesion that occupies space and has a convex outward contour. The following features are used to characterize a mass:

- Shape
  – Oval (elliptical shape that also includes lobulated shape)
  – Round (spherical or circular shape)
  – Irregular (neither round nor oval)
- Margin
  – Circumscribed (sharply demarcated with abrupt transition between the lesion and background parenchyma)
  – Irregular (margin is composed of edges)
  – Spiculated (margin with lines radiating from the mass)

Enhancement kinetics (see Figure 3-15) are used to further characterize lesions on MRI and can be classified as initial phase and delayed phase. Initial phase describes enhancement within the first 2 minutes or when the curve starts to change (Ikeda, 2011) and is characterized as follows:

- Slow—more than 50% increase in signal intensity
- Medium—50%–100% increase in signal intensity
- Fast—greater than 100% increase in signal intensity

Delayed phase is the enhancement pattern after two minutes or when the curve starts to change, and is described as follows:

- Persistent—continued greater than 10% increase in signal over time
- Plateau—no change in signal intensity over time after its initial rise
- Washout—signal intensity decreases more than 10% after its highest point from initial rise

Enhancement can also be characterized as follows:

- Homogenous (uniform enhancement of the mass)
- Heterogeneous (nonuniform enhancement of the mass)
- Rim enhancement (enhancement more pronounced at the periphery of the mass)
- Dark internal septations (dark, nonenhancing lines within a mass, suggestive of benign fibroadenoma)

Masses with the following features are suggestive of a benign process:

- High signal on bright fluid sequences (e.g., T2-weighted sequences)
- Fatty central component (indicative of fatty hilum of lymph node)
- Persistent delayed kinetics

Figure 3-12. Examples of Magnetic Resonance Imaging With Contrast

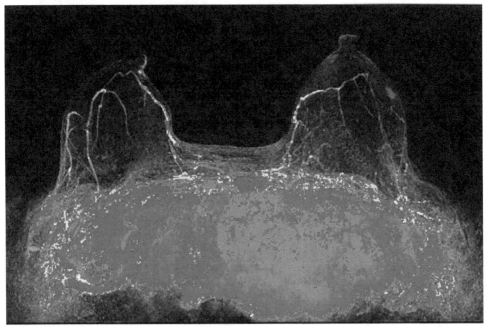

Minimal background enhancement < 25% glandular tissue

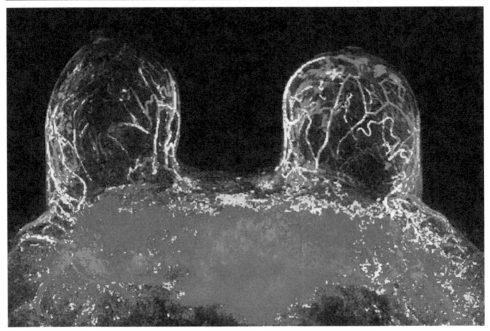

Mild background enhancement 25%–50% glandular tissue

(Continued on next page)

Figure 3-12. Examples of Magnetic Resonance Imaging With Contrast *(Continued)*

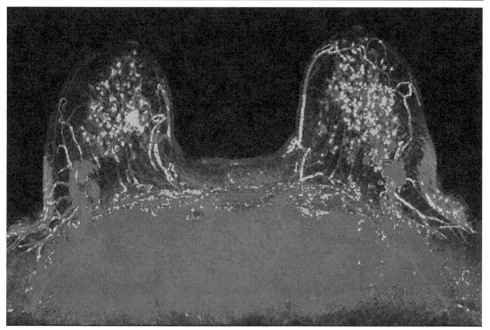

Moderate background enhancement 50%–75% glandular tissue

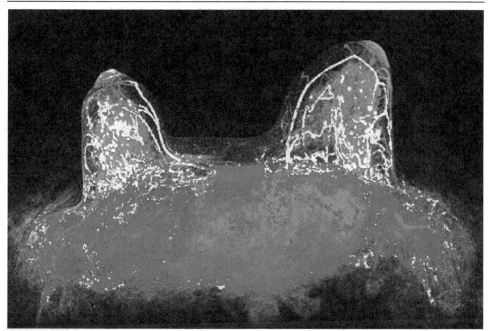

Marked background enhancement > 75% glandular tissue

Note. Figures courtesy of City of Hope. Used with permission.

Figure 3-13. Irregularly Shaped Heterogeneous Enhancing Carcinoma

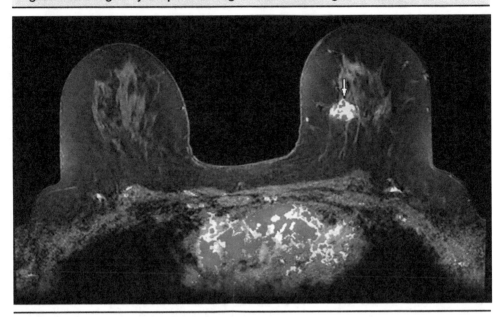

Note. Figure courtesy of City of Hope. Used with permission.

Figure 3-14. Postcontrast Nonenhancing Cyst, Oval Circumscribed

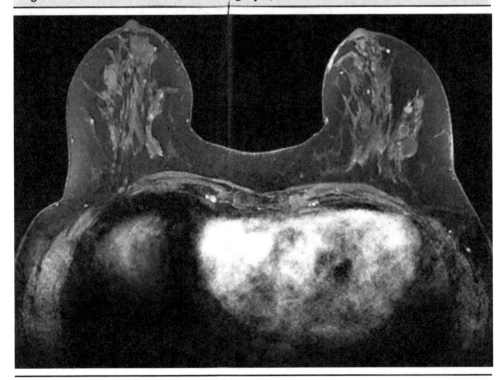

Note. Figure courtesy of City of Hope. Used with permission.

Figure 3-15. Enhancement Kinetics Graphic

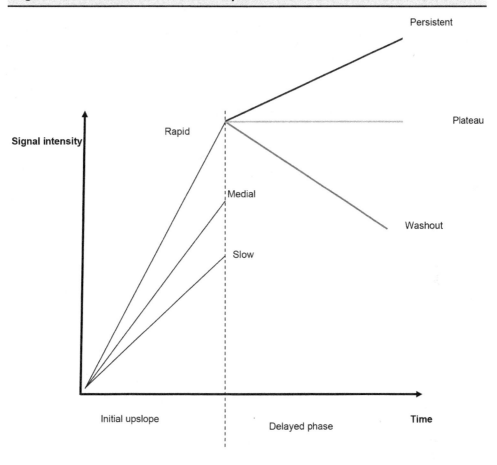

Initial phase: Enhancement within the first 2 minutes or when the curve starts to change. Slow = < 50% increase in signal intensity; medium = 50%–100% increase in signal intensity; fast = > 100% increase in signal intensity

Delayed phase: Enhancement pattern after 2 minutes or when the curve starts to change. Persistent = continued > 10% increase in signal over time; plateau = no change in signal intensity over time after its initial rise; washout = signal intensity decreases > 10% after its highest point from initial rise

- Stable since the prior examination(s)
   Masses with the following features are suggestive of a suspicious focus:
- Not bright on bright fluid sequences
- No fatty hilum
- Washout delayed kinetics
- Increased in size or new focus since prior examination(s)

   A *focus* is a dot of enhancement so small that margins and shape cannot be fully characterized (see Figure 3-16). In general, margins and shape cannot be visualized clearly or are below the resolution of MRI. This does not represent a space-occupying lesion or mass and is unique from surrounding background parenchyma enhancement.

Figure 3-16. Focus of Enhancement

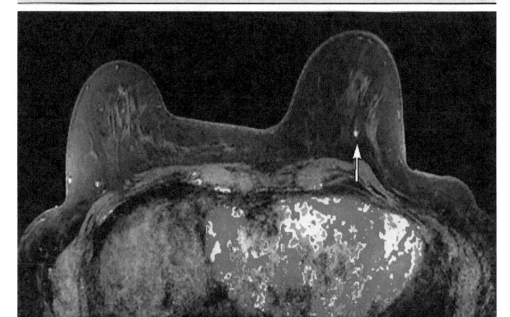

Note. Figure courtesy of City of Hope. Used with permission.

A *non–mass enhancement* (see Figure 3-17) pattern is neither mass nor focus and is separate from background enhancement. The following features are used to characterize non–mass enhancement:
• Distribution
  – Focal—enhancement confined to an area that occupies less than a breast quadrant and has fat or normal fibroglandular tissue interspersed between abnormal enhancing components
  – Linear—enhancement in a line or line that is branching and is suggestive of enhancement in duct
  – Segmental—enhancement in a triangular or cone shape with the apex toward the nipple and is suggestive of enhancement within or around ducts
  – Regional—enhancement that involves a region and therefore more than one ductal system
• Internal enhancement pattern
  – Homogenous—confluent uniform enhancement
  – Heterogeneous—nonuniform enhancement in a random pattern
  – Clumped—cobblestone enhancement of varying sizes and shapes
  – Clustered ring—rings of enhancement clustered together around ducts

Figure 3-17. Postcontrast Non–Mass Enhancement

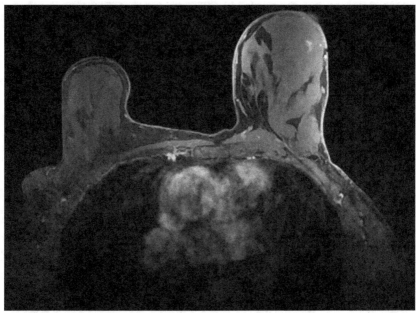

T1 postcontrast focal non–mass enhancement biopsy-proven carcinoma

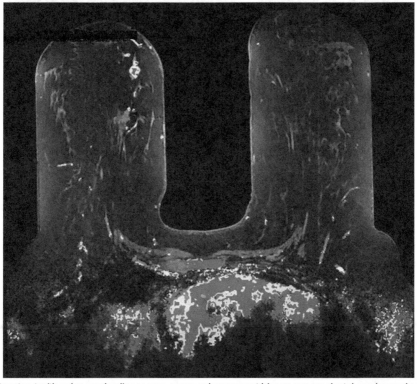

T1 postcontrast with color overlay linear non–mass enhancement biopsy-proven ductal carcinoma in situ

(Continued on next page)

Figure 3-17. Postcontrast Non–Mass Enhancement *(Continued)*

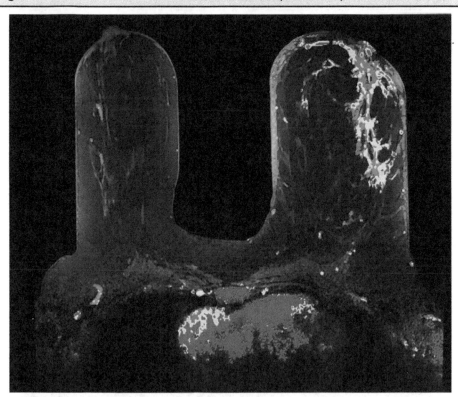

Postcontrast with color overlay segmented enhancement biopsy-proven cancer

Note. Figures courtesy of City of Hope. Used with permission.

Ultrasound

Ultrasound is a useful complement to mammography in detecting and characterizing breast masses. Handheld, high-frequency (central frequency of at least 10 MHz) ultrasound should be utilized in breast imaging (Ikeda, 2011). Ultrasound findings and reporting include tissue composition and masses (D'Orsi et al., 2013).

Tissue composition is the background echotexture of the breast parenchyma. Homogenous background echotexture includes fat lobules and echogenic bands of supporting structures and comprises the majority of the breast parenchyma. Homogenous echogenic fibroglandular parenchyma is present under the layer of fat lobules. Heterogeneous background echotexture is defined as when focal or diffuse heterogeneity is present with increased or decreased echogenicity and superimposed shadowing at interfaces.

A *mass* is a space-occupying lesion seen in three planes (see Figures 3-18, 3-19, and 3-20). Similar to mammogram and MRI, the following features are used to characterize a mass on ultrasound:

• Shape—oval, round, or irregular
• Orientation—unique feature of mass to ultrasound and is defined in reference to skin surface

- – Parallel—long axis of the mass is parallel to skin surface
- – Not parallel—long axis of the mass is not parallel to the skin surface; usually a sign of malignancy
- Margin
  - – Circumscribed or not circumscribed
  - – Echo pattern—echogenicity of the lesion as compared to mammary fat (a unique feature of ultrasound)
  - – Anechoic—without internal echoes; suggestive of a cystic lesion
  - – Hyperechoic—increased echogenicity relative to fat or equal to fibroglandular tissue
  - – Complex cystic and solid—complex mass containing both anechoic (cystic) and echogenic (solid) components
  - – Hypoechoic—decreased echogenicity in relation to fat
  - – Isoechoic—same echogenicity as subcutaneous fat
- Posterior features—attenuation characteristics of a mass in respect to its acoustic transmission and unique to ultrasound
- No posterior features—no shadowing or enhancement present posterior to the mass
- Enhancement—enhancement posterior to the lesion in a column distribution that is more echogenic deep to the mass; one of the criteria for cyst diagnosis
- Shadowing—area posterior to the mass appears darker
- Combined pattern—more than one pattern of posterior attenuation
- Calcifications—generally poorly visualized and characterized with ultrasound; at times can be seen as echogenic foci within mass, duct, or cyst (see Figure 3-21)

Figure 3-18. Ultrasound of Oval Circumscribed Mass With Orientation Parallel to Skin Surface, Benign

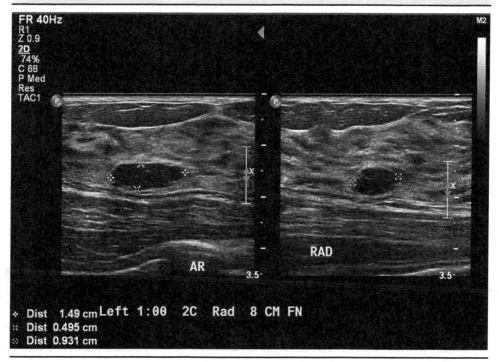

Figure 3-19. Ultrasound of Oval Circumscribed Anechoic Simple Cyst With Orientation Parallel to Skin Surface

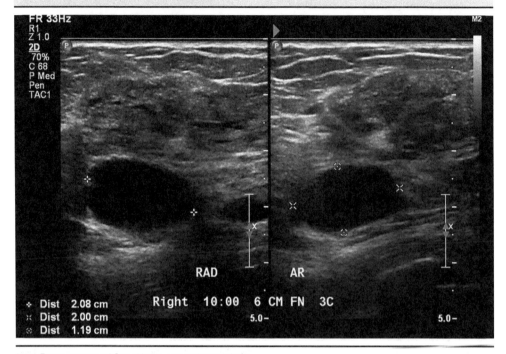

Note. Figure courtesy of City of Hope. Used with permission.

Figure 3-20. Ultrasound of Spiculated Mass With Posterior Shadowing Not Parallel to Skin Surface

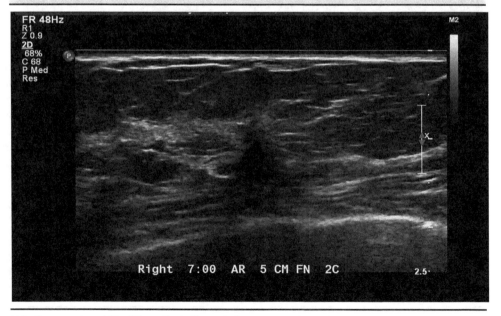

Note. Figure courtesy of City of Hope. Used with permission.

Figure 3-21. Ultrasounds of Pre-Fire and Post-Fire Biopsies

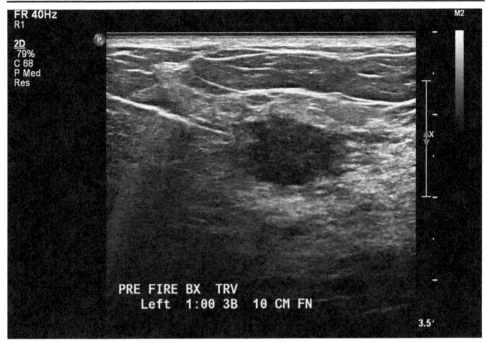

Ultrasound biopsy of mass pre-fire image

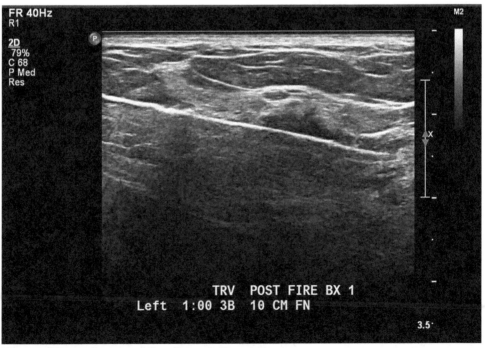

Ultrasound biopsy of mass post-fire with needle through the mass

Note. Figures courtesy of City of Hope. Used with permission.

Breast Imaging Reporting and Data System

The American College of Radiology's Breast Imaging Reporting and Data System (BI-RADS®) is an assessment and quality assurance tool in mammography, ultrasound, and breast MRI (D'Orsi et al., 2013). Report structure must include the indication for examination, statement on technique, and description of overall breast composition. The description indicates relative possibility that a lesion could be obscured by overlying fibroglandular parenchyma and, therefore, the sensitivity of mammography can be compromised by dense breast tissue. The denser the breast, the lower the sensitivity of mammography. Four categories are defined by visual estimation of fibroglandular tissue within the breast: breast is almost entirely fatty, scattered areas of fibroglandular density are indicated, breasts are heterogeneously dense (which may obscure small masses), and breasts are extremely dense, which lowers the sensitivity of mammography. The report must also include clear description of findings, assessment, management, and classification, with concordance between assessment categories and management recommendations as depicted in Table 3-1 (D'Orsi et al., 2013).

Table 3-1. Concordance Between Assessment Categories and Recommendations

Assessment	Management	Likelihood of Cancer
Category 0: Need additional imaging evaluation	Recall for additional imaging	N/A
Category 1: Negative	Routine screening	Essentially 0% likelihood of malignancy
Category 2: Benign	Routine screening	Essentially 0% likelihood of malignancy
Category 3: Probably benign	Short-interval (6-month) follow-up or continued surveillance	> 0% but ≤ 2% likelihood of malignancy
Category 4: Suspicious	Tissue diagnosis	> 2% but < 95% likelihood of malignancy
• Category 4A: Low suspicion for malignancy		> 2% but ≤ 10% likelihood of malignancy
• Category 4B: Moderate suspicion for malignancy		> 10% to ≤ 50% likelihood of malignancy
• Category 4C: High suspicion for malignancy		> 50% to < 95% likelihood of malignancy
Category 5: Highly suggestive of malignancy	Tissue diagnosis	≥ 95% likelihood of malignancy
Category 6: Known biopsy-proven malignancy	Surgical excision when clinically appropriate	N/A

Note. From *ACR BI-RADS® Atlas: Breast Imaging Reporting and Data System* (5th ed., p. 135), by C.J. D'Orsi, E.A. Sickles, E.B. Mendelson, and E.A. Morris, 2013, Reston, VA: American College of Radiology. Copyright 2013 by American College of Radiology. Reprinted with permission.

Breast Biopsies and Interventions

Fine Needle Aspiration and Core Needle Biopsy

Fine needle aspiration sensitivity and specificity are reported to be 75%–99% and 56%–99%, respectively (Bassett, Jackson, Fu, & Fu, 2004). Fine needle aspiration has a high rate of insufficient or nondiagnostic samples. The wide variability of fine needle aspiration is related to operator experience and training, presence of an onsite, trained cytopathologist, different sizes of needles, and number of passes.

Core needle biopsy is the preferred method of breast biopsy. It has higher sensitivity and specificity than fine needle aspiration (Moschetta et al., 2014; Willems, van Deurzen, & van Diest, 2012).

Stereotactic Core Needle Biopsy

Stereotactic core needle biopsy (see Figure 3-22) is used to biopsy lesions or calcifications best visualized with mammogram (Bassett et al., 2004). Lesions that can be sampled with stereotactic core needle biopsy include masses, calcifications, and architectural distortions with suspicious features. Two general categories of stereotactic biopsy units are available. The first is a smaller add-on upright unit that is attached to conventional mammography equipment and is either a vacuum-assisted device or a spring-loaded, automated, large core biopsy device used during biopsy. A stand-alone digital mammography unit with a prone biopsy table and vacuum-assisted directional cutting device is also used. With this device, the patient is placed prone on the biopsy table, and the breast is suspended through an opening in the table. The breast is positioned against the image receptor plate, and compression is applied. The location of the lesion is marked, and the coordinates are calculated. With use of sterile technique and after local infiltration of anesthesia, the vacuum-assisted biopsy device is advanced into the lesion, and multiple core samples are obtained. Once sampling is determined to be adequate, a stainless steel or titanium microclip is often placed at the biopsy site via a hollow biopsy needle.

Ultrasound-Guided Core Needle Biopsy

This imaging method (see Figure 3-23) is used to biopsy lesions best visualized with ultrasound. Lesions can be sampled with ultrasound-guided core needle biopsy, including various masses such as architectural distortions with suspicious features and rare calcifications that are visualized on ultrasound. The patient is appropriately positioned to enable percutaneous access by shortest distance and with the needle parallel to the chest wall throughout the procedure. With use of sterile technique and after application of local anesthesia, multiple core samples are obtained with either a vacuum-assisted device or a spring-loaded, automated core biopsy device. Once sampling is determined to be adequate, a stainless steel or titanium microclip is often placed at the biopsy site.

Magnetic Resonance Imaging–Guided Core Needle Biopsy

This imaging method is used to biopsy lesions best visualized with MRI. Lesions that can be sampled with MRI-guided core needle biopsy include masses, non–mass

Figure 3-22. Stereotactic Images

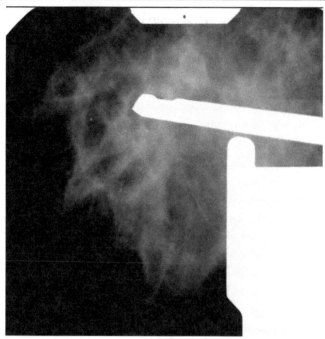

Stereotactic image of needle in the area of calcifications

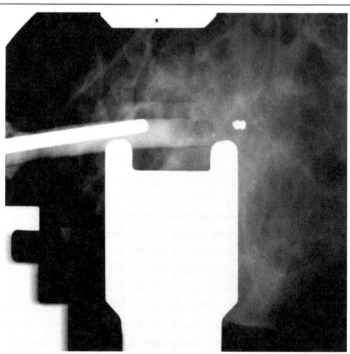

Stereotactic postbiopsy image with clip in place

Note. Figures courtesy of City of Hope. Used with permission.

Figure 3-23. Localization Images

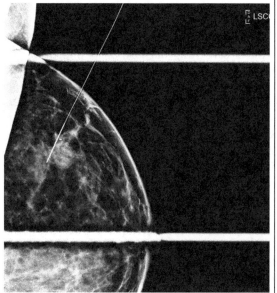

Hawkins localization wire adjacent to postbiopsy microclip

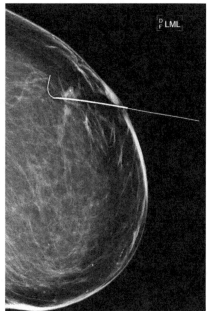

Homer localization needle and wire through the mass with clip

Note. Figures courtesy of National Cancer Institute. Illustrations created by Alan Hoofring. Retrieved from https://visualsonline.cancer.gov/details.cfm?imageid=9405 and https://visualsonline.cancer.gov/details.cfm?imageid=4361.

enhancement, focus of enhancement, and architectural distortion with suspicious features. The patient is appropriately positioned prone on the MRI table, the breast is placed in a biopsy coil, and the lesion is identified after contrast administration.

The lesion is triangulated, and coordinates are calculated either manually or by commercially available software. As in the other procedures, a sterile technique is used, and after administration of local anesthesia, a vacuum-assisted automated core biopsy device is advanced to the lesion. Once sampling is determined to be adequate, a stainless steel or titanium microclip is often placed at the biopsy site.

Presurgical Image-Guided Needle Localization

This type of needle localization is important in providing guidance for nonpalpable lesions to undergo surgical excision. Imaging techniques used for needle localization include mammography, ultrasound, or MRI (Bassett et al., 2004). Under image guidance, a localization wire or wire/needle system is placed in the appropriate position, demarcating the lesion of interest. Two types of hook wire systems are available: a needle and wire system with a J-type curved wire extending from the needle; and a wire system where the barb-type hook wire remains in the breast. Once the surgeon removes the appropriate tissue, as demarcated by the localization wire, an x-ray of the specimen typically is obtained to confirm presence of the lesion, which is communicated to the surgeon in the operating room.

Emerging Breast Imaging Techniques

Digital Breast Tomosynthesis

Digital breast tomosynthesis (three-dimensional mammography) is emerging as the new standard of care for breast cancer screening because of its improved cancer detection rate coupled with reduction in recall rate compared to standard two-dimensional digital mammography (Gilbert, Tucker, & Young, 2016). During this type of screening, digital breast tomosynthesis obtains multiple low-dose tomographic projections of the breast by moving the x-ray tube in an arc. The images are subsequently reconstructed and viewed on the workstation. Digital breast tomosynthesis overcomes the primary limitation of overlapping tissue inherent to standard two-dimensional mammography. Multiple recent studies report increased sensitivity and specificity of digital tomosynthesis when compared to standard two-dimensional mammography (Gilbert et al., 2016).

Molecular Breast Imaging

Molecular breast imaging uses a dedicated gamma camera or dedicated positron-emission tomography unit to visualize preferential uptake of a radiopharmaceutical (such as ^{99m}Tc-sestamibi or ^{18}F-FDG) in tumors relative to normal breast parenchyma. Studies show that molecular breast imaging can be effective for detection of breast cancer, particularly in women with dense breast parenchyma, in comparison to standard two-dimensional mammography. Currently, the American College of Radiology does not recommend molecular breast imaging for routine screening because most studies to date have limited sample sizes or are retrospective analyses (Holbrook & Newel, 2015).

Breast Computed Tomography

Cone-beam breast computed tomography technology has been explored as an alternative to mammography. However, it has been challenging to balance radiation dose with imaging quality. Currently, only research prototypes are available (O'Connell et al., 2010).

Summary

Breast imaging techniques are used for both screening and diagnostic purposes. People undergoing breast imaging can find the procedures stressful. Careful patient education on the rationale for various procedures and the implications of the findings is important to reduce stress and help patients make good decisions about care. Oncology nurses working with radiologists can provide excellent patient education and support.

References

American College of Radiology. (2014). *ACR practice parameter for the performance of contrast-enhanced magnetic resonance imaging (MRI) of the breast.* Retrieved from https://www.acr.org/~/media/ACR/Documents/PGTS/guidelines/MRI_Breast.pdf

Bassett, L.W., Jackson, V.P., Fu, K.L., & Fu, Y.S. (2004). *Diagnosis of diseases of the breast* (2nd ed.). Philadelphia, PA: Saunders.

D'Orsi, C.J., Sickles, E.A., Mendelson, E.B., & Morris, E.A. (2013). *ACR BI-RADS® atlas: Breast Imaging Reporting and Data System* (5th ed.). Reston, VA: American College of Radiology.

Gilbert, F.J., Tucker, L., & Young, K.C. (2016). Digital breast tomosynthesis (DBT): A review of the evidence for use as a screening tool. *Clinical Radiology, 71,* 141–150. doi:10.1016/j.crad.2015.11.008

Holbrook, A., & Newel, M.S. (2015). Alternative screening for women with dense breasts: Breast-specific gamma imaging (molecular breast imaging). *American Journal of Roentgenology, 204,* 252–256. doi:10.2214/AJR.14.13525

Ikeda, D.M. (2011). *Breast imaging: The requisites* (2nd ed.). St. Louis, MO: Elsevier Mosby.

Morris, E.A. (2007). Diagnostic breast MR imaging: Current status and future directions. *Radiologic Clinics of North America, 45,* 863–880. doi:10.1016/j.rcl.2007.07.002

Moschetta, M., Telegrafo, M., Carluccio, D.A., Jablonska, J.P., Rella, L., Serio, G., ... Angelelli, G. (2014). Comparison between fine needle aspiration cytology (FNAC) and core needle biopsy (CNB) in the diagnosis of breast lesions. *Giornale di Chirurgia, 35,* 171–176. doi:10.11138/gchir/2014.35.7.171

O'Connell, A., Conover, D.L., Zhang, Y., Seifert, P., Logan-Young, W., Lin, C.F., ... Ning, R. (2010). Cone-beam CT for breast imaging: Radiation dose, breast coverage, and image quality. *American Journal of Roentgenology, 195,* 496–509. doi:10.2214/AJR.08.1017

Saslow, D., Boetes, C., Burke, W., Harms, S., Leach, M.O., Lehman, C.D., ... Russell, C.A. (2007). American Cancer Society guidelines for breast screening with MRI as an adjunct to mammography. *CA: A Cancer Journal for Clinicians, 57,* 75–89. doi:10.3322/canjclin.57.2.75

Telegrafo, M., Rella, L., Ianora, A.A.S., Angelelli, G., & Moschetta, M. (2016). Effect of background parenchymal enhancement on breast cancer detection with magnetic resonance imaging. *Diagnostic and Interventional Imaging, 97,* 315–320. doi:10.1016/j.diii.2015.12.006

Warren, R.M.L., Pointon, L., Thompson, D., Hoff, R., Gilbert, F.J., Padhani, A., ... Leach, M.O. (2005). Reading protocol for dynamic contrast-enhanced MR images of the breast: Sensitivity and specificity analysis. *Radiology, 236,* 779–788. doi:10.1148/radiol.2363040735

Willems, S.M., van Deurzen, C.H.M., & van Diest, P.J. (2012). Diagnosis of breast lesions: Fine-needle aspiration cytology or core needle biopsy? A review. *Journal of Clinical Pathology, 65,* 287–292. doi:10.1136/jclinpath-2011-200410

CHAPTER 4

Pathology and Staging

Joanne Lester, PhD, CRNP, ANP-BC, AOCN®

Introduction

The visualization of breast anatomy (see Figure 4-1) is essential to the understanding of breast anatomic landmarks and standard breast surgical interventions. Breast anatomy includes the pair of complex mammary organs with extensive networks of hematologic and lymphatic vessels (Carlson et al., 2011). The lobules are essential to the production of breast milk and linked to the widespread ductal system, which carries milk to the nipple. The ductal system is the more common site of breast abnormalities, including premalignant and malignant tumors. The lymphatic system removes toxins and byproducts and consists of three levels of axillary lymph nodes that may or may not be removed in breast cancer surgeries. Additional breast components are found in the glandular and connective tissues, subcutaneous fat, and supportive Cooper ligaments. The anatomic landmarks of the breast include the underlying pectoralis major muscle, which lies below the layers of the skin, subcutaneous fat, and overlying fascia; the posterior margin of the clavicle (i.e., top margin of the breast); the inframammary fold on the anterior chest wall (i.e., lower margin of the breast); and horizontal markers extending from the mediolateral edge of the sternum to midaxillary line bilaterally (National Comprehensive Cancer Network® [NCCN®], 2017).

The female breasts evolve from the anterior chest wall in an early embryonic cycle and reach final developmental stages when pregnancy and breast-feeding ensue. Over a lifetime, the components of the breast continue to change, responding to the person's hormonal environment (exogenous and endogenous hormones) and body weight (Canadian Cancer Society, n.d.).

Breast Lesions

Breast lesions that are noted on physical examination or imaging studies often warrant a biopsy to determine whether they are benign, premalignant, or malignant. The majority of breast lesions are benign (Dyrstad, Yan, Fowler, & Colditz, 2015). Biopsy results often provide a snapshot of a woman's breast tissue and potential risk for developing breast cancer in the future. Incidental microscopic findings may guide lifestyle

---

Figure 4-1. Breast Anatomy and Lymphatic System

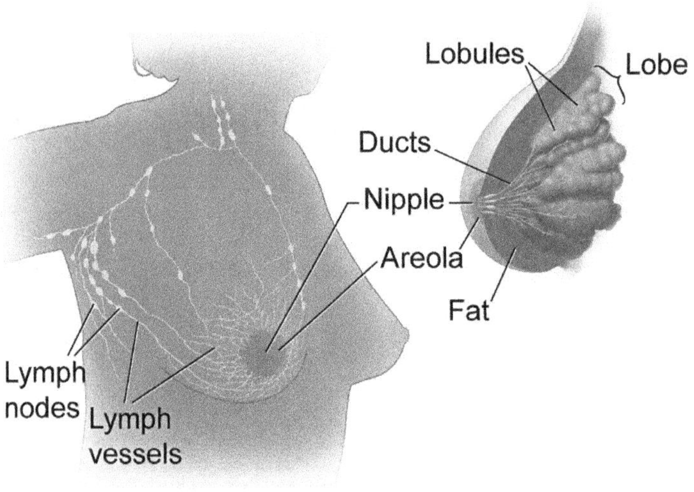

Lobules
Lobe
Ducts
Nipple
Areola
Fat
Lymph nodes
Lymph vessels

Note. Figure courtesy of National Cancer Institute. Illustration created by Don Bliss.

changes and future decision making based on personal and family breast or ovarian cancer history.

Benign Breast Lesions

Benign breast lesions represent a heterogeneous group of normal and abnormal breast tissue. Lesions may contain a combination of benign, premalignant, and malignant cells (Aumann et al., 2016; Carney et al., 2016; Neal et al., 2014). Generated by hormonal imbalances of estrogen (primarily) and progesterone, benign breast lesions tend to arise in the second and third decades of life, following puberty. The occurrence of lesions peaks during the fourth and fifth decades of life during perimenopausal years. The mean age at a woman's first breast biopsy is 46.6 years; while the mean age at diagnosis of breast cancer is 55.9 years (Dyrstad et al., 2015). This gap indicates the involution of breast tissue that occurs over time with normal changes that indicate fibrocystic disease. Changes in the breast may initially warrant a biopsy with continual close follow-up (i.e., annual mammography with possible tomography or magnetic resonance imaging [MRI], and annual or biannual clinical examination). Tissue changes also can include atypia, ductal carcinoma in situ, or invasive breast cancer, which underlines the importance of breast biopsies. The mean duration from initial pathologically defined benign breast lesion to diagnosis of breast cancer is 9.4 years (Dyrstad et al., 2015).

Various types of benign pathology, termed *fibrocystic disease*, exist. Nonproliferative lesions present no significant risk for future breast cancer development (Dyrstad et al., 2015). Fluid-filled cysts can be a very painful component of fibrocystic breast disease. Cysts disappear with aspiration, while fluid-filled cysts with a septum are difficult to resolve with aspiration alone. Therefore, these cysts may require biopsy or short-term follow-up with imaging. Complex cysts with debris may require a biopsy or short-term follow-up with imaging to monitor any changes. This type of cyst may have a malignant component and should not be ignored.

Fibroadenoma is another type of benign lesion. Occurring in early reproductive years, a fibroadenoma is the most common benign breast lesion. Oral contraceptive use prior to age 20 may be a causative factor of fibrocystic lesions in younger women, while the Epstein-Barr virus may be a causative factor in immunosuppressed women. The treatment of benign lesions such as fibroadenomas is based on physical examination, age, and imaging studies. A lesion suspicious for a fibroadenoma may require a core needle biopsy, an excisional biopsy, or follow-up examination. Current scientific knowledge suggests that fibroadenomas will not transform into breast cancer.

Lipomas are lesions composed of mature fat cells. They may require a core needle biopsy, an excisional biopsy, or follow-up examination depending on their anatomic location and personal discomfort. Lipomas represent no potential cancer risk to the patient, although a person with multiple lipomas may harbor a genetic risk for other types of cancers.

There is a long list of benign pathologic findings that are part of the fibrocystic process. These findings are generally inconsequential in women without risk factors for breast cancer. In women at risk for breast cancer (e.g., familiar or hereditary risk or previous abnormal biopsy), these changes may cause increased concern of cellular changes and risk for future development of breast cancer. These additional pathologic changes can include papillary apocrine changes, epithelial-related calcifications, mild epithelial hyperplasia, ductal ectasia, and columnar cell changes. These cellular changes all fall in the category of benign lesions and indicate normal involution that occurs in the breast cells during the pre- or perimenopausal periods.

Nonsclerosing adenosis, another component of fibrocystic disease, occurs during the reproductive ages as described previously. These lesions also are benign, although in women at risk for breast cancer development, these cellular findings may represent concerning changes.

An epithelial benign neoplasm often mimics a malignant neoplasm on imaging. Therefore, an excisional biopsy is typically recommended with or without previous core biopsy of the lesion.

Adenomas are also included in the components of fibrocystic disease and include tubular adenoma, lactating adenoma, nipple adenoma, apocrine adenosis, ductal adenosis, and pleomorphic adenomas (mixed). These findings often are seen on benign breast pathology reports and indicate fibrocystic disease in the average woman with no other risk factors.

Preductal fibrosis is another type of benign, nonsclerosing adenosis. It is a form of fibrocystic disease and not associated with an increased risk of developing breast cancer in women of average risk.

Hamartomas are benign lesions composed of glandular, adipose, and fibrous tissues. Hamartomas typically are found on imaging studies and designated as lesions of concern. They are removed from the breast with an excisional biopsy to differentiate between benign tissue and an invasive cancer.

Granular cell tumors originate from Schwann cells (Schwannoma) and, like hamartomas, require excisional biopsy to differentiate between benign tissue and invasive cancer. Although these lesions may cause concern on mammography, once they are removed they pose no specific risk to the woman.

Proliferative stromal lesions require excisional biopsy to exclude invasive cancer. One type of stromal lesion is a diabetic fibrous mastopathy, occurring in premenopausal women with type 1 diabetes but rarely found in men with type 1 diabetes.

Pseudoangiomatous stromal hyperplasia is a benign proliferation of mammary stroma that mimics a fibroadenoma or phyllodes tumor. Phyllodes tumor and cystosarcoma phyllodes are rare tumors that originate in the connective tissue/stroma of the breast (Adesoye et al., 2016). These tumors must be removed with clear margins of benign tissue. Phyllodes tumors may carry a low malignant potential, although most have benign tendencies. This type of tumor requires close follow-up with frequent clinical examinations and annual mammography.

Proliferative lesions without atypia represent another category of relatively benign lesions that may indicate a slightly increased relative risk for future breast cancer development. These lesions, as noted on imaging studies, require a core or an excisional biopsy to exclude a premalignant or invasive cancer. These pathologic changes include moderate or florid ductal hyperplasia, sclerosing adenosis, radial scar, and benign pseudoinfiltrative lesions.

Intraductal papilloma or papillomatosis is another category of benign tissue. It is typically found in breast ductal excisions, a procedure performed in cases of spontaneous bloody nipple discharge.

Findings also may show proliferative lesions with atypia. Atypia in breast tissue indicates that a progression of cellular changes has occurred with abnormal cellularity and premalignant characteristics. Atypia is found on core or excisional biopsy and confirms significant changes in breast tissue. In the event of a core biopsy, a subsequent excisional biopsy must be performed to exclude adjacent malignant changes.

It is important to differentiate atypical ductal hyperplasia from ductal carcinoma in situ (DCIS), a somewhat common discrepancy among pathologists. Atypical ductal hyperplasia occurs in the ductal tissue of the breast and bodes a higher risk for breast cancer development in the biopsied (ipsilateral) breast. Proliferative lesions with atypia have a fourfold relative increased risk for future breast cancer development in either breast (Dyrstad et al., 2015; Hartmann et al., 2014; Neal et al., 2014; Renshaw & Gould, 2016). This risk is higher in premenopausal women than in postmenopausal women who have no other personal risk factors. Atypical lobular hyperplasia occurs in the lobules of the breast and must be differentiated from lobular carcinoma in situ (LCIS).

Malignant Breast Lesions

Advanced premalignant breast lesions are also termed *noninvasive* or *in situ* breast cancer (American Cancer Society, n.d.; Gipponi et al., 2015; Nimptsch & Pischon, 2015; Roetzheim et al., 2015). If a premalignant breast lesion is found on a core biopsy, a subsequent excisional biopsy is necessary to exclude the possibility of an adjacent invasive cancer. As discussed previously, atypical cells occur in the ductal system of the breast (DCIS) or in the lobules (LCIS). DCIS is primarily diagnosed in a pathologic sample that includes an abnormal cluster of microcalcifications (i.e., before the abnormality forms a malignant nodule). Contrarily, LCIS is typically an incidental finding concomitant with a biopsy for a different lesion. LCIS can be multicentric (50%) and may involve the contralateral breast (30%) (Capobianco et al., 2014; Hartmann et al., 2014; Renshaw & Gould, 2016).

The primary difference between DCIS and LCIS is that DCIS, if left alone, can advance to invasive breast cancer (ductal or lobular cancer, or both), whereas LCIS will never turn into a cancer and remains a risk factor only (Breastcancer.org., 2017; Capobianco et al., 2014; Lange, Reimer, Hartmann, Glass, & Stachs, 2016). Instead, the abnormal cells remain in the lobules. In LCIS, significant risk (relative risk increase of 7%–12%) of breast cancer development (e.g., ductal or lobular) exists for either or both breasts (Nimptsch & Pischon, 2015; Roetzheim et al., 2015), although the relative risk is higher in the ipsilateral breast.

DCIS originates in the epithelial lining of ductal cells (see Figure 4-2) and remains inside the milk duct. Because DCIS has no access to either the hematologic or lymphatic systems from within the milk duct, there is no mechanism for the development

Figure 4-2. Breast Duct With Ductal Carcinoma in Situ (DCIS)

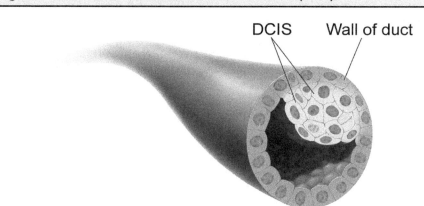

Note. Figure courtesy of National Cancer Institute. Illustration created by Don Bliss.

of metastatic disease. Therefore, ductal carcinoma itself is a noninvasive breast cancer as compared to an invasive cancer, which has the ability to spread to distant organs. DCIS can be categorized as low-, intermediate-, or high-grade cellularity. These levels are comparable to the ability of DCIS to continue to progress into invasive ductal or lobular carcinoma. Hence, a high-grade DCIS is treated aggressively in an attempt to prevent further progression to invasive cancer. It is unknown if DCIS precedes all invasive breast cancers, or if DCIS occurs after invasive breast cancer development.

Paget disease of the nipple often is diagnosed with findings of DCIS alone. Evidence of Paget disease must be completely removed, as residual cells may allow for continued cellular changes and growth outside the duct. Findings of high-grade DCIS/Paget disease are most worrisome because an invasive component may be involved, carrying the short- or long-term threat of metastatic disease.

Invasive Breast Cancer

Invasive breast cancer is the most common female cancer in the United States and throughout the world (American Cancer Society, n.d.; Gipponi et al., 2015; Nimptsch

& Pischon, 2015; Roetzheim et al., 2015). Invasive breast cancer is a group of 30 or more breast cancers with significant heterogeneity and diverse phenotypes of cells. Invasive (or infiltrating) breast cancer defines cells that have broken through their cellular wall of origin (duct or lobule) and invaded, or infiltrated, surrounding tissues. Of concern is the potential to shed cells into the lymphatic channels or blood vessels. A tumor may include invasive and noninvasive cells with various combinations that invoke the saying, "Which came first, the chicken or the egg?" It remains relatively unknown whether the presence of DCIS promotes the development of invasive breast cancer or if they are unrelated.

A breast cancer can have mixed cellular features of invasive lobular and invasive ductal carcinoma. Termed *invasive mammary cancer* or *infiltrating mammary carcinoma*, this mixed breast cancer is treated as an invasive ductal carcinoma and includes more than one tumor in the breast. *Multifocal breast cancer* refers to more than one lesion within the same quadrant of the breast, with all tumors theoretically arising from the original tumor. *Multicentric breast cancer* refers to different tumors in more than one quadrant of the breast, with tumors arising from different lesions.

Invasive ductal carcinoma comprises 70%–80% of all breast cancers (NCCN, 2017) (see Figure 4-3). Various invasive ductal carcinoma subtypes exist, including tubular, medullary, mucinous, papillary, cribriform, and micropapillary.

Invasive lobular carcinoma comprises 10%–15% of breast cancers (NCCN, 2017). The relative difference between invasive ductal and invasive lobular carcinoma is the pathologic presentation. Invasive ductal carcinoma tends to form an ovoid shape, with a size consistent with clinical examination and imaging studies, whereas lobular carcinoma tends to have multiple microscopic fingers reaching out from its central tumor. Typically, the measurement of an invasive lobular tumor on imaging or clinical examination is not consistent with its increased size on pathologic examination.

Inflammatory breast cancer is rare, accounting for only 2% of all breast cancers (Goldner, Behrendt, Schoellhammer, Lee, & Chen, 2014). Inflammatory breast cancer is confirmed by clinical presentation and includes diffuse erythema, diffuse lymphedema of the breast and possibly the arm, and diffuse thickening of breast skin

Figure 4-3. Invasive Ductal Cancer

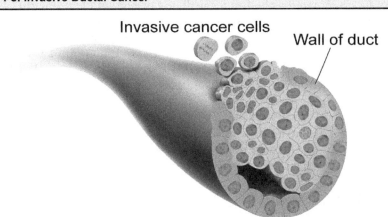

Note. Figure courtesy of National Cancer Institute. Illustration created by Don Bliss.

overlying the mass (*peau d'orange*). This type of breast cancer is confirmed by pathologic testing, including a punch biopsy of erythematous skin overlying the mass and removal of a piece of skin at the time of surgery.

Pathology Report Components and Prognostic Indicators

The grade of the tumor predicts how likely the malignancy is to grow and spread, considering details such as tubule formation, nuclear grade, and mitotic count. The lower the grade, the lower the growth curve and the better the prognosis. Conversely, the higher the grade, the higher the growth curve and poorer the prognosis. The term *grade* has synonymous terms:

- Grade 1 = low grade = well differentiated
- Grade 2 = intermediate grade = moderately differentiated
- Grade 3 = high grade = poorly differentiated

Histologic grade, Nottingham grade, and Elston-Ellis grade are other ways to describe tumor grade. Numbers are assigned to various features of tumor: score of 3–5 = grade 1; score of 6–7 = grade 2; and score of 8–9 = grade 3.

Tumor Cellularity

A number of notations may be included on the preliminary or final pathology reports that identify components of tumor cellularity. Ki-67 is a numeric value represented by a percentage that indicates how fast the cells are growing in vivo. Although the exact cutoff is not clear, values greater than 15%–20% indicate a higher degree of cell division and represent a poorer prognosis as compared to values less than 15%–20% (Ács et al., 2017; Soliman & Yussif, 2016). Additional notations may be made about tumor cellularity, although their true value and contribution to scientific knowledge remain under consideration.

Tumor Margins

The pathologic tumor size describes the largest span from one malignant cell to another. Invasive ductal carcinoma has a rather predictive tumor size with a fairly circumscribed shape. The size of invasive lobular carcinoma can be quite unpredictable and large with the measurement of malignant cells from one spindle to the one furthest away. The true tumor size is not attained until negative surgical margins in a three-dimensional fashion are identified by the pathologist. Negative margins indicate that there is no evidence of invasive or noninvasive (DCIS) malignant cells from the two farthest points of the tumor in all three dimensions.

Ex vivo (e.g., removed) margin status of a noninvasive or invasive tumor can be defined as close, positive, or negative. Close margins equate with less than 2 mm from the tumor, whereas positive margins equate with malignant cells at the surgical margin. Negative margins equate with more than 2 mm from any malignant cells. Negative margins are considered essential for both DCIS as well as invasive cancers for optimal outcomes (Rarick, Kimler, & Tawfik, 2016; Shaikh et al., 2016).

Ultimately, the surgeon must determine the location of the tumor, the markings with ink or sutures, and the use of intraoperative ultrasonography or radioactive seeds (Rarick et al., 2016; Volders, Haloua, Krekel, Meijer, & van den Tol, 2016). The pathologist relies on the surgeon to thoroughly examine the tumor bed for any palpable or visible tumor and to meticulously tag and label each surgically excised piece of tissue. This is of utmost importance not only to ensure negative margins, but also to determine where to reexcise in the case of one or two positive margins.

When three or more positive margins are identified with invasive carcinoma following a lumpectomy, most likely the woman will require a mastectomy unless the surgeon is confident that more tissue can be removed with retained cosmetic integrity of the breast. In the case of multiple positive margins following a mastectomy, sometimes additional surgery can be performed, or radiation therapy is given to the area of concern to prevent a local recurrence.

Tumor Invasion

Tumor invasion is described by several indices particular to each tumor. The presence or absence of vascular, lymphovascular, or angiolymphatic invasion is a cellular indicator of tumor aggressiveness (Shah, Djisam, Damulira, Aganze, & Danquah, 2016). The presence of vascular invasion indicates microscopic evidence that cells have invaded the hematologic system. The presence of lymphovascular invasion indicates invasion of the tumor in the lymphatic channels. Angiolymphatic invasion provides evidence that tumor cells are growing in the lymph channels and hematologic system.

Oncogene Typing

Oncogene typing is a procedure to identify personalized characteristics about the genes within a tumor. These characteristics are specific to each person and the person's tumor profile. Oncogene typing can provide adjunct information to the pathologic findings, with improvements in stratification of prognostic markers (Lynch, Venne, & Berse, 2015). Oncogene typing is relevant in the following tumor characteristics:
- Tumor size T1 or T2
- Nodal status of N0 only (i.e., negative lymph nodes)
- Estrogen/progesterone positive (either or both)
- Ability to take antiestrogen or aromatase inhibitor

Evidence from clinical studies supports that people with a low oncogene score may not require chemotherapy for their systemic treatment; an aromatase inhibitor or antiestrogen is used instead (Lynch et al., 2015). A moderate or high oncogene score indicates increased cellularity and activity of the tumor and typically requires chemotherapy followed by years of antiestrogen and/or aromatase inhibitors. Oncogene typing individualizes care for each person and guides the most appropriate treatment with intended optimal outcomes.

Lymph Nodes

The lymph node status remains the most important indicator of tumor invasion and prognosis. It is ascertained by sentinel lymph node biopsy, axillary node dissection, or both. In addition, a supraclavicular or infraclavicular node biopsy may indicate the presence of regional metastatic disease. The number of lymph nodes involved and their impact on prognosis is further discussed below in the explanation of the tumor-node-metastasis (TNM) staging process.

Staging of Invasive Breast Cancer

Breast cancer staging is documented in a systematic manner in concordance with the most recent published universal method (American Joint Committee on Cancer, n.d.). Staging is another individualized entity that correlates pathology and radiology results, physical examination, and the patient's personal history. Each of the items can be considered individually, but when considered together, they create the TNM staging report (Carney et al., 2016; Sparano, 2016).

The clinical stage at diagnosis is based on the interprofessional team's estimation and clinical measurement of the tumor size in centimeters or millimeters. The estimated clinical size of the tumor is determined by clinical examination and imaging studies with documentation in two or three dimensions. The location by quadrants (e.g., upper inner, upper outer, lower inner, lower outer) or central under the nipple-areolar complex is noted, as well as centimeters from the nipple. Imaging studies such as mammography, three-dimensional tomosynthesis, ultrasonography, and MRI also can be used to determine tumor size.

Clips may be present in the breast tissue following a core needle or open breast biopsy. Their placement may mark the tumor size prior to neoadjuvant treatment or surgery. If only one clip is present, as in the case of most core needle biopsies, a clip is generally ineffective in determining tumor size, although it marks the location of the original lesion. Radioactive seeds can be inserted prior to surgery to facilitate clear margins when seeking a lumpectomy for definitive surgery.

Other factors taken into consideration include assessment of lymph node status, absence or presence of palpable axillary lymph nodes, palpable supra- and infraclavicular lymph nodes, visual or measured arm lymphedema, and assessment of breast skin. Breast skin is assessed for the following symptoms: absence or presence of erythema, firm skin with peau d'orange changes, or breast edema. The assessment also includes examination of the contralateral breast and axilla.

Radiology imaging can include a mammogram (digital or analog), ultrasound of the tumor mass and axilla (Diaz-Ruiz et al., 2016), digital tomosynthesis, MRI, and the use of imaging guidance to insert metallic clips to mark the size of the mass (essential when neoadjuvant chemotherapy is planned). Additional imaging may be required to identify regional or distant metastasis.

Proper notation of the clinical breast cancer stage has several variables to consider. The clinical presentation prior to any treatment is noted as cTNM. Pathologic staging using pTNM is the pathologic designation of a tumor following surgery and without systemic treatment (e.g., no neoadjuvant treatment using chemotherapy or hormonal therapy), whereas ypT ypN ypM is the pathologic designation following neoadjuvant treatment and surgical removal of the tumor (Park, Jung, & Koo, 2016).

In the TNM staging system, T indicates tumor size and is the clinical or pathologic assessment, citing the largest dimension of the tumor. The notations of T include the following:

- TX = primary tumor cannot be assessed
- T0 = no evidence of primary tumor
- Tis = noninvasive disease, carcinoma in situ (e.g., DCIS, Paget disease)
- Tmic = microscopic tumor, ≤ 1 mm
- T1 = tumor measures up to 20 mm (2 cm) in size
  - T1a = > 1 mm but ≤ 5 mm (0.5 cm)
  - T1b = > 5 mm (0.5 cm) but ≤ 10 mm (1 cm)
  - T1c = > 10 mm (1 cm) but ≤ 20 mm (2 cm)

- T2 = tumor is > 20 mm (2 cm) but ≤ 50 mm (5 cm)
- T3 = tumor is > 50 mm (5 cm)
- T4 = tumor is any size with direct adherence to skin (inflammatory breast cancer) or chest wall

N indicates nodal status and is the clinical assessment of the lymph nodes in the axilla. In the clinical setting, it is difficult to know exactly how many nodes may be positive, although ultrasound may be helpful in the assessment. Methods to determine the malignant potential include fine needle aspiration or core needle biopsy of a palpable adenopathy. Sentinel lymph node biopsy may be performed to determine axillary status prior to neoadjuvant treatment.

Notations of *N* include the following:
- NX = regional lymph nodes cannot be assessed
- N0 = no regional lymph node metastasis
- N1 = metastasis to 1–3 ipsilateral lymph nodes
- N2 = metastasis to 4–9 ipsilateral lymph nodes
- N3 = metastasis to 10 or more ipsilateral lymph nodes; matted nodes

A notation of cN1/N2 may indicate an axilla with multiple clinically evident lymph nodes, yet unknown pathologic status.

M indicates metastatic status and is the clinical assessment of suspicious distant metastases. Estimations may be made of possible distant metastasis based on patient-stated symptoms pending imaging studies. Notations of *M* include the following:
- MX = metastatic disease has not been assessed
- M0 = no evidence of metastatic disease
- M1 = evidence of distant metastatic disease

The clinical description of a tumor may not be as detailed as the pathologic report, as some factors may be unknown or inexact. It is important to obtain the most precise clinical assessment to accurately stage the cancer prior to neoadjuvant therapy because the initial clinical stage will stand as the final tumor stage regardless of whether neoadjuvant treatment was effective or if disease progression occurs (Bossuyt & Symmans, 2016). The components of each stage are shown in Figures 4-4 to 4-10.

Figure 4-4. Stage 1A and 1B Breast Cancer

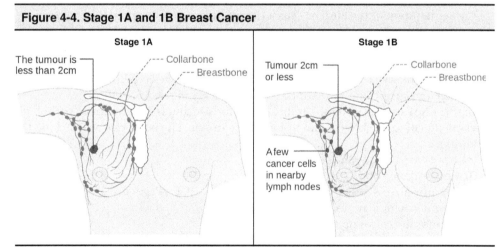

Stage 1A

The tumour is less than 2cm — ---Collarbone --- Breastbone

Stage 1B

Tumour 2cm or less — --- Collarbone --- Breastbone

A few cancer cells in nearby lymph nodes

Note. Figures courtesy of Cancer Research UK/Wikimedia Commons, 2016. Retrieved from http://www .cancerresearchuk.org/about-cancer/breast-cancer/stages-types-grades/number-stages/stage-1.

Figure 4-5. Stage 2A Breast Cancer

Stage 2A—Tumour is 2 cm or smaller and cancer cells are found in 1–3 lymph nodes in the armpit or near the breastbone.

Stage 2A—Tumour is larger than 2 cm but not larger than 5 cm and there is no cancer in the lymph nodes.

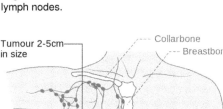
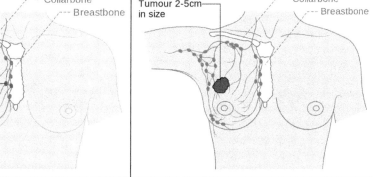

Note. Figures courtesy of Cancer Research UK/Wikimedia Commons, 2016. Retrieved from http://www.cancerresearchuk .org/about-cancer/breast-cancer/stages-types-grades/number-stages/stage-2.

When neoadjuvant chemotherapy is effective, the tumor will shrink or be clinically undetectable. Changes in tumor size after neoadjuvant therapy are based on interprofessional providers' measurements (Park et al., 2016) and findings from surgical removal. A TNM staging pathology report should always include the tumor size, nodal status, and metastatic status.

The synoptic report (see Figure 4-11) complies, in slightly modified form, with the guidelines of the College of American Pathologists and the Association of Directors of Anatomic and Surgical Pathology for the reporting of cancer specimens. Additional paragraphs may describe the type of testing done on various specimens.

The pathologist describes the specimens that were sent to the laboratory, including the number of sentinel lymph nodes (or axillary dissection), lumpectomy, mastectomy, or radical mastectomy (with lymph nodes), skin plastic repair, and gross description of specimen. The specimen description includes the number of containers with confirmation of the patient's name and medical record number, description/ size (cm) of each of the sentinel lymph nodes, and breast specimen. The report identifies the breast specimen using the following indices: laterality, presence of stitch/ clip, time removed, weight in grams, size of breast and skin in centimeters, description of nipple, margins as described by surgeon's markings, size of mass, distance from margins, description of lymph node(s), description of remaining breast parenchyma, summary of cassettes of tissue, time specimen was placed in formalin, cold ischemia time, and the time specimen was removed from formalin with notation of total fixation time. Pathologic tumor margins are examined to determine the presence or absence of macroscopic (visible tumor) or microscopic disease along the various tumor margins. Skilled pathologic measurements may indicate marked tumor reduction yet significant pathologic evidence of residual microscopic tumor.

Documentation of the pathologic stage of breast cancer with or without neoadjuvant treatment includes access of films to the pathologist and acknowledgment of radiographic results, and pre- and post-treatment clinical size of the tumor

Figure 4-6. Stage 2B Breast Cancer

Stage 2B—Tumour is larger than 2 cm but not larger than 5 cm (small areas of cancer in the lymph nodes).

Stage 2B—Tumour is larger than 2 cm but not larger than 5 cm and cancer cells are found in 1–3 lymph nodes in the armpit or near the breastbone.

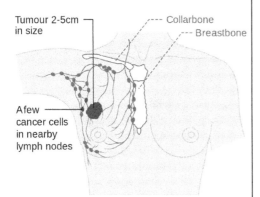

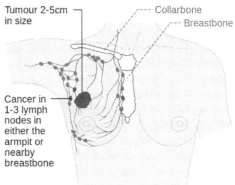

Stage 2B—Tumour is larger than 5 cm and hasn't spread to the lymph nodes.

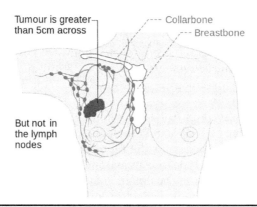

Note. Figures courtesy of Cancer Research UK/Wikimedia Commons, 2016. Retrieved from http://www .cancerresearchuk.org/about-cancer/breast-cancer/stages-types-grades/number-stages/stage-2.

and lymph node status (Aumann et al., 2016; Bossuyt & Symmans, 2016). The tumor or tumor cavity is identified with close examination of fresh pathology specimens. The presence of metallic clips inserted at the time of biopsy or preoperatively using radiographic clips helps to identify the gross tumor bed and should be noted.

The pathologist will examine peritumoral tissue and slice surgical specimens into sections 5 mm or smaller. Additional measures include documentation of any evidence of macroscopic tumor, microscopic foci, or absence of malignant cells (e.g., pathologic complete response, noted as pCR). Documentation includes indices such as absence or presence of DCIS, LCIS, lymphovascular invasion, and disease in lymph nodes, including evidence of micrometastasis or isolated tumor cells (Bossuyt & Symmans, 2016). The pathologic size of the tumor is the largest contiguous foci of invasive carcinoma, including DCIS. Other measures may include cellularity with comparison to pretreatment tumor (e.g., estrogen and progesterone receptors, HER2 receptors), tumor bed or tumor margins, lymph node metastasis with size of largest foci, and treatment effect (breast and lymph nodes). Changes in axillary assessment are based on previous documentation of palpable adenopathy and results of previous fine needle, core biopsy, or sentinel lymph node biopsy (Bossuyt & Symmans, 2016). Axillary node dissection is conducted with definitive surgery for failure of sentinel lymph node biopsy, questionable nodal status on imaging studies, or palpable adenopathy. Results of the axillary node dissection only change the presumed stage from N1 to N2 or N3 if 4–9 or 10 or more positive nodes, respectively, are found (Tadayyon et al., 2016).

Example: Mary is a 34-year-old Caucasian woman diagnosed with a left breast cancer. Upon clinical presentation, she had a palpable breast mass of 2.4 cm × 2.8 cm ×

Figure 4-7. Stage 3A Breast Cancer

Stage 3A—Tumour can be of any size, or no tumour is seen in the breast, and cancer is found in 4–9 lymph glands under the arm or near the breastbone.

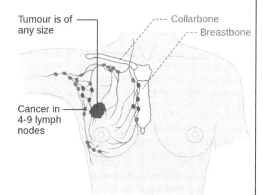

Stage 3A—Tumour is larger than 5 cm and small clusters of breast cancer cells are found in the lymph nodes.

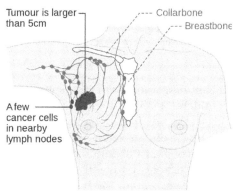

Stage 3A—Tumour is larger than 5 cm and cancer cells have spread into up to 3 lymph nodes in the armpit or near the breastbone.

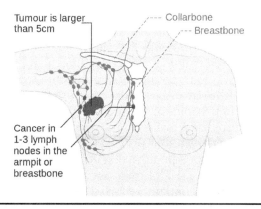

Note. Figures courtesy of Cancer Research UK/Wikimedia Commons, 2016. Retrieved from http://www.cancerresearchuk.org/about-cancer/breast-cancer/stages-types-grades/number-stages/stage-3.

Figure 4-8. Stage 3B Breast Cancer

Stage 3B—Tumour has spread to the skin of the breast or the chest wall, causing swelling or ulceration.

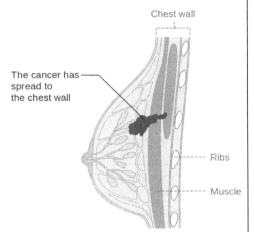

Chest wall

The cancer has spread to the chest wall

------ Ribs

------ Muscle

Stage 3B—Cancer may have spread to up to 9 lymph nodes in the armpit or near the breastbone.

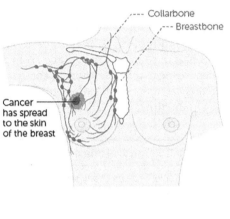

---- Collarbone

---- Breastbone

Cancer has spread to the skin of the breast

Note. Figures courtesy of Cancer Research UK/Wikimedia Commons, 2016. Retrieved from http://www .cancerresearchuk.org/about-cancer/breast-cancer/stages-types-grades/number-stages/stage-3.

1.6 cm (consistent with ultrasound) and five palpable axillary nodes that were also considered malignant on ultrasound. An ultrasound-guided core needle biopsy confirmed the breast malignancy; a fine needle aspiration of one axillary node confirmed metastatic disease to an axillary node. Mary had no complaints of bone pain, headaches, cough, or abdominal pain. Because neoadjuvant chemotherapy was planned, she underwent computed tomography scans of her chest and abdomen, which were negative (except for the breast mass and multiple axillary nodes), and an MRI of her head, which was likewise negative. Therefore, her clinical stage was cT2 N2 M0. Mary underwent neoadjuvant chemotherapy.

After four cycles of dose-dense doxorubicin and cyclophosphamide, and 12 consecutive weeks of docetaxel, Mary's mass and axillary nodes were no longer palpable. Mary underwent surgery and had no pathologic residual tumor in her lumpectomy specimen; none of the 24 axillary nodes contained malignant disease. Her surgical staging was pyT0 pyN0 pyM0 (*py* stands for "pathologic" and "after neoadjuvant therapy"). Mary remains free of symptoms related to bone pain, cough, abdominal pain, or headaches, so the scans were not repeated at this time. Therefore, Mary's cancer is stage IIIA because of the size of her initial tumor (2.8 cm, T2) and positive lymph nodes (4–9, N2) prior to neoadjuvant chemotherapy. The number of positive lymph nodes (4–9 clinically suspicious) pushes Mary's stage of disease to IIIA.

Staging of a breast cancer without prior neoadjuvant chemotherapy is described only as the surgical stage. A preoperative diagnosis of a breast cancer, laterality, and potential clinical or radiologic size of the mass are provided to the radiologist. The sentinel lymph node status is initially reported as a frozen section during surgery. Finally, the tumor size and numbering, laterality, and location (e.g., axilla) of each removed and identified sentinel lymph node are noted.

Figure 4-9. Stage 3C Breast Cancer

Stage 3C—Tumour can be of any size, or there may be no tumour, and cancer has spread to the skin of the breast or the chest wall, causing swelling or ulceration, and 10 or more lymph nodes in the armpit.

Stage 3C—Tumour can be of any size, or there may be no tumour, and cancer has spread to the skin of the breast or the chest wall, causing swelling or ulceration, and lymph nodes above and below the collarbone.

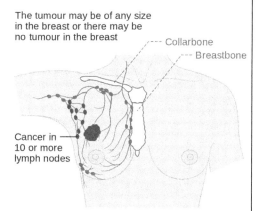

The tumour may be of any size in the breast or there may be no tumour in the breast

Collarbone

Breastbone

Cancer in 10 or more lymph nodes

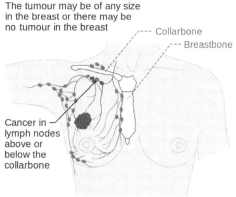

The tumour may be of any size in the breast or there may be no tumour in the breast

Collarbone

Breastbone

Cancer in lymph nodes above or below the collarbone

Stage 3C—Tumour can be of any size, or there may be no tumor, and cancer has spread to the skin of the breast or the chest wall, causing swelling or ulceration, and lymph nodes in the armpit and near the breastbone.

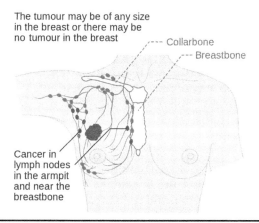

The tumour may be of any size in the breast or there may be no tumour in the breast

Collarbone

Breastbone

Cancer in lymph nodes in the armpit and near the breastbone

Note. Figures courtesy of Cancer Research UK/Wikimedia Commons, 2016. Retrieved from http://www.cancerresearchuk.org/about-cancer/breast-cancer/stages-types-grades/number-stages/stage-3.

Lymph nodes are numbered sequentially, with identification of sentinel or nonsentinel lymph nodes designating the presence or absence of breast cancer cells. The sum of lymph nodes is described by a ratio of positive to negative, with a notation that sentinel lymph nodes were examined in multiple ways. Lymph node negativity or positivity is one of the most important prognostic factors (Harlow & Weaver, 2016); therefore, it is imperative that the pathologist find and note any malignant cells. In lymph

Figure 4-10. Stage 4 Breast Cancer

Stage 4—Tumour can be of any size, lymph nodes may or may not contain cancer cells, and the cancer has spread (metastasised) to other parts of the body.

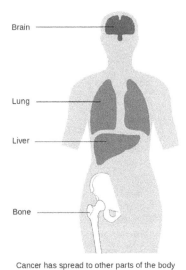

Cancer has spread to other parts of the body

Note. Figure courtesy of Cancer Research UK. Retrieved from http://www.cancerresearchuk.org/about-cancer/breast -cancer/stages-types-grades/number-stages/stage-4. Reprinted with permission.

node examination, the analysis includes macroscopic and microscopic evidence of disease and any tumor cell cluster larger than 2 mm (Harlow & Weaver, 2016). Isolated tumor cells are defined as small clusters of cells no greater than 0.2 mm or clusters larger than 0.2 mm but no greater than 2 mm.

Occult disease is also examined. This information may be of importance to planned systemic treatment. Nodal metastases that are not seen on initial examination but are detected subsequently by other means, including hematoxylin and eosin, immunohistochemistry, and reverse transcriptase polymerase chain reaction, must be reported.

Example: Rachel is a 58-year-old Asian woman who noted a mass in her right breast during breast self-examination in the shower. Rachel saw her gynecologist, who ordered an updated mammogram and right breast ultrasound. The radiologist spoke with Rachel and her gynecologist and recommended a right breast ultrasound-guided core needle biopsy to determine the diagnosis of this 1.5 cm lesion. Prior to the procedure, Rachel was examined by the institution's nurse practitioner, who noted the small, hard mass in her right breast with an estimated size of 1.5 cm. Rachel's ipsilateral axilla was free of any suspicious nodes. Likewise, her left breast and axilla were within normal limits. Therefore, Rachel underwent ultrasound-guided core needle biopsy of the right breast.

The diagnosis of Rachel's right breast mass was consistent with infiltrating ductal carcinoma. Rachel underwent a lumpectomy with sentinel lymph node biopsy. Three days later, her surgeon called and stated she had a stage I breast cancer with negative lymph nodes. This information was noted in her chart as pT1 N0 M0.

Figure 4-11. Components of a Pathology Report

Synoptic Report
- Specimen (P = partial resection, M = mastectomy)
- Location in the breast
- Laterality (R = right, L = left)
- Focality (unifocal or multifocal)
- Tumor size (cm)
- Histologic type (ductal or lobular)
- Nottingham grade
  - Tubule score (1–3)
  - Nuclear score (1–3)
  - Mitotic score (1–3)
- Involvement of skin, nipple epidermis, skeletal muscle (yes or no)
- Lymphovascular invasion (P = present, N = not identified)
- Margins of main specimen (P = positive, N = negative)
  - Distance to closest margin of main specimen (cm)
  - Designation of closest margin of main specimen
  - Re-resection margin status (P = positive, N = negative, NA = not applicable)
- DCIS (P = present, N = not identified)
  - Nuclear grade
  - Comedo necrosis (P = present, N = not identified)
  - Extensive intraductal component (P = present, N = not identified)
  - Margins of main specimen (P = positive, N = negative)
  - Distance to closest margin of main specimen
  - Designation of closest margin of main specimen
  - Re-resection margin status (P = positive, N = negative, NA = not applicable)
- LCIS/ALH (P = present, N = not identified)
- Regional lymph nodes: axillary node dissection
  - Total number of lymph nodes (sentinel and nonsentinel)
  - Number of sentinel lymph nodes
  - Number of lymph nodes with macrometastases (> 2 cm)
  - Number of lymph nodes with micrometastases (> 0.2 mm and < 2 mm)
  - Number of lymph nodes with isolated tumor cells (< 0.2 mm)
  - Size of largest nodal metastasis (mm)
  - Size of extranodal extension (mm) (N = not identified)
- Markers
  - Estrogen receptor (positive or negative)
  - Progesterone receptor (positive or negative)
  - HER2 IHC (1+ [negative], 2+ [borderline], 3+ [positive])
  - HER2 FISH (definitive "tie-breaker" for above IHC HER2 with positive or negative results)

ALH—atypical lobular hyperplasia; DCIS—ductal carcinoma in situ; FISH—fluorescence in situ hybridization; IHC—immunohistochemistry; LCIS—lobular carcinoma in situ

Note. The above synoptic report complies, in slightly modified form, with the guidelines of the College of American Pathologists and the Association of Directors of Anatomic and Surgical Pathology for the reporting of cancer specimens. Additional paragraphs of pathology reports measure (in three dimensions) and weigh (in kilograms) each segment of resected tissue. A summary of all tissue cassettes is also noted for future reference.

Summary

Histologic and pathologic review and classification of surgical breast specimens are essential to the prognosis and treatment of breast cancer for all men and women. Frequently, neoadjuvant chemotherapy is administered prior to surgery with the goals of shrinking the tumor, observing the effect of specific chemotherapy agents, and reducing the impact of surgical intervention. The order and components of pathology reports may vary among institutions, although the multiple segments as described in this chapter are ideally necessary to understand components of the breast cancer. The recommendations for systemic treatment (e.g., neoadjuvant or adjuvant) depend on an accurate pathology report. The stage of disease and various pathologic indices are crucial to determine the prognosis of a new breast cancer diagnosis and possible timeline of disease progression. Oncology nurses need to be comfortable reading pathology reports, anticipating the expected components of a synoptic report, understanding how staging influences treatment decisions, and helping patients to understand the information on pathology and staging reports.

References

Ács, B., Zámbó, V., Vízkeleti, L., Szász, A.M., Madaras, L., Szentmártoni, G., ... Tőkés, A.-M. (2017). Ki-67 as a controversial predictive and prognostic marker in breast cancer patients treated with neoadjuvant chemotherapy. *Diagnostic Pathology, 12,* 20. doi:10.1186/s13000-017-0608-5

Adesoye, T., Neuman, H.B., Wilke, L.G., Schumacher, J.R., Steiman, J., & Greenberg, C.C. (2016). Current trends in the management of phyllodes tumors of the breast. *Annals of Surgical Oncology, 23,* 3199–3205. doi:10.1245/s10434-016-5314-0

American Cancer Society. (n.d.). Breast pathology. Retrieved from https://www.cancer.org/treatment/understanding-your-diagnosis/tests/understanding-your-pathology-report/breast-pathology.html

American Joint Committee on Cancer. (n.d.). General education. Retrieved from https://cancerstaging.org/CSE/general/Pages/articles.aspx

Aumann, K., Niermann, K., Asberger, J., Wellner, U., Bronsert, P., Erbes, T., ... Werner, M. (2016). Structured reporting ensures complete content and quick detection of essential data in pathology reports of oncological breast resection specimens. *Breast Cancer Research and Treatment, 156,* 495–500. doi:10.1007/s10549-016-3769-0

Bossuyt, V., & Symmans, W.F. (2016). Standardizing of pathology in patients receiving neoadjuvant chemotherapy. *Annals of Surgical Oncology, 23,* 3153–3161. doi:10.1245/s10434-016-5317-x

Breastcancer.org. (2017). Getting your pathology report. Retrieved from http://www.breastcancer.org/symptoms/diagnosis/getting_path_report

Canadian Cancer Society. (n.d.). Breast cancer: The breasts. Retrieved from http://www.cancer.ca/en/cancer-information/cancer-type/breast/breast-cancer/the-breasts/?region=on

Capobianco, G., Simbula, L., Soro, D., Meloni, F., Cossu-Rocca, P., Dessole, S., ... Meloni, G.B. (2014). Management of breast lobular carcinoma in situ: Radio-pathological correlation, clinical implications, and follow-up. *European Journal of Gynaecological Oncology, 35,* 157–162.

Carlson, R.W., Allred, D.C., Anderson, B.O., Burstein, H.J., Carter, W.B., Edge, S.B., ... Zellars, R. (2011). Invasive breast cancer. *Journal of the National Comprehensive Cancer Network, 9,* 136–222.

Carney, P.A., Allison, K.H., Oster, N.V., Frederick, P.D., Morgan, T.R., Geller, B.M., ... Elmore, J.G. (2016). Identifying and processing the gap between perceived and actual agreement in breast pathology interpretation. *Modern Pathology, 29,* 717–726. doi:10.1038/modpathol.2016.62

Diaz-Ruiz, M.J., Arnau, A., Montesinos, J., Miguel, A., Culell, P., Solernou, L., ... Salvador-Tarrasón, R. (2016). Diagnostic accuracy and impact on management of ultrasonography-guided fine-needle aspiration to detect axillary metastasis in breast cancer patients: A prospective study. *Breast Care, 11,* 34–39. doi:10.1159/000442481

Dyrstad, S.W., Yan, Y., Fowler, A.M., & Colditz, G.A. (2015). Breast cancer risk associated with benign breast disease: Systematic review and meta-analysis. *Breast Cancer Research and Treatment, 149,* 569–575. doi:10.1007/s10549-014-3254-6

Gipponi, M., Fregatti, P., Garlaschi, A., Calabrese, M., Baccini, P., Gallo, M., ... Friedman, D. (2015). Clinical decision-making in atypical and suspicious categories in fine-needle aspiration cytology of the breast. *Anticancer Research, 35,* 2369–2374.

Goldner, B., Behrendt, C.E., Schoellhammer, H.F., Lee, B., & Chen, S.L. (2014). Incidence of inflammatory breast cancer in women, 1992–2009, United States. *Annals of Surgical Oncology, 21,* 1267–1270. doi:10.1245/s10434-013-3439-y

Harlow, S.P., & Weaver, D.L. (2016, December 12). Overview of sentinel lymph node biopsy in breast cancer [Literature review current through August 2017]. Retrieved from http://www.uptodate.com/contents/overview-of-sentinel-lymph-node-biopsy-in-breast-cancer

Hartmann, L.C., Radisky, D.C., Frost, M.H., Santen, R.J., Vierkant, R.A., Benetti, L.L., ... Degnim, A.C. (2014). Understanding the premalignant potential of atypical hyperplasia through its natural history: A longitudinal cohort study. *Cancer Prevention Research, 7,* 211–217. doi:10.1158/1940-6207.CAPR-13-0222

Lange, M., Reimer, T., Hartmann, S., Glass, A., & Stachs, A. (2016). The role of specimen radiography in breast-conserving therapy of ductal carcinoma in situ. *Breast, 26,* 73–79. doi:10.1016/j.breast.2015.12.014

Lynch, J.A., Venne, V., & Berse, B. (2015). Genetic tests to identify risk for breast cancer. *Seminars in Oncology Nursing, 31,* 100–107. doi:10.1016/j.soncn.2015.02.007

National Comprehensive Cancer Network. (2017). *NCCN Clinical Practice Guidelines in Oncology (NCCN Guidelines®): Breast cancer* [v.2.2017]. Retrieved from https://www.nccn.org/professionals/physician_gls/pdf/breast.pdf

Neal, L., Sandhu, N.P., Hieken, T.J., Glazebrook, K.N., Mac Bride, M.B., Dilaveri, C.A., ... Visscher, D.W. (2014). Diagnosis and management of benign, atypical, and indeterminate breast lesions detected on core needle biopsy. *Mayo Clinic Proceedings, 89,* 536–547. doi:10.1016/j.mayocp.2014.02.004

Nimptsch, K., & Pischon, T. (2015). Body fatness, related biomarkers and cancer risk: An epidemiological perspective. *Hormone Molecular Biology and Clinical Investigation, 22,* 39–51. doi:10.1515/hmbci-2014-0043

Park, C.K., Jung, W.-H., & Koo, J.S. (2016). Pathologic evaluation of breast cancer after neoadjuvant therapy. *Journal of Pathology and Translational Medicine, 50,* 173–180. doi:10.4132/jptm.2016.02.02

Rarick, J., Kimler, B.F., & Tawfik, O. (2016). Comparison of margin status and lesional size between radioactive seed localized vs conventional wire localized breast lumpectomy specimens. *Annals of Diagnostic Pathology, 21,* 47–52. doi:10.1016/j.anndiagpath.2016.01.003

Renshaw, A.A., & Gould, E.W. (2016). Long term clinical follow-up of atypical ductal hyperplasia and lobular carcinoma *in situ* in breast core needle biopsies. *Pathology, 48,* 25–29. doi:10.1016/j.pathol.2015.11.015

Roetzheim, R.G., Lee, J.-H., Fulp, W., Gomez, E.M., Clayton, E., Tollin, S., ... Kiluk, J.V. (2015). Acceptance and adherence to chemoprevention among women at increased risk of breast cancer. *Breast, 24,* 51–56. doi:10.1016/j.breast.2014.11.006

Shah, P., Djisam, R., Damulira, H., Aganze, A., & Danquah, M. (2016). Embelin inhibits proliferation, induces apoptosis and alters gene expression profiles in breast cancer cells. *Pharmacological Reports, 68,* 638–644. doi:10.1016/j.pharep.2016.01.004

Shaikh, T., Li, T., Murphy, C.T., Zaorsky, N.G., Bleicher, R.J., Sigurdson, E.R., ... Anderson, P. (2016). Importance of surgical margin status in ductal carcinoma in situ. *Clinical Breast Cancer, 16,* 312–318. doi:10.1016/j.clbc.2016.02.002

Soliman, N.A., & Yussif, S.M. (2016). Ki-67 as a prognostic marker according to breast cancer molecular subtype. *Cancer Biology and Medicine, 13,* 496–504. doi:10.20892/j.issn.2095-3941.2016.0066

Sparano, J.A. (2016, December 5). Breast cancer staging. Retrieved from http://emedicine.medscape.com/article/2007112-overview

Tadayyon, H., Sannachi, L., Gangeh, M., Sadeghi-Naini, A., Tran, W., Trudeau, M.E., ... Czarnota, G.J. (2016). Quantitative ultrasound assessment of breast tumor response to chemotherapy using a multiparameter approach. *Oncotarget, 7,* 45094–45111. doi:10.18632/oncotarget.8862

Volders, J.H., Haloua, M.H., Krekel, N.M., Meijer, S., & van den Tol, P.M. (2016). Current status of ultrasound-guided surgery in the treatment of breast cancer. *World Journal of Clinical Oncology, 7,* 44–53. doi:10.5306/wjco.v7.i1.44

CHAPTER 5

Surgical Care

Joanne Lester, PhD, CRNP, ANP-BC, AOCN®

Introduction

Surgery is an essential component of care for both nonmalignant and malignant breast tumors. It is the oldest treatment modality for breast cancer and is provided through multiple services and at different time points in the cancer trajectory (see Figure 5-1). The surgical team offers a broad spectrum of services and is an important member of the interprofessional breast cancer team (Neuman et al., 2016).

Indications for Surgery

Individuals may be referred to a breast surgeon for multiple reasons. Individuals with increased risk due to known or suspected genetic risk may be referred for closer surveillance and possibly prophylactic surgery. Breast surgeons may also follow individuals with pathologic findings on core biopsy, such as atypical ductal or lobular hyperplasia, as well as a pathologic diagnosis of breast cancer. Postmastectomy breast malignancy can still occur (3%–10%) despite removal of all visible breast tissue (Li et al., 2016; Manning & Sacchini, 2016). Therefore, individuals who have completed treatment for breast cancer should have long-term follow-up with the breast oncology team to detect changes. Women should also be educated about the signs of local breast cancer recurrence. The anatomic edges are the probable sites of disease recurrence at the lateral chest wall, midaxillary line, or below the clavicle on the anterior chest wall.

Diagnosis of Breast Cancer

The surgical diagnosis of breast cancer employs innovative diagnostic and imaging techniques that can identify early-stage cancers. Once cancer is identified by physical examination or imaging, various biopsy options are discussed among the surgical oncology team, breast radiologist, and the patient (Carlson et al., 2011; National Comprehensive Cancer Network® [NCCN®], 2017).

Figure 5-1. Roles of Surgery in the Treatment of Breast Cancer

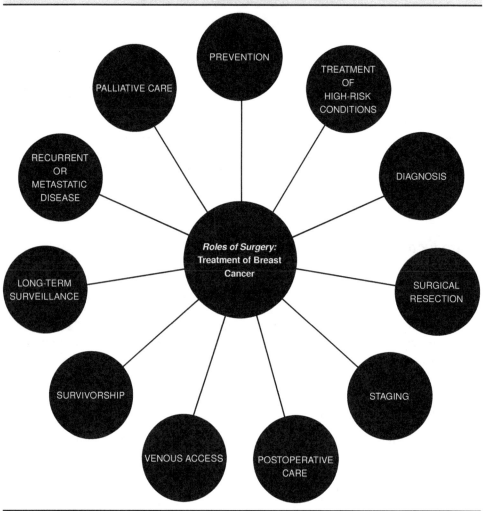

Palpable Tumors

Fine needle aspiration (FNA) can be used to diagnose a palpable lesion (Saha et al., 2016). The benefit of FNA is that it provides quick turnaround of the results if a pathologist is available to identify the presence or absence of malignant cells. Contrarily, FNA only provides a "yes" or "no" result. Therefore, a subsequent core biopsy is required as a definitive biopsy to inform the surgical team of multiple pathologic factors to individualize care. FNA is performed using a 20-gauge needle and 10 ml syringe. The goal is to obtain cells from the palpable mass by moving the needle up and down briskly for several passes. At times, the tumor is so hard that penetration is difficult to achieve.

A core needle biopsy can be performed by the surgeon for palpable lesions or by the radiologist for palpable lesions or abnormal imaging. A core needle biopsy uses a 12–14-gauge needle in a spring-loaded biopsy gun. The superficial area of the breast is aseptically cleansed and anesthetized with a wheal of injectable anesthetic; additional anesthetic is placed deep at the tumor edge. A small incision (3–5 mm) is made in the skin overlying the area of clinical or radiographic concern (Neal et al., 2014). Following several biopsy passes, a metal clip is placed in the deep biopsy site to designate the biopsy location. Unless the tissue is subsequently removed (e.g., lumpectomy or mastectomy), this tiny metal clip will remain in the breast and be visualized on subsequent breast imaging. Subsequent core needle biopsies can be performed as a follow-up biomarker to measure chemotherapeutic response in neoadjuvant chemotherapy studies (i.e., chemotherapy before surgery).

Other biopsy techniques include incisional, excisional, and punch biopsies. An incisional biopsy requires a skin incision (i.e., 3–5 cm) over the palpable area of concern. During the procedure, a segment of the visible mass is removed for pathologic review, and the area is closed with sutures. Excisional biopsy also requires a skin incision of 3–5 cm during which the entire mass is removed for pathologic review. If a cancer diagnosis is confirmed, this type of biopsy will require lumpectomy or mastectomy to establish clear margins. Finally, a punch biopsy is used to determine the presence of cancer cells in the skin. Clinicians often order punch biopsies when diagnosing inflammatory breast cancer or evaluating questionable (i.e., metastatic) lesions at the mastectomy site.

Nonpalpable Tumors

Nonpalpable breast masses are typically biopsied using image-guided (e.g., ultrasound-guided) core needle biopsy (Houssami & Turner, 2014; Saha et al., 2016). This technique uses a 12–14-gauge needle in a spring-loaded biopsy gun. This procedure offers easy access in a radiology setting, with the support of guidance systems such as ultrasound, mammography, magnetic resonance imaging (MRI), or computed tomography guidance. In this procedure, minimal to no scarring results when obtaining tissue cores for diagnosis. A metal clip is placed to designate the location of the lesion where tissue was removed.

Stereotactic breast biopsy is another method for biopsy of nonpalpable lesions (Mayo Foundation for Medical Education and Research, n.d.). During this procedure, the woman lies prone on a table in the radiology laboratory. The breast hangs through an opening in the table and is compressed between two plates. The radiologist uses mammography to guide the core needle biopsy and makes several passes to obtain tissue. Stereotactic breast biopsies are often used to biopsy the areas adjacent to microcalcifications as noted on imaging studies (Rominger, Steinmetz, Westerman, Ramaswamy, & Albert, 2015). A metal clip is inserted into the breast to designate the location of the lesion.

Similar to ultrasound-guided core needle biopsy is the vacuum-assisted core biopsy. In this procedure, a large, hollow-core needle is inserted at the site of the lesion with guided imaging. A rotating knife with an attached vacuum pulls tissue into the probe. This procedure obtains multiple tissue cores with only one pass into the breast. Often, very small lesions are completely removed. This technique is used to remove benign masses and to verify no evidence of malignancy.

Needle localization biopsy (Chan, Wiseberg-Firtell, Jois, Jensen, & Audisio, 2015) uses radiographic imaging to locate the lesion. The radiologist inserts one or two guide wires to localize the lesion (see Figure 5-2). Once the sheath is removed from the guide wire, a thin wire remains and is hooked to ensure placement (see Figure

Figure 5-2. Using Mammography to Place Wire Adjacent to Lesion

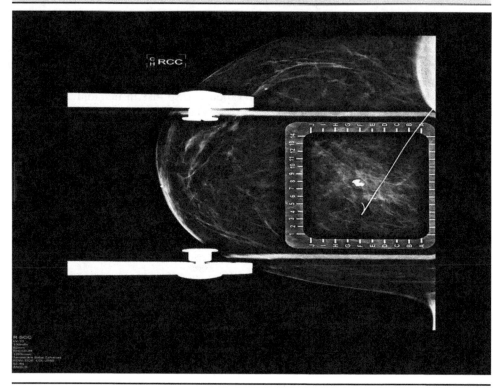

Note. Figure copyright 2015 by Adele Lipari. Used with permission.

5-3). Mammography or ultrasound is used for guidance of wire placement. Finally, bracketed needle localization (see Figure 5-4) enables a surgeon to follow two or more wires down to the lesion. Excisional biopsy is used to remove the tracks of the needles and the lesion or area of concern.

Radioactive seeds provide yet another method to target the lesion or area of concern. Radioactive seeds are inserted prior to surgery to target the lesion instead of needle localization (Cox et al., 2016). At the time of surgery, a probe is used to locate the radioactive seeds and guide the surgeon in the excision of tissue for clear margins.

Side Effects of Breast Biopsy

Breast biopsies sometimes present negative side effects for patients. Prior to the biopsy, the patient's medications should be reviewed. The patient should be instructed to refrain from aspirin or nonsteroidal anti-inflammatory drugs for 5–10 days prior to biopsy. Anticoagulants should be held at least three to five days or until laboratory tests confirm normal coagulability (Cuker & Siegal, 2015; Olson, 2015).

The patient should be instructed to bring a supportive brassiere or sports bra. Despite interventions, hematoma formation can occur with any biopsy (Sun et al.,

Figure 5-3. Mediolateral Mammographic View

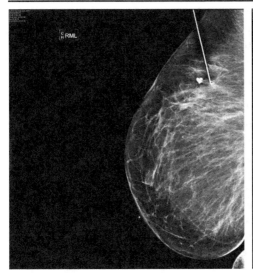 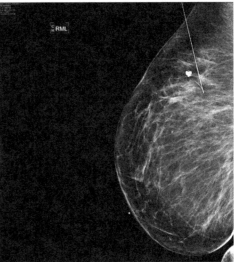

Using a mediolateral mammographic view, needle is placed (left), sheath withdrawn (right), and hook deployed, holding wire in place for biopsy or lumpectomy.

Note. Figure copyright 2015 by Adele Lipari. Used with permission.

Figure 5-4. Using Mammography for Double-Bracketed Needle Localization

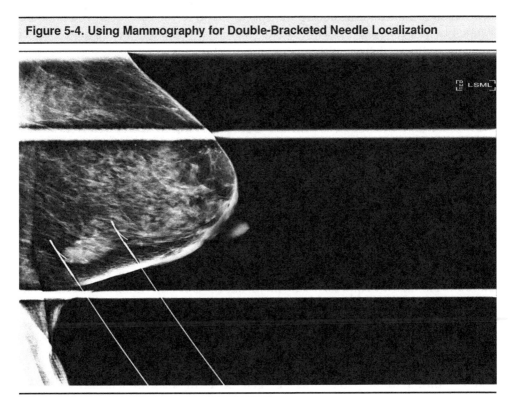

Note. Figure copyright 2015 by Adele Lipari. Used with permission.

2014) and may delay definitive surgery (Fu, Wang, Yin, & Song, 2015). If a hematoma is evident, several steps may minimize the eventual size. The risk of hematoma can be reduced by applying firm pressure and ice to the site for 15–20 minutes immediately after the biopsy. Following the application of pressure, a sterile pressure dressing is applied to the insertion site. The woman should don her supportive brassiere and place a disposable ice pack on top of the dressing. The patient should be instructed to apply ice intermittently and rest quietly for the remainder of the day. The patient should be educated about potential hematoma formation and care. This includes instruction to intermittently apply ice for the next 48 hours and, if a hematoma forms, to apply intermittent heat to accelerate blood flow and healing.

Hematoma prevention is a substantial challenge when patients are receiving anticoagulants (Cuker & Siegal, 2015; Olson, 2015). With consideration of comorbid conditions and reasons for anticoagulation, patients may be converted from oral anticoagulants to IV heparin for both the biopsy and definitive surgery. Heparin enables real-time control of anticoagulation without risk to the patient's underlying condition. Following the biopsy, firm pressure should be applied at the site for at least 20 minutes. Sutures are necessary if the site oozes for more than 30 minutes. The patient should apply ice to the dressing intermittently after the procedure and throughout the day.

Preoperative Considerations for Breast Surgery

The surgical algorithm and subsequent interventions for breast cancer are dependent on several factors, including the specific type of breast cancer, presentation, symptoms, and characteristics inherent to the individual patient (Chagpar, Babiera, Aguirre, Hunt, & Hughes, 2016). The specific surgical approach varies according to the skill and experience level of the surgical team, equipment availability, regional practices that affect decision making, evidence-based practice, and the interprofessional team (Sofocleous, Sideras, & Petre, 2013). Surgical approaches are also tailored to each person with cancer. Assessment and possible biopsy of the axilla must occur prior to neoadjuvant therapy to provide an accurate stage of disease (Diaz-Ruiz et al., 2016; Gahlaut et al., 2016).

Preoperative assessment and evaluation are valuable for safe completion of the surgical intervention and to decrease postoperative complications. In preoperative assessment, the surgical team weighs the operative risk versus the potential benefit to the patient. In assessing, the team examines past and current health history; medical, surgical, and psychosocial histories; current physical status; and vital signs (Drummond, Blake, Patel, Copton, & Schulteis, 2013). Comorbid conditions and concomitant diagnoses are considered, including the date of onset. The team must weigh resolution of the diagnosis versus seriousness of comorbid conditions and concomitant illnesses. The surgical approach may vary from the norm in order to maximize outcomes for the patient.

Family history of breast, ovarian, or other cancers is another consideration in preoperative assessment. Clinicians consider the family or personal history of breast or ovarian malignancies and the presence or absence of a known genetic mutation. This assessment includes the primary site of the cancer's origin, as well as the relative's age and relationship to the patient. Because genetic testing may influence surgical decisions when choosing between lumpectomy and mastectomy, a consultation with a credentialed genetics professional should occur as soon as possible after the diagnosis is made, as test results might take two to three weeks to obtain.

The healthcare team will assess the patient's medications at each visit. The surgical team must check the use of prescription drugs and over-the-counter medications, vitamins, and herbs. Current and past tobacco, alcohol, and recreational drug use is monitored as well.

Prior to surgery, the team assesses morbidity and mortality risks and measures them against predictive outcomes. If a patient has a history of congestive heart failure, the hospital stay is likely to increase. A history of hypertension represents a twofold increase in intraoperative risk of a cardiac event (Huang & Camp, 2016). Active smokers have a fourfold increase in the likelihood of postoperative respiratory difficulties, and obesity represents a fourfold increase in intra- and postoperative respiratory events (Huang & Camp, 2016). Finally, a history of uncontrolled reflux allows for an eightfold increase in intubation events, including aspiration. Preoperative consultations with interprofessional services are conducted (Kwaan et al., 2013), and teaching needs are assessed. The mental health status of all patients is also assessed.

Laboratory and imaging studies are integral in preoperative assessment (Patterson, 2013). Baseline orders include a complete blood count, liver function studies, electrolytes, mammogram, and other imaging studies as necessary, such as three-dimensional tomosynthesis, MRI, ultrasound, and chest x-ray.

Geriatric considerations include safety issues, functional status, frailty, polypharmacy, comorbid conditions, nutritional status, current and serial weights, serum protein level, and serum glucose level (Mohanty et al., 2016; Mrózek, Povoski, & Shapiro, 2013; O'Donovan, Mohile, & Leech, 2015; Robinson et al., 2013).

The clinical stage before and after neoadjuvant chemotherapy is based on the interprofessional providers' measurements (Park, Jung, & Koo, 2016). Measurements encompass breast and nodal characteristics as previously described, imaging with mammogram, MRI, quantitative ultrasound (Tadayyon et al., 2016), and pathologic tumor margins. Skilled measurements may indicate marked tumor reduction, yet significant pathologic evidence of residual tumor may still exist.

A tumor board review is conducted on a regular basis with representation from the surgical teams, radiology, pathology, and medical oncology, as well as oncology nursing and other interprofessional team members (Broglio et al., 2016; Capobianco et al., 2014; Carney et al., 2016; Chen et al., 2014; Eccles et al., 2013; Lamb et al., 2013). Various members of the team discuss the case and offer opinions on evidence-based approaches to care.

Perioperative Surgical Care

The surgical team considers core measures with evidence-based surgical interventions as monitored by the Joint Commission (2017):

- Administer broad-spectrum prophylactic antibiotics within one hour of surgical incision.
- Perform glucose monitoring with 6 am sample on postoperative day 1, as indicated.
- Avoid preoperative hair removal with a razor.
- Remove urinary catheters on postoperative day 1 or 2.
- Maintain perioperative core temperature with warming blankets.
- Administer beta-blockers the morning of the surgery.

- Implement venous thromboembolic prophylaxis measures:
  - Lower limb compression pumps
  - Anticoagulant prophylaxis with heparin or low-molecular-weight blood thinners, as needed

Surgical site infection (SSI) is a major cause of morbidity and mortality in surgical cases. SSI can result in increased healthcare costs and may affect the length of hospital stay (Godfrey, Villa, Dawson, Swindells, & Schouten, 2013). The infection matrix comprises various factors, including the patient's current health status, the physical environment of the surgery, and clinical risks such as clean or clean-contaminated surgery (Kataria, Badgia, & Srivastava, 2015). Bacteria are the common sources of infection, whether endogenous or exogenous, with myriad potential carriers. Patient selection can play a role, with a focus on timing and preparation for surgery, antibiotic prophylaxis, hand hygiene of the surgical team, and the facility's use of universal precautions (Huntington, Strayer, Huynh, & Green, 2015).

Risks of infection are relative to each patient and important to predict potential infection. Risk factors include suboptimal nutritional states, nitrogen balance and protein stores, and control of metabolic diseases such as diabetes. Tight control of serum blood sugars with a sliding scale for insulin may improve the infection threshold (Schroeder, 2014). Other risk factors include recent chemotherapy, use of immunosuppressive drugs, chronic steroid use, previous and current drug use, and the use of nicotine. The patient should abstain from nicotine for at least one week prior to surgery. A review of all drugs and abstinence from at-risk drugs may prevent an infection or breakdown of the skin and incision. Taking time to enrich nitrogen balance and protein stores in a nonurgent surgery may significantly improve the outcome (Bottorff, Seaton, & Lamont, 2015). Avoidance of a preoperative admission may decrease nosocomial bacterial exposure. Review of the patient's personal hygiene habits should be conducted, encouraging the use of institutional soapy preparation the night prior and the morning of the surgery.

The type and dosage of medications that a patient takes can also affect surgery. Clinicians should pay attention to preoperative drug dosing. Patients should be advised to discontinue certain medications to avoid anesthesia-related complications or excessive bleeding. In addition, detailed personal or family history of difficulties with anesthesia, specifically anesthesia-induced hyperthermia, is crucial information to obtain preoperatively. Rare, often hereditary conditions can occur after exposure to certain anesthetic agents, such as volatile gases and muscle relaxants (Schuster, Johannsen, Schneiderbanger, & Roewer, 2013). Symptoms in these extreme cases include increased fever, hypoxia, circulatory collapse, and death.

Avoidance of abrupt changes to the following medications is prudent:

- Alpha-agonists
- Angiotensin-converting enzyme inhibitors
- Barbiturates
- Beta-blockers
- Calcium channel blockers
- Corticosteroids
- Monoamine oxidase inhibitors
- Opioids
- Oral hypoglycemics and insulin

Drugs that alter platelet aggregation or prolong bleeding should be evaluated several weeks before surgery (Lyman et al., 2013). These include herbal remedies, antithrombotic agents, and antiplatelet agents. In addition to evaluating drugs that affect bleeding and alter platelet aggregation, diagnoses of related conditions should be evaluated. Patients with the following conditions or diagnoses should be particularly monitored: artificial cardiac valves, atrial fibrillation, history of hypercoagulable state, significant cardiac valvular disease, and thrombotic events such as deep vein thrombosis or pulmonary embolism.

Anticoagulation is done for a number of reasons, some more serious than others. In some diagnoses, the specific anticoagulation medications can be temporarily stopped and then restarted immediately after surgery. One such example is atrial fibrillation, as anticoagulation is prescribed as a preventive mechanism. Consultation with the ordering physician is prudent prior to the surgical team stopping any drugs. A significant history of clotting disorders may require bridge therapy, which includes preoperative hospital admission with a shift from oral anticoagulants to short-acting, low-molecular-weight heparin (Cuker & Siegal, 2015; Olson, 2015). In the case of urgent surgery, often the only option is to forge ahead with surgery (Curtis, Schweitzer, & van Vlymen, 2015). The use of vitamin K injections is contraindicated in these settings.

Surgical Treatment Options

Surgical treatment of breast cancer involves decision making from the patient's perspective with education and support from the surgical oncology team, caregivers, and family (Lamb et al., 2013; Litsas, 2013; Shen & Cai, 2016). Prior to surgery, patients require information about their cancer with an individualized approach and explanation (Covelli, Baxter, Fitch, McCready, & Wright, 2015; Litsas, 2013; Shen & Cai, 2016; Toi et al., 2015). Clinicians should present patients with information on their treatment options and related treatment trajectory, anticipated outcomes, long-term prognosis, and explanation about systemic treatment. A discussion of neoadjuvant chemotherapy (i.e., prior to surgery) and adjuvant chemotherapy (i.e., after surgery) is important, when appropriate. The concept of micrometastasis can be difficult for patients to understand and may need to be explained several times. Women are often well versed about surgical options as compared to systemic treatment options. Surgical and systemic options vary for each individual. Therefore, interprofessional consultations prior to surgery will be unique to each patient.

Surgery, otherwise termed *local treatment*, requires a detailed explanation and discussion with patients and families. A lumpectomy can be performed if the surgeon anticipates an acceptable cosmetic result. When cosmesis may be significantly altered because of tumor size in relation to breast size, perioperative oncoplasty may be an option. Otherwise, a mastectomy is in order, with or without reconstruction. Neoadjuvant chemotherapy may be considered to shrink the tumor prior to surgery, with a postchemotherapy option of lumpectomy. Patients must understand that a lumpectomy requires radiation therapy, which provides treatment to the entire breast. The surgical option of mastectomy is still considered local treatment, with or without radiation therapy. Immediate or delayed reconstruction is nearly always a consideration to provide symmetry.

Evaluation of the axilla is required with any invasive cancer and high-risk noninvasive cancer, as lymph node status is one of the most important and reliable prognostic measures. Most common is the sentinel lymph node biopsy (SLNB), a sampling of targeted nodes in the axilla. When the SLNB is not evaluable or shows positive lymph nodes, an axillary node dissection is performed to remove involved nodes. Most common is removal of the lower two levels in the axilla. Removal of the third level (i.e., deep) of lymph nodes only occurs in the case of extensive disease.

Prior to surgery, patients should be aware of the goals of any surgical intervention. Examples of specific goals for a cancer surgery include removal of the cancer, maintenance of normal function of related organs, removal of tissue as necessary to avoid local recurrence, and attainment of negative margins as determined by pathology (Hargreaves, Mohamed, & Audisio, 2014; Rarick, Kimler, & Tawfik, 2016). The goal of negative margins is to decrease the risk of local recurrence of tumor in the breast (Ang et al., 2016; Bodilsen et al., 2016). The American Society of Breast Surgeons (2013) proposed an algorithm recommending the need for reexcision based on surgical margin status. Wide speculation exists of the exact measurements that define clear margins (Ang et al., 2016), although tumor at the inked margin is unacceptable, and one or more positive margins requires additional surgery. Lumpectomy reexcision is essential for 1 or 2 positive margins, and a mastectomy is typically recommended for multiple positive margins (Ang et al., 2016; Bodilsen et al., 2016; NCCN, 2017).

The recommendation of local and systemic therapies is dependent on several factors, including the type of breast cancer, the size of the tumor, the size of the breast, and the presence or absence of axillary metastasis. Other factors include the oncogenetic factors of the tumor (Litsas, 2013) and patient characteristics. Local treatment comprises lumpectomy plus postoperative radiation therapy, or mastectomy with or without reconstruction. Chest wall radiation therapy is recommended after a mastectomy for tumors greater than 5 cm, positive margins, or inflammatory breast cancer. Consideration of chemotherapy before surgery (i.e., neoadjuvant chemotherapy) or chemotherapy after surgery (i.e., adjuvant chemotherapy) is also discussed (Broglio et al., 2016; Chen et al., 2014). Neoadjuvant chemotherapy may be helpful to decrease the size of the tumor, enable breast-conserving surgery (Zervoudis et al., 2014), and provide evidence of the efficacy of chemotherapy.

Following neoadjuvant chemotherapy, the patient may undergo breast-conserving treatment with a lumpectomy or quadrantectomy and evaluation of the lymph nodes (unless SLNB was performed prior to neoadjuvant chemotherapy). A mastectomy is performed if the patient chooses that option, or when pathology identifies multifocal or multicentric disease. In the case of palpable axillary lymph nodes, or concerning axillary nodes on imaging, an axillary dissection is necessary.

If the patient is not satisfied with the aesthetic outcome of surgery, they can opt to undergo oncoplastic surgery. Oncoplastic surgery can be a planned procedure during the primary surgery (Hoy, 2016) or delayed until after completion of the primary surgery. The outcome of perioperative oncoplastic surgery may be altered by postsurgical radiation therapy. The addition of a radiation boost at the site of tumor origin decreases the risk of local recurrence, although it may darken the skin and tighten the lumpectomy scar. The boost may be an important factor in younger women because of their longer life span (Cao et al., 2014; Carlson et al., 2011; NCCN, 2017), although it may increase scarring.

Sentinel Lymph Node Biopsy

SLNB is performed to assess the axilla and has a lower rate of complications and discomfort than axillary node dissection (Bertozzi & Londero, 2016; Canavese et al.,

2016; Reintgen, Kerivan, Reintgen, Swaninathan, & Reintgen, 2016; Wallace et al., 2013). With SLNB, there is less chance for issues such as seroma, infection, arm stiffness, pain, paresthesia, or lymphedema. SLNB increases findings of micrometastatic nodal involvement that ultimately may upgrade the stage of disease, which is important to determine appropriate systemic treatment (Giuliano & Gangi, 2015). Extra stains often are required to evaluate microscopic disease, including hematoxylin and eosin staining.

During SLNB, the affected breast is intradermally injected with technetium-99m sulfur colloid at least two hours prior to surgery. At the time of surgery, 1% isosulfan blue dye is injected near the known breast cancer, and the breast is gently massaged in the operating room. Both technetium-99m sulfur colloid and 1% isosulfan blue dye are recommended for injection within the surgical skin ellipse or centrally around the nipple (see Figure 5-5A). A handheld gamma detection probe is used to transcutaneously identify the location of the underlying sentinel lymph nodes within the corresponding axillary region, as well any extra-axillary sites (see Figure 5-5B). A skin incision is made in the axilla at the area of maximum transcutaneous gamma counts. Sentinel lymph nodes are found using visual identification of blue dye and highest gamma counts (see Figure 5-5C, D). Each sentinel lymph node is dissected out, and its lymphovascular pedicle (representing the vascular and lymphatic inflow and outflow vessels) is ligated and divided (see Figure 5-5E). A handheld gamma detection probe is used to record counts for each excised sentinel lymph node (see Figure 5-5F). All attempts are made to identify any axillary sentinel lymph node candidates that contain radioactive counts to ensure adequate assessment of the axilla for the absence or presence of metastatic disease.

The pathologist reviews the sentinel lymph node or nodes during surgery to determine the need for further axillary surgery. A negative SLNB indicates a negative axilla, whereas a positive SLNB indicates potential disease in the axilla, likely requiring axillary dissection. Microscopic disease in the sentinel node indicates that no further axillary surgery may be necessary (Tallet et al., 2016), whereas macrometastatic disease found in the sentinel node or axilla will lead to an axillary node dissection (e.g., levels I and II) (Verheuvel, Ooms, Tjan-Heijnen, Roumen, & Voogd, 2016). Performance of SLNB after neoadjuvant chemotherapy is feasible (El Hage Chehade, Headon, Kasem, & Mokbel, 2016; Enokido et al., 2016). SLNB after a previous SLNB may also be possible (Kothari, Rusby, Agusti, & MacNeill, 2012), although SLNB is not possible after previous axillary node dissection.

Axillary Node Dissection

In an axillary node dissection, lumpectomy is performed in the same manner and goals are similar as previously stated in this chapter (Cox et al., 2016). An axillary node dissection (e.g., levels I and II) is a planned procedure for palpable adenopathy in the axilla or if there is a failed SLNB at the time of surgery. In addition, an axillary node dissection is indicated in inflammatory breast cancer because of its virulent nature and potential for positive nodes even after neoadjuvant treatment. Following axillary node dissection, a postoperative drain/suction apparatus is placed in the axilla. The drain is removed when serous drainage decreases to 30 ml or less per 24-hour period.

Figure 5-5. Steps Involved in Sentinel Lymph Node Biopsy

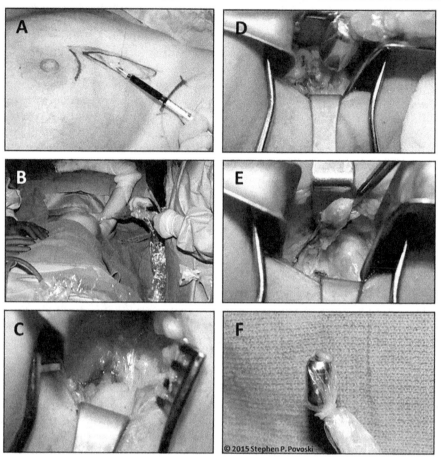

(A) The breast is intradermally injected with technetium-99m sulfur colloid and 1% isosulfan blue dye within the same geographic location as the known breast cancer. Both the technetium-99m sulfur colloid and 1% isosulfan blue dye are recommended to be injected within the skin ellipse that is planned for surgical excision as part of the resected breast tissue, either by breast-conserving surgery or mastectomy.
(B) A handheld gamma detection probe is used to transcutaneously identify the location of the underlying sentinel lymph node(s) within the corresponding axilla region, as well as within any extra-axillary locations.
(C, D) A skin incision is made over the area of maximum transcutaneous counts within the axillary region. Using visual identification of the blue dye and handheld gamma detection probe identification of the technetium-99m sulfur colloid, the subcutaneous tissues and axillary tissues are divided and the underlying sentinel lymph nodes are identified.
(E) Each sentinel lymph node is dissected out, and its lymphovascular pedicle (representing the vascular and lymphatic inflow and outflow vessels) is ligated and divided.
(F) The handheld gamma detection probe is used to record the ex vivo counts for each excised sentinel lymph node. It is recommended that the probe head of the handheld gamma detection probe be directed away from the technetium-99m sulfur colloid primary injection site of the breast during acquisition of the ex vivo sentinel lymph node counts to obtain the most representative maximum ex vivo counts for each excised sentinel lymph node. All attempts are made to identify any axillary sentinel lymph node candidates that contain radioactive counts down to 10% of the maximum radiative counts found within the "hottest" (i.e., most radioactive) axillary sentinel lymph node to ensure adequate assessment of the axilla for the absence or presence of metastatic disease.

Note. Figure copyright 2015 by Stephen P. Povoski. Used with permission.

Lumpectomy

Nearly 30 years of research studies have documented that a lumpectomy with radiation therapy is as effective as mastectomy (NCCN, 2017), although exceptions exist that should be considered. Contraindications to lumpectomy alone include history of previous radiation therapy to the chest or breast, current pregnancy, diffuse suspicious-appearing microcalcifications, widespread disease, or positive margins that were not cleared with repeat lumpectomy (Carlson et al., 2011; NCCN, 2017). Breast-conserving treatment may be suboptimal in women with connective tissue disorders that involve the skin (e.g., scleroderma, lupus). Individuals with known or suspected genetic risk may not be candidates for lumpectomy because of the increased risk of second primary cancers.

Mastectomy

Total Mastectomy

A total mastectomy is indicated when chosen by the individual or to control significant disease burden that cannot be surgically removed with a lumpectomy. A total mastectomy is also indicated when the tumor is comparably larger than the breast or a lumpectomy would result in poor cosmetic outcome. The total mastectomy removes all breast tissue from the landmarks as previously described (e.g., posterior clavicle to inframammary fold, midsternal border to midaxillary line). SLNB will be performed to assess the lymph node status, and some nodes may be identified in the tail of Spence.

A total mastectomy manages multicentric ductal carcinoma in situ and essentially cures this premalignant change in the breast. Mastectomy is indicated for prophylactic removal of contralateral (or bilateral) breast tissue, in the case of contraindications to radiation therapy, or in the case of recurrence in the ipsilateral breast with previous radiation therapy. During the procedure, a postoperative suction apparatus is placed under the skin along the posterior border of the chest wall. The drain is removed when serous drainage decreases to 30 ml or less per 24-hour period (Lester, 2015).

Modified Radical Mastectomy

A modified radical mastectomy (e.g., total mastectomy and axillary node dissection) is indicated to treat a large invasive tumor with palpable nodes, positive margins after lumpectomy, or recurrence in the ipsilateral breast with previous radiation (in this case, clinicians may try SLNB) (Rezai, Kraemer, Kimmig, & Kern, 2015). The presence of two invasive carcinomas in separate quadrants is another indication for a modified radical mastectomy, as the use of SLNB may be contraindicated.

The difference between a total mastectomy and modified radical mastectomy is the surgical evaluation of the ipsilateral axillary lymph nodes. In a total mastectomy, SLNB is typically used, whereas in a modified radical mastectomy, the axillary lymph nodes are removed. A modified radical mastectomy removes all breast tissue on the chest wall as well as the lower two levels (I and II) of the axillary lymph nodes, with dissection and sparing of the axillary vein main trunk, long thoracic nerve, and thoracodorsal neurovascular bundle. The level III lymph nodes are only removed in the case of advanced and diffuse disease. Two postoperative suction apparatuses are placed—one in the axilla and the other along the posterior border of the chest wall.

The drain is removed when serous drainage decreases to 30 ml or less per 24-hour period.

Total Skin-Sparing Mastectomy

A total skin-sparing mastectomy is performed when reconstruction is occurring concurrently with the surgery or planned for the future. The provision of extra skin for the oncoplastic surgeon specifically enables the placement of saline expanders, or a pocket for the variety of tissue-moving surgeries.

Sparing of Nipple-Areolar Complex

Before mastectomy is performed, a bilateral breast MRI is obtained to evaluate the nipple-areolar complex (Peled et al., 2012). The patient must have absence of disease within 2 cm of the nipple-areolar complex. A preoperative subareolar biopsy is recommended to ensure the area is free of disease. Potential complications of this surgery include findings of occult ductal carcinoma in situ in the nipple-areolar complex, implant loss, skin flap necrosis, and infection. Any of these situations may cause loss of the spared nipple-areolar complex. A postoperative suction apparatus is placed under the skin on the posterior border of the chest wall. If an axillary node dissection was performed, a second drain is placed in the axilla. The drain or drains are removed when serous drainage decreases to 30 ml or less per 24-hour period. The nipple-areolar complex–sparing surgery may also be possible in locally advanced disease depending on the depth of disease (Peled et al., 2016). Despite frequent nipple-sparing surgeries, NCCN (2016, 2017) continues to recommend complete removal of the nipple-areolar complex with mastectomy and advises nipple-areolar complex–sparing surgery only be performed in patients carefully selected by an experienced interprofessional team. Figure 5-6 shows a nipple-sparing mastectomy and implant reconstruction.

Bilateral Mastectomy

A bilateral mastectomy is performed in a similar surgical procedure as the total or modified radical mastectomy if axillary lymph nodes need to be removed. This procedure will require a postoperative suction apparatus with bilateral drains under the skin on the posterior chest wall and in the axilla when an axillary dissection is performed. Each drain is removed when serous drainage decreases to 30 ml or less per 24-hour period.

Lumpectomy Versus Mastectomy

To assist in the education of their patients, nurses must learn the difference between lumpectomy and mastectomy (Lester, 2015). Patients may desire a lumpectomy, immediate mastectomy, or delayed mastectomy, with or without reconstruction. Women often state they want to undergo a bilateral mastectomy (e.g., "so I never have to deal with this again"), with the unilateral (i.e., ipsilateral) and prophylactic (i.e., contralateral) surgeries. These procedures may be done before or after radiation therapy and with or without chemotherapy. To undergo SLNB or axillary node dissection is yet another topic of discussion, although most patients desire an SLNB and are gravely concerned if they must undergo an axillary dissection or modified radical mastectomy. The underlying concern is the potential development of lymphedema in the ipsilateral (i.e., affected) arm.

Figure 5-6. Nipple-Sparing Mastectomy and Implant Reconstruction

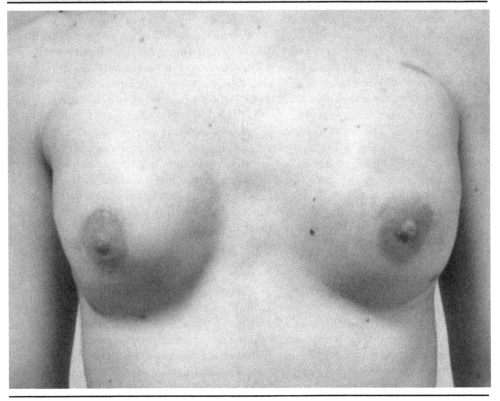

Note. From "Oncological Outcome and Patient Satisfaction With Skin-Sparing Mastectomy and Immediate Breast Reconstruction: A Prospective Observational Study," by S. Reefy, N. Patani, A. Anderson, G. Burgoyne, H. Osman, and K. Mokbel, 2013, *BMC Cancer, 10,* 171, p. 5. Copyright 2010 by Reefy et al.; licensee BioMed Central Ltd. This is an Open Access article distributed under the terms of the Creative Commons Attribution License (http://creativecommons .org/licenses/by/2.0), which permits unrestricted use, distribution, and reproduction in any medium, provided the original work is properly cited.

The explanation of a lumpectomy includes a discussion about radiation. In a lumpectomy, the radiation type and schedule can vary significantly and are determined by the radiation oncologist. Following a lumpectomy, patients may receive accelerated partial breast irradiation, whole breast irradiation, or prone breast irradiation. Likewise, the radiation type and schedule may vary following a mastectomy.

Another intense discussion between the oncology team and the patient and family is the topic of chemotherapy and whether the patient wants chemotherapy prior to surgery (i.e., neoadjuvant) or after surgery (i.e., adjuvant). Some patients want surgery first, as they are hoping to avoid chemotherapy despite indications that they will require it. Neoadjuvant chemotherapy is used to decrease the size of the tumor; this is important for women who hope to have a lumpectomy.

The timing of local and systemic treatments, including adjuvant chemotherapy, neoadjuvant chemotherapy, or mixed neoadjuvant and adjuvant therapies, and recovery from multiple surgeries can interfere with life and create much consternation (Lester et al., 2015; Petty & Lester, 2014). Nurses should discuss with patients and families issues such as working during this process versus taking a leave of absence, child-care responsibilities, responsibilities to older adult patients, fatigue, financial issues, menopausal symptoms, family planning, and emotional reactions such as anxiety, depression, distress, fear, sleep deprivation, self-image, and worry (Lester et al., 2015). Optimal outcomes can be reached with detailed planning prior to the first surgery or round of chemotherapy (Jacob, 2016). The nurse and nurse practitioner are integral team members who are often readily available to answer patients' questions.

Women and men diagnosed with breast cancer require intense and ongoing supportive care from their diagnosis forward (Kiely, 2014). The diagnosis of breast cancer forces patients to gain an understanding of breast cancer and its related treatment in order to make numerous cancer-related decisions. One major decision is whether to undergo a lumpectomy or mastectomy. Patients and families have multiple pathways to consider and much to learn. These challenges are intermingled with the intense fear of the cancer diagnosis and fear of what may happen to them and their families. The oncology nurse and nurse practitioner are essential to patient and family understanding of the disease process and cancer trajectory.

Postoperative Care

The goals of postoperative care include prevention of surgical complications and surgical wound infection, as well as maintenance of overall body homeostasis in healthy persons. Symptom management is an ongoing process with realistic goals for the patient, caregiver, and family. Breast cancer surgeries are typically short compared to other types of cancer surgeries, except for bilateral mastectomies with immediate reconstruction. Depending on the type of reconstruction and the variables for each person, bilateral mastectomies with tissue reconstruction can last up to 20 hours. Long and detailed surgeries such as these are targets for significant postoperative issues.

Care of the Surgical Site

Nursing considerations for surgical site care are varied. Nurses must administer and care for dressings on incisions. They must practice and teach aseptic care, use appropriate dressing supplies, and provide caregiver instructions. Nurses must also manage drainage devices associated with the surgical site, use the correct aseptic technique when caring for the dressing, empty drainage devices, record drainage amounts, and provide caregiver instructions. Caregivers differ widely from visiting home nurses. The caregiver is typically the significant other and has an intense desire to "do it right." It is vital to support caregivers with proper instructions and a 24-hour telephone number.

Pain Management

Pain management is a primary element of pre- and postoperative care. The goal of pain control is to restore function with both objective and subjective improvement. Pain can manifest in several pathways: sensory pain is an autonomic response, whereas emotional pain comes from a patient's psychological responses, and mental pain evokes a behavioral response. The understanding of pain medications and their potential side effects is a crucial nursing consideration (Bonomi, Salval, & Crippa, 2016). The use of adjunct medications for symptom management includes opioids, nonsteroidal anti-inflammatory drugs, selective serotonin reuptake inhibitors, gabapentin, pregabalin, muscle relaxants, anxiolytics, and sleep aids. Patients and clinicians must balance addiction concerns against the need for pain relief. When pain medication is needed pre- or postoperatively, the clinician and the patient must resolve to gradually decrease administration of medications (Khan, Zhang, Sollazzo, Mohammed, & Gui, 2016). Women who are undergoing extensive chemotherapy, radiation therapy, and bilateral reconstruction may be in treatment for longer than 20 months. Therefore, ongoing symptom management is an important role of the nurse and nurse practitioner. Nurses must acquire or finesse their knowledge of breast cancer care to prepare patients with decision-making skills for the type of treatment needed throughout their cancer trajectory (Khan et al., 2016).

Nausea and Vomiting

Uncontrolled nausea and vomiting can result in several negative outcomes, including unplanned hospital admission from ambulatory surgery, delay in hospital discharge, and significant discomfort, with patient dissatisfaction. Risk factors for nausea include female gender, prior history of nausea and vomiting with anesthesia, history of motion sickness, ingestion of food too quickly after surgery, side effects of pain medication, duration of surgery, and breast augmentation procedures. Postoperative control of nausea and vomiting requires a combination of serotonin antagonists and other antiemetic agents to control vomiting and spasms.

Fever and Infection

Fever is common in the immediate postoperative setting and typically is not associated with an infectious process. Fevers of concern occur days after surgery with a persistent pattern. The absence of fever does not rule out infection. This is especially true in immunocompromised patients, whose host defense mechanisms, including temperature response, are altered. The most common sites of postoperative infection include the pulmonary system secondary to atelectasis or aspiration; the urinary tract secondary to a urinary catheter; the operative site; and phlebitis (Godfrey et al., 2013). Postoperative bacterial infections occur due to preexisting symptoms or conditions, intubation for anesthesia, the surgical procedure, and nosocomial risk from rotating staff.

SSIs typically occur in either superficial or deep incisions (Matsumura et al., 2016). They can also occur in the organ space, specifically in areas such as a pocket at the mastectomy site, a pocket in the axilla, or a pocket at the lumpectomy site. If an SSI occurs at a drain site, prompt removal is recommended. Risks for developing infections at the drain site include the number of drains, the duration of placement, and the type of drainage apparatus. The longer the drains are in place, the higher the risk of infection. Fluid can form in the spaces because of overuse of the ipsilateral extremity or early removal of drains and subsequent fluid accumulation, which are risks for infection. Chronic illnesses such as diabetes require close attention with avoidance of hypo- or hyperglycemic events, specifically ketoacidosis. Dehydration has an effect on glucose level and wound healing. A sliding scale of regular insulin may aid in tighter control.

Thromboembolism

Thromboembolism can manifest as either a pulmonary embolism or a deep vein thrombosis (Barber & Clarke-Pearson, 2016). Multiple risk factors are associated with clotting disorders, including immobility with varicosities, obesity, age older than 40 years, and extended prolonged breast surgery. People with Virchow triad, history of previous venous embolic event, venous access devices, pregnancy, and history of hormonal drug usage (e.g., use of birth control pills; exogenous hormone usage; current or past use of raloxifene, tamoxifen, or aromatase inhibitors) are at higher risk. Prophylactic measures include elevation of the legs with knee flexion, early mobilization after surgery, and leg exercises to improve circulation. Pneumatic compression boots and elastic stockings are also used. Anticoagulation is a key preventive measure, with the use of heparin (i.e., for abrupt anticoagulation) and low-molecular-weight heparin for four to eight weeks, pending the health of the patient. Low-molecular-weight heparin (e.g., enoxaparin) can be administered at home by the patient or caregiver.

Complications

Formation of fluid in surgical spaces may require aspiration. This fluid collection can occur due to overuse of the ipsilateral extremity or early removal of drains. These fluid collections are termed *seromas* and, if not drained, may fester and become infected. On the other hand, if aseptic technique is not used for seroma aspiration, bacteria transmission may occur.

Pneumonia can occur and is most common in immunocompromised patients, including those with a cancer diagnosis. Other risk factors include intubation for general anesthesia, several surgeries with repeated intubation, nosocomial exposure with rotating staff, and inactivity. Patients with diabetes also require close attention. Clinicians must take care to avoid hypo- or hyperglycemia, with special attention to conditions such as ketoacidosis and dehydration. These conditions may affect wound healing and may require a sliding scale of regular insulin with frequent glucose monitoring to manage tight control (Schroeder, 2014).

Breast Reconstruction

Oncoplastic procedures for restoration of tissue have expanded and changed exponentially over the past 20 years, providing pleasing aesthetic outcomes, improved patient satisfaction, and greater overall quality of life for both men and women (Cemal et al., 2013; Piper, Peled, & Sbitany, 2015; Reeder-Hayes, Wheeler, & Mayer, 2015).

Oncoplastic surgery following lumpectomy or partial mastectomy requires interprofessional pre-, peri-, and postoperative evaluations and a decision between surgery or neoadjuvant chemotherapy as the first treatment and between immediate or delayed reconstruction (Piper et al., 2015). The oncoplastic team performs a number of assessments with attention to the degree of ptosis of the affected and unaffected breasts, overall skin quality, and the skin before and after radiation therapy. A woman's overall breast size includes the tumor-to-breast ratio before and after chemotherapy, intended and desired breast size, availability of adjacent tissue rearrangement versus flap, desirability of reduction mammoplasty/mastopexy, use of local or regional flaps, condition of the nipple-areolar complex, and reduction mammoplasty/mastopexy of the contralateral breast.

Intraoperative oncoplastic procedures allow for preservation of normal parenchymal tissue and control over surgical margins with complete resection (Ang et al., 2016; Piper et al., 2015). Procedures use local or regional tissue for immediate reconstruction and are dependent on the type of available tissue. Options include complete tumor extirpation, partial reconstruction of wide local excisions, and immediate or delayed procedures to achieve symmetry for the contralateral breast. Oncoplastic reconstruction of the breast during a surgical lumpectomy is a novel concept and provides an excellent opportunity to reconstruct the affected and unaffected breasts to provide symmetry prior to radiation therapy. If radiation therapy is planned, as with a tumor larger than 5 cm or multiple positive lymph nodes, immediate oncoplastic procedures may need to be reconsidered. Radiation therapy may contract and ruin tissue reconstruction. When it is known that cancer treatment will include radiation therapy, delayed reconstruction is planned to take place after all treatments have been completed. One exception to these rules is if the patient desires a saline expander.

Autologous Reconstructive Procedures

Autologous reconstructive procedures, either immediate (e.g., during mastectomy) or delayed, following mastectomy are some of the most popular reconstructive techniques (Motakef, Mountziaris, Ismail, Agag, & Patel, 2015). The deep inferior epigastric perforator (DIEP) flap is an example of autologous reconstruction.

Prior to surgery, a computed tomography angiogram is obtained to identify adequate donor and recipient vessels. Following a skin-sparing mastectomy, a flap is formed from extra skin and fat of the external abdomen with attached single or multiple perforator vessels (e.g., artery, vein) connected to the inferior epigastric artery. The blood supply (e.g., artery and vein) and tissue are removed from donor site with anastomosis to vessels at the site of the absent breast. Meticulous postoperative surveillance is necessary to ensure a viable flap (Long & Israelian, 2013); patients are often placed on a special unit immediately out of surgery with specially trained nurses. Examination of the anastomosis with perfusion checks of the flap is required every 15 minutes for 24–48 hours. Visual examination is used, as well as Doppler readings and tissue oximetry. These checks are crucial to an excellent outcome after surgery. Loss of arterial supply or venous congestion may require emergent surgery to revitalize the flap. The special unit is set up to accommodate an emergent surgery to reattach the vessels or drain the venous congestion. Multiple additional surgeries may need to be performed over the next 12–18 months to ensure tailoring of the site and symmetry with the contralateral breast. This type of procedure provides a comparable pre- and postsurgical look. Cosmetic outcomes are typically excellent with DIEP flap reconstruction, with the aim of looking normal in a brassiere or tailored clothing.

This type of reconstructive procedure provides a long-lasting, more natural breast mound. Total flap failure is rare, although devastating. Complications include flap loss due to lack of circulation (despite emergent surgery to save the flap), donor site necrosis due to impaired healing and death of tissue, seroma (i.e., accumulation of fluid under flap), and sensory deficits (i.e., paresthesias). Negative outcomes that may require additional surgery include delayed healing, infection, necrosis of the incision or flap, weakness of the abdominal wall, and possible ventral hernia.

Similar to DIEP, the superficial inferior epigastric artery (SIEA) flap is an abdominal flap with donor vessels from superficial inferior epigastric vessels. The SIEA flap can be raised without involving the rectus muscle or sheath, providing an advantage for overall quality of life. The risk of abdominal hernia is less than with other types of abdominal transfers, and there is minimal involvement with the rectus muscle, ensuring strength of this important core muscle. Potential complications are the same as with other surgical interventions discussed earlier in this chapter.

Gluteal artery perforator (GAP) flap is another option. In this surgical intervention, the superior (SGAP) or inferior (IGAP) arteries are used as the reconstructive flaps. Previous abdominal liposuction may be a contraindication to GAP flaps. Potential complications are the same as with other surgical interventions described in this chapter. This reconstructive approach is used to compensate for previous long abdominal incisions that scar the abdominis muscle. The procedure allows for removal of a significant amount of abdominal fat. Although some of the fat is discarded and sent to pathology labs for testing, most of the fat is used to create one or two breast mounds on the upper chest wall. The breast mounds can be created to match a patient's desired cup size.

In another flap technique, the profunda femoris artery perforator flap, vessels from the posterior compartment of the thigh are used. The immediate care and potential complications are the same as with the procedures described previously.

Another type of flap is the pedicled transverse rectus abdominis myocutaneous (TRAM) flap. The TRAM flap is a free flap formed using the transverse rectus abdominis muscle, abdominal tissue, and skin. The pedicled flap leaves blood supply at the original site. In this procedure, tissue is tunneled under the anterior abdominal muscle to the site of the absent breast. The TRAM flap uses one-half of the abdominal rectus muscle, thus reducing the strength of the remaining abdominal muscle. This procedure could result in an abdominal bulge or could weaken the abdominal muscle, resulting in a hernia. The muscle provides support for a fat mound that is reconstructed into the new breast, but this results in a large, horizontal incision across the lower abdomen. Surgeons have used this muscle to create a double TRAM reconstruction, which results in a pleasing outcome. The TRAM flap had been used for quite some time until oncoplastic surgeons started using pedicled or free flaps. The TRAM flap is still a reconstructive option, although it is used less often than previously. It is still a viable option if the perforator vessel options are not ideal as visualized on computed tomography angiogram. A muscle-sparing TRAM flap can also be prepared. In this case, some of the fat is discarded, but most of the fat is used to create one or two mounds on the upper chest wall, matching the desired cup size of the patient.

Allogeneic Reconstructive Procedures

Allogeneic, or alloplastic, surgery involves implanting an artificial prosthesis under the native chest wall skin and muscle. Typically, this process is a two-stage procedure using a saline expander followed by insertion of permanent implant (Quinn et al., 2016). This is the most common type of breast reconstruction and can be performed at the time of mastectomy. The implant is serially inflated over six to eight weeks to stretch the muscle and skin. It can also be inflated during chemotherapy at times of optimal white blood cell and platelet counts. The implant must be fully inflated prior to radiation therapy to avoid the risk of contracture. Finally, the implant is over-expanded prior to replacement to ultimately decrease final skin tension. Once full expansion has been completed with extra stretching of the skin, the permanent saline or silicone implant is inserted. The implant is not an optimal option if the patient has had previous radiation to the breast (i.e., previous lumpectomy or chest wall irradiation). It also is not the optimal option if neoadjuvant chemotherapy is given and shortly thereafter definitive surgery is completed. Because radiation therapy is ideally started six weeks after surgery, not enough time is available for wound healing and implant expansion. Therefore, this procedure is best done when chemotherapy is given postoperatively.

In small-breasted women, an immediate saline or silicone implant may be placed under the chest wall muscle following the mastectomy if the patient has, and desires, a small breast size (e.g., A or AA cup). This type of procedure does not require expansion of the skin and muscle as with a saline expander. The saline or silicone implant is symmetrical to the contralateral breast, although additional surgery, such as a contralateral breast lift or reduction, may be required.

Silicone gel–filled implants received U.S. Food and Drug Administration approval in 2012 for use in breast reconstruction. As with the saline implant, this type of implant requires expansion of the skin and muscle with a saline expander. The silicone implant may provide symmetry to the contralateral breast, although additional surgery, such as a contralateral breast lift or reduction, may be required. The silicone gel implant offers a more natural feel and appearance of breast tissue than does the saline implant and is a safe alternative to a saline implant.

Implants are not guaranteed for lifetime duration and can be interchanged with a minor surgical procedure. Loss of saline is a common cause for replacing saline implants. The loss can be gradual or immediate, and the saline is absorbed by the body. Because saline is nontoxic, absorption is harmless. However, implants can present complications. Patients can develop capsular contracture around the implant. Infections can also occur.

Mixed Methods: Allogeneic and Autologous Reconstruction

Mixed reconstruction techniques using both allogeneic and autologous procedures are not as common as saline expanders or tissue implants but can be used when these methods are not available or viable. The latissimus dorsi flap in combination with a saline or silicone implant can provide a natural-appearing breast reconstruction. This flap is created by pulling the latissimus dorsi muscle to the front and moving it forward under the skin to serve as a muscular sling for an implant. The latissimus dorsi is commonly used when the mastectomy site has been irradiated and the native skin is not amenable to surgery for a saline expander (with saline or silicone) implant or pedicle flap (Agarwal et al., 2015). A permanent saline or silicone implant often is inserted at the time of surgery.

Additional Reconstructive Procedures

Additional reconstruction includes creation of a nipple and areola tattoo (see Figure 5-7). This can be performed after breast reconstruction has completely healed. Multiple steps are involved in the formation of the nipple, followed by the areolar tattoo. This multistep procedure involves removing tissue from the inner thigh, or fashioning the nipple from the excess tissue on the breast flap, and then coloring the areola with a tattoo or micropigmentation. Typically, the areola tattoo is a one-step procedure, although it may require additional coloring.

Fat transfer is another intervention used to fill defects caused by tissue death from the initial reconstruction. Vessel-rich adipose tissue is harvested and then inserted

Figure 5-7. Nipple Reconstruction Followed by Tattooing

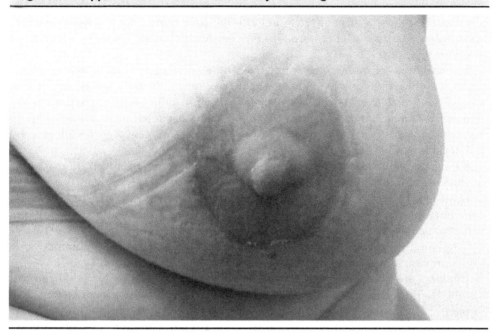

Note. From "Oncological Outcome and Patient Satisfaction With Skin-Sparing Mastectomy and Immediate Breast Reconstruction: A Prospective Observational Study," by S. Reefy, N. Patani, A. Anderson, G. Burgoyne, H. Osman, and K. Mokbel, 2013, *BMC Cancer, 10,* 171, p. 6. Copyright 2010 by Reefy et al.; licensee BioMed Central Ltd. This is an Open Access article distributed under the terms of the Creative Commons Attribution License (http://creativecommons .org/licenses/by/2.0), which permits unrestricted use, distribution, and reproduction in any medium, provided the original work is properly cited.

into defects caused by tumor and tissue removal. Biologic materials can also be used as an adjunct to human tissue. Biologic matrix agents can recreate tissue or bone, although this remains in clinical trials.

Discussion With the Oncoplastic Surgical Team

Regardless of age, all patients should be offered a consult with a plastic surgery team prior to definitive breast cancer surgery (Sisco et al., 2015). When discussing outcomes with the plastic surgery team, women should understand that breast reconstruction is intended to look normal in a bra and clothing, not naked. Individualized reconstruction options are dependent on several factors, including the disease stage and the treatment of the disease in relation to the timing of the reconstruction (Duxbury, Gandhi, Kirwan, Jain, & Harvey, 2015; Eltahir et al., 2015).

Research data related to immediate reconstruction indicate a positive effect for women as compared to delayed reconstruction (Metcalfe et al., 2015). Immediate reconstruction improves psychological issues related to body habitus and the removal of one or two breasts. It also improves self-esteem and can decrease overall stress, improve anxiety and depression, and improve freedom of dress. Immediate reconstruction can also improve sexuality and satisfaction as related to the cancer diagnosis and removal of the breast or breasts as compared to delayed reconstruction.

All women should be informed of the Women's Health and Cancer Rights Act of 1998, which requires insurance companies to provide coverage for restorative surgery in connection with a mastectomy throughout a woman's life (U.S. Department of Labor, 2014). Therefore, a woman can choose immediate or delayed reconstruction or be reassured that she needs additional surgeries, they will be covered. Reconstruction is most cost-effective when done immediately following the cancer surgery, although additional surgery or surgeries are necessary after any type of reconstruction. Reconstruction of the contralateral breast is also covered when seeking a lift or other procedure, or prophylactic surgery and reconstruction for symmetry to the ipsilateral breast.

Delayed reconstruction is another option for patients to discuss with the plastic surgery team. Delayed reconstruction allows patients more time to consider their options and enables women to obtain their genetic status, if desired. However, delayed reconstruction also comes with increased distress (Metcalfe et al., 2015) and increased body stigma. Some women have difficulty dealing with a mastectomy without reconstruction or desire a bilateral mastectomy to deal with clothing. These times are when the cancer diagnosis and its implications are not foremost. Rather, the woman is learning to deal with physical changes created by the cancer or the comorbid conditions caused by the cancer. Women who are obese (e.g., body mass index greater than 30 kg/m^2) may struggle with reconstructive options. Although a tummy tuck may sound enticing, it does not reduce fat in other parts of the body. Distress surrounds women when considering reconstruction options, yet they have limitations that change their options, such as large abdominal scars from prior surgeries. These scars may limit reconstructive options and may negate many of the autologous reconstruction surgeries.

The use of tobacco products also may negatively influence reconstructive surgery. The patient's smoking history will be scrutinized, and smoking cessation will be imperatively recommended prior to surgery. This cessation is a serious commitment between the patient and the oncoplastic surgeon. Laboratory values of systemic cotinine are measured pre- and postoperatively. Should cotinine values indicate recent use of tobacco products, the patient's surgery will likely be postponed or canceled indefinitely.

Comorbid conditions are another consideration, especially if they interfere with reconstruction. In patients with significant cardiac or pulmonary disease, extended anesthesia time may not be possible or recommended. Women who have pacemakers may require a change to the opposite chest wall to prevent issues with surgery, radiation therapy, or reconstructive surgery. Previous breast surgery may alter reconstruction options. Patients are also evaluated based on their history of breast-altering surgery, such as breast augmentation with implants, breast reduction, previous or contralateral skin-sparing mastectomy, or nipple-sparing mastectomy. Previous radiation therapy is yet another consideration (including previous history of Hodgkin lymphoma or breast cancer) (Duxbury et al., 2015). For patients with a history of radiation therapy, factors that may affect reconstruction options include tightened skin due to scarring and ischemic skin edges secondary to radiation.

Factors that are significant in women choosing bilateral mastectomy with or without reconstruction include age of the patient and ethnic variations (Covelli et al., 2015). Younger women and those of Asian descent are more apt to choose bilateral mastectomies with bilateral reconstruction. Some women choose prophylactic surgery because of their family history or known breast cancer–related genetic mutations.

Factors to discuss with patients prior to seeking bilateral mastectomy for a unilateral noninvasive or invasive breast cancer include the following:

- Knowledge that another person's breast cancer trajectory cannot be compared to the current status of patient (e.g., bilateral cancer, recurrence, death). Bilateral breast cancer is not common, and removal of the contralateral breast does not augment or reduce the length of life from the current cancer.
- Removal of all breast tissue does not guarantee elimination of future breast cancer occurrence, as it is nearly impossible to remove all breast cells from the chest wall. Recurrence can occur along the medial, lateral, superior, or posterior aspects of the chest wall.
- The risk of metastatic disease is higher than the risk of contralateral breast cancer in women with an invasive cancer diagnosis.
- Bilateral surgery significantly increases anesthesia time, depending on the choice of reconstruction. Bilateral skin and tissue transfers are very extensive when done at the same time.
- Bilateral surgery increases wound size, healing time, and the risk of infection and complications from surgery (e.g., flap necrosis).
- Bilateral surgery may delay the start of systemic therapy and negatively affect overall survival. Therefore, bilateral reconstruction may be delayed in women with locally advanced disease that will also require chest wall or axillary radiation therapy (Duxbury et al., 2015; Rudolph, 2015).

External Prostheses

External prostheses are used to provide adjustment to body changes, cosmesis, and symmetry. This is an option for women who are unwilling or unable to undergo oncoplastic procedures. All patients with planned unilateral or bilateral mastectomy should be referred preoperatively for their first visit. After surgery, patients will be given temporary postoperative garments, including a soft, padded bra or camisole. Postoperative garments contain multiple pockets for drains. A permanent prosthesis cannot be worn until the chest wall completely heals and remodeling of the tissue has occurred. A permanent prosthesis purchased before healing has occurred may not fit appropriately, and the woman's size may change over time. It is important for the cancer care team to know what Medicare and private insurance companies offer so that they can purchase reimbursable products each year.

Summary

The surgical team is part of a patient's breast cancer journey, from surveillance of high-risk status and hereditary syndromes to breast cancer diagnosis, surgical treatment, survivorship, long-term surveillance, and surgical palliation. The interprofessional team that serves women and men with breast cancer includes RNs and nurse practitioners that are integral to optimal outcomes and emotional support. Lengthy discussions occur about the cancer itself, potential surgical and reconstructive options, and systemic treatment options. The surgical nursing team provides an ongoing support system throughout the cancer trajectory.

References

Agarwal, S., Kidwell, K.M., Farberg, A., Kozlow, J.H., Chung, K.C., & Momoh, A.O. (2015). Immediate reconstruction of the radiated breast: Recent trends contrary to traditional standards. *Annals of Surgical Oncology, 22,* 2551–2559. doi:10.1245/s10434-014-4326-x

American Society of Breast Surgeons. (2013). Position statement on breast cancer lumpectomy margins. Retrieved from https://www.breastsurgeons.org/new_layout/about/statements/PDF_Statements /Lumpectomy_Margins.pdf

Ang, S.C., Tapia, G., Davidson, E.J., Kahramangil, B., Mak, C., Carmalt, H., & Warrier, S. (2016). Positive anterior margins in breast conserving surgery: Does it matter? A systematic review of the literature. *Breast, 27,* 105–108. doi:10.1016/j.breast.2015.12.013

Barber, E.L., & Clarke-Pearson, D.L. (2016). The limited utility of currently available venous thromboembolism risk assessment tools in gynecological oncology patients. *American Journal of Obstetrics and Gynecology, 215,* 445.e1–445.e9. doi:10.1016/j.ajog.2016.04.034

Bertozzi, S., & Londero, A.P. (2016). The sentinel lymph node biopsy for breast cancer over the years. *European Journal of Gynaecological Oncology, 37,* 13–16.

Bodilsen, A., Bjerre, K., Offersen, B.V., Vahl, P., Amby, N., Dixon, J.M., ... Christiansen, P. (2016). Importance of margin width in breast-conserving treatment of early breast cancer. *Journal of Surgical Oncology, 113,* 609–615. doi:10.1002/jso.24224

Bonomi, S., Salval, A., & Crippa, S. (2016). Ultrasound-guided thoracic wall nerve blocks to reduce postoperative pain and eliminate opioid consumption in patients undergoing implant-based breast reconstruction. *Plastic and Reconstructive Surgery, 138,* 543e–544e. doi:10.1097/PRS.0000000000002436

Bottorff, J.L., Seaton, C.L., & Lamont, S. (2015). Patients' awareness of the surgical risks of smoking: Implications for supporting smoking cessation. *Canadian Family Physician, 61,* e562–e569.

Broglio, K.R., Quintana, M., Foster, M., Olinger, M., McGlothlin, A., Berry, S.M., ... Berry, D.A. (2016). Association of pathologic complete response to neoadjuvant therapy in HER2-positive breast cancer with long-term outcomes: A meta-analysis. *JAMA Oncology, 2,* 751–760. doi:10.1001/jamaoncol.2015 .6113

Canavese, G., Bruzzi, P., Catturich, A., Tomei, D., Carli, F., Garrone, E., ... Dozin, B. (2016). Sentinel lymph node biopsy versus axillary dissection in node-negative early-stage breast cancer: 15-year follow-up update of a randomized clinical trial. *Annals of Surgical Oncology, 23,* 2494–2500. doi:10.1245 /s10434-016-5177-4

Cao, J.Q., Truong, P.T., Olivotto, I.A., Olson, R., Coulombe, G., Keyes, M., ... Tyldesley, S. (2014). Should women younger than 40 years of age with invasive breast cancer have a mastectomy? 15-year outcomes in a population-based cohort. *International Journal of Radiation Oncology, Biology, Physics, 90,* 509–517. doi:10.1016/j.ijrobp.2014.06.041

Capobianco, G., Simbula, L., Soro, D., Meloni, F., Cossu-Rocca, P., Dessole, S., ... Meloni, G.B. (2014). Management of breast lobular carcinoma in situ: Radio-pathological correlation, clinical implications, and follow-up. *European Journal of Gynaecological Oncology, 35,* 157–162. doi:10.12892/ejgo25012014

Carlson, R.W., Allred, D.C., Anderson, B.O., Burstein, H.J., Carter, W.B., Edge, S.B., ... Zellars, R. (2011). Invasive breast cancer. *Journal of the National Comprehensive Cancer Network, 9,* 136–222. doi:10.6004/ jnccn.2011.0016

Carney, P.A., Allison, K.H., Oster, N.V., Frederick, P.D., Morgan, T.R., Geller, B.M., ... Elmore, J.G. (2016). Identifying and processing the gap between perceived and agreement in breast pathology interpretation. *Modern Pathology, 29,* 717–726. doi:10.1038/modpathol.2016.62

Cemal, Y., Albornoz, C.R., Disa, J.J., McCarthy, C.M., Mehrara, B.J., Pusic, A.L., ... Matros, E. (2013). A paradigm shift in U.S. breast reconstruction: Part 2. The influence of changing mastectomy patterns on reconstructive rate and method. *Plastic and Reconstructive Surgery, 131,* 320e–326e. doi:10.1097/PRS .0b013e31827cf576

Chagpar, A.B., Babiera, G.V., Aguirre, J., Hunt, K.K., & Hughes, T. (2016). Variation in practice of the diagnostic workup of asymptomatic patients diagnosed with invasive breast cancer. *Frontiers in Oncology, 11*(6), 56. doi:10.3389/fonc.2016.00056

Chan, B.K.Y., Wiseberg-Firtell, J.A., Jois, R.H.S., Jensen, K., & Audisio, R.A. (2015). Localization techniques for guided surgical excision of non-palpable breast lesions. *Cochrane Database of Systematic Reviews, 2015*(12). doi:10,1002/14651858.CD009206.pub2

Chen, S., Liu, Y., Huang, L., Chen, C.-M., Wu, J., & Shao, Z.-M. (2014). Lymph node counts and ratio in axillary dissections following neoadjuvant chemotherapy for breast cancer: A better alternative to traditional pN staging. *Annals of Surgical Oncology, 21*, 42–50. doi:10.1245/s10434-013-3245-6

Covelli, A.M., Baxter, N.N., Fitch, M.I., McCready, D.R., & Wright, F.C. (2015). 'Taking control of cancer': Understanding women's choice for mastectomy. *Annals of Surgical Oncology, 22*, 383–391. doi:10.1245/s10434-014-4033-7

Cox, C.E., Garcia-Henriquez, N., Glancy, M.J., Whitworth, P., Cox, J.M., Themar-Geck, M., … Shivers, S.C. (2016). Pilot study of a new nonradioactive surgical guidance technology for locating nonpalpable breast lesions. *Annals of Surgical Oncology, 23*, 1824–1830. doi:10.1245/s10434-015-5079-x

Cuker, A., & Siegal, D. (2015). Monitoring and reversal of direct oral anticoagulants. *Hematology: American Society of Hematology Education Book, 2015*, 117–124. doi:10.1182/asheducation-2015.1.117

Curtis, R., Schweitzer, A., & van Vlymen, J. (2015). Reversal of warfarin anticoagulation for urgent surgical procedures. *Canadian Journal of Anesthesia, 62*, 634–649. doi:10.1007/s12630-015-0366-3

Diaz-Ruiz, M.J., Arnau, A., Montesinos, J., Miguel, A., Culell, P., Solernou, L., … Salvador-Tarrasón, R. (2016). Diagnostic accuracy and impact on management of ultrasonography-guided fine-needle aspiration to detect axillary metastasis in breast cancer patients: A prospective study. *Breast Care, 11*, 34–39. doi:10.1159/000442481

Drummond, J.C., Blake, J.L., Patel, P.M., Copton, P., & Schulteis, G. (2013). An observational study of the influence of "white-coat hypertension" on day-of-surgery blood pressure determinations. *Journal of Neurosurgical Anesthesiology, 25*, 154–161. doi:10.1097/ANA.0b013e31827a0151

Duxbury, P.J., Gandhi, A., Kirwan, C.C., Jain, Y., & Harvey, J.R. (2015). Current attitudes to breast reconstruction surgery for women at risk of post-mastectomy radiotherapy: A survey of UK breast surgeons. *Breast, 24*, 502–512. doi:10.1016/j.breast.2015.05.002

Eccles, S.A., Aboagye, E.O., Ali, S., Anderson, A.S., Armes, J., Berditchevski, F., … Thompson, A.M. (2013). Critical research gaps and translational priorities for the successful prevention and treatment of breast cancer. *Breast Cancer Research, 15*, R92. doi:10.1186/bcr3493

El Hage Chehade, H., Headon, H., Kasem, A., & Mokbel, K. (2016). Refining the performance of sentinel lymph node biopsy post-neoadjuvant chemotherapy in patients with pathologically proven pre-treatment node-positive breast cancer: An update for clinical practice. *Anticancer Research, 36*, 1461–1471. Retrieved from http://ar.iiarjournals.org/content/36/4/1461.long

Eltahir, Y., Werners, L.L., Dreise, M.M., Zeijlmans van Emmichoven, I.A., Werker, P.M., & de Bock, G.H. (2015). Which breast is the best? Successful autologous or alloplastic breast reconstruction: Patient-reported quality-of-life outcomes. *Plastic and Reconstructive Surgery, 135*, 43–50. doi:10.1097/PRS.0000000000000804

Enokido, K., Watanabe, C., Nakamura, S., Ogiya, A., Osako, T., Akiyama, F., … Sato, N. (2016). Sentinel lymph node biopsy after neoadjuvant chemotherapy in patients with an initial diagnosis of cytology-proven lymph node-positive breast cancer. *Clinical Breast Cancer, 16*, 299–304. doi:10.1016/j.clbc.2016.02.009

Fu, S.-M., Wang, X.-M., Yin, C.-Y., & Song, H. (2015). Effectiveness of hemostasis with Foley catheter after vacuum-assisted breast biopsy. *Journal of Thoracic Disease, 7*, 1213–1220. doi:10.3978/j.issn.2072-1439.2015.05.17

Gahlaut, R., Bennett, A., Fatayer, H., Dall, B.J., Sharma, N., Velikova, G., … Shaaban, A.M. (2016). Effect of neoadjuvant chemotherapy on breast cancer phenotype, ER/PR and HER2 expression—Implications for the practicing oncologist. *European Journal of Cancer, 60*, 40–48. doi:10.1016/j.ejca.2016.03.006

Giuliano, A.E., & Gangi, A. (2015). Sentinel node biopsy and improved patient care. *Breast Journal, 21*, 27–31. doi:10.1111/tbj.12365

Godfrey, C., Villa, C., Dawson, L., Swindells, S., & Schouten, J.T. (2013). Controlling healthcare-associated infections in the international research setting. *Journal of Acquired Immune Deficiency Syndromes, 62*, e115–e118. doi:10.1097/QAI.0b013e3182845b95

Hargreaves, A.C., Mohamed, M., & Audisio, R.A. (2014). Intra-operative guidance: Methods for achieving negative margins in breast conserving surgery. *Journal of Surgical Oncology, 110*, 21–25. doi:10.1002/jso.23645

Houssami, N., & Turner, R.M. (2014). Staging the axilla in women with breast cancer: The utility of preoperative ultrasound-guided needle biopsy. *Cancer Biology and Medicine, 11*, 69–77. doi:10.7497/j.issn.2095-3941.2014.02.001

Hoy, E. (2016). State of the art: Reconstructing partial mastectomy defects with autologous fat grafting. *Delaware Medical Journal, 88,* 20–23.

Huang, B.Z., & Camp, M.S. (2016). Burden of preoperative cardiovascular disease risk factors on breast cancer surgery outcomes. *Journal of Surgical Oncology, 114,* 144–149. doi:10.1002/jso.24298

Huntington, C.R., Strayer, M., Huynh, T., & Green, J.M. (2015). A multidisciplinary approach to improving SCIP compliance. *American Surgeon, 81,* 687–692.

Jacob, J.A. (2016). More women with breast cancer opt for bilateral mastectomy despite lack of survival benefit. *JAMA, 315,* 2154–2156. doi:10.1001/jama.2016.3584

Joint Commission. (2017). Joint Commission FAQ page: eCQM. Retrieved from http://www .jointcommission.org/about/jointcommissionfaqs.aspx#180

Kataria, K., Bagdia, A., & Srivastava, A. (2015). Are breast surgical operations clean or clean contaminated? *Indian Journal of Surgery, 77* (Suppl. 3), 1360–1362. doi:10.1007/s12262-015-1252-5

Khan, A., Zhang, J., Sollazzo, V., Mohammed, K., & Gui, G. (2016). Sensory change of the reconstructed breast envelope after skin-sparing mastectomy. *European Journal of Surgical Oncology, 42,* 973–979. doi:10.1016/j.ejso.2016.03.018

Kiely, D. (2014). Timeliness in breast cancer care as an indicator of quality. *Clinical Journal of Oncology Nursing, 18,* 82–88. doi:10.1188/14.CJON.82-88

Kothari, M.S., Rusby, J.E., Agusti, A.A., & MacNeill, F.A. (2012). Sentinel lymph node biopsy after previous axillary surgery: A review. *European Journal of Surgical Oncology, 38,* 8–15. doi:10.1016/j.ejso.2011 .10.003

Kwaan, M.R., Vogler, S.A., Sun, M.Y., Sirany, A.M.E., Melton, G.B., Madoff, R.D., & Rothenberger, D.A. (2013). Readmission after colorectal surgery is related to preoperative clinical conditions and major complications. *Diseases of the Colon and Rectum, 56,* 1087–1092. doi:10.1097/DCR.0b013e31829aa758

Lamb, B.W., Green, J.S.A., Benn, J., Brown, K.F., Vincent, C.A., & Sevdalis, N. (2013). Improving decision making in multidisciplinary tumor boards: Prospective longitudinal evaluation of a multicomponent intervention for 1,421 patients. *Journal of the American College of Surgeons, 217,* 412–420. doi:10.1016 /j.jamcollsurg.2013.04.035

Lester, J. (2015). Local treatment of breast cancer. *Seminars in Oncology Nursing, 31,* 122–133. doi:10.1016 /j.soncn.2015.02.001

Lester, J., Crosthwaite, K., Stout, R., Jones, R.N., Holloman, C., Shapiro, C., & Andersen, B.L. (2015). Women with breast cancer: Self-reported distress in early survivorship [Online exclusive]. *Oncology Nursing Forum, 42,* E17–E23. doi:10.1188/15.ONF.E17-E23

Li, X., You, R., Wang, X., Liu, C., Xu, Z., Zhou, J., … Zou, Q. (2016). Effectiveness of prophylactic surgeries in *BRCA1* or *BRCA2* mutation carriers: A meta-analysis and systematic review. *Clinical Cancer Research, 22,* 3971–3981. doi:10.1158/1078-0432.CCR-15-1465

Litsas, G. (2013). Individualizing care for women with early-stage breast cancer: The role of molecular assays. *Clinical Journal of Oncology Nursing, 17,* 332–334. doi:10.1188/13.CJON.332-334

Long, L., & Israelian, A. (2013). Care of patients with deep inferior epigastric perforator reconstruction. *Plastic Surgical Nursing, 33,* 63–68. doi:10.1097/PSN.0b013e31828dc73a

Lyman, G.H., Khorana, A.A., Kuderer, N.M., Lee, A.Y., Arcelus, J.L., Balaban, E.P., … Falanga, A. (2013). Venous thromboembolism prophylaxis and treatment in patients with cancer: American Society of Clinical Oncology clinical practice guideline update. *Journal of Clinical Oncology, 31,* 2189–2204. doi:10 .1200/JCO.2013.49.1118

Manning, A.T., & Sacchini, V.S. (2016). Conservative mastectomies for breast cancer and risk-reducing surgery: The Memorial Sloan Kettering Cancer Center experience. *Gland Surgery, 5,* 55–62. doi:10 .3978/j.issn.2227-684X.2015.10.02

Matsumura, M., Saiura, A., Inoue, Y., Ishizawa, T., Mise, Y., & Takahashi, Y. (2016). High rate of organ/ space surgical site infection after hepatectomy with preexisting bilioenteric anastomosis. *World Journal of Surgery, 40,* 937–945. doi:10.1007/s00268-015-3340-x

Mayo Foundation for Medical Education and Research. (n.d.). Stereotactic breast biopsy. Retrieved from http://www.mayoclinic.org/tests-procedures/breast-biopsy/multimedia/stereotactic-breast-biopsy /img-20008883

Metcalfe, K.A., Zhong, T., Narod, S.A., Quan, M.-L., Holloway, C., Hofer, S., … Semple, J. (2015). A prospective study of mastectomy patients with and without delayed breast reconstruction: Long-term psychosocial functioning in the breast cancer survivorship period. *Journal of Surgical Oncology, 111,* 258–264. doi:10.1002/jso.23829

Mohanty, S., Rosenthal, R.A., Russell, M.M., Neuman, M.D., Ko, C.Y., & Esnaola, N.F. (2016). Optimal perioperative management of the geriatric patient: A best practices guideline from the American College of Surgeons NSQIP and the American Geriatrics Society. *Journal of the American College of Surgeons, 222,* 930–947. doi:10.1016/j.jamcollsurg.2015.12.026

Motakef, S., Mountziaris, P.M., Ismail, I.K., Agag, R.L., & Patel, A. (2015). Emerging paradigms in perioperative management for microsurgical free tissue transfer: Review of the literature and evidence-based guidelines. *Plastic and Reconstructive Surgery, 135,* 290–299. doi:10.1097/PRS.0000000000000839

Mrózek, E., Povoski, S.P., & Shapiro, C.L. (2013). The challenges of individualized care for older patients with localized breast cancer. *Expert Review of Anticancer Therapy, 13,* 963–973. doi:10.1586/14737140.2013.820568

National Comprehensive Cancer Network. (2016). *NCCN Clinical Practice Guidelines in Oncology (NCCN Guidelines®): Breast cancer risk reduction* [v.1.2017]. Retrieved from https://www.nccn.org/professionals/physician_gls/pdf/breast_risk.pdf

National Comprehensive Cancer Network. (2017). *NCCN Clinical Practice Guidelines in Oncology (NCCN Guidelines®): Breast cancer* [v.2.2017]. Retrieved from http://www.nccn.org/professionals/physician_gls/pdf/breast.pdf

Neal, L., Sandhu, N.P., Hieken, T.J., Glazebrook, K.N., Mac Bride, M.B., Dilaveri, C.A., … Visscher, D.W. (2014). Diagnosis and management of benign, atypical, and indeterminate breast lesions detected on core needle biopsy. *Mayo Clinic Proceedings, 89,* 536–547. doi:10.1016/j.mayocp.2014.02.004

Neuman, H.B., Steffens, N.M., Jacobson, N., Tevaarwerk, A., Anderson, B., Wilke, L.G., & Greenberg, C.C. (2016). Oncologists' perspectives of their roles and responsibilities during multi-disciplinary breast cancer follow-up. *Annals of Surgical Oncology, 23,* 708–714. doi:10.1245/s10434-015-4904-6

O'Donovan, A., Mohile, S.G., & Leech, M. (2015). Expert consensus panel guidelines on geriatric assessment in oncology. *European Journal of Cancer Care, 24,* 574–589. doi:10.1111/ecc.12302

Olson, J.D. (2015). Chapter one–D-dimer: An overview of hemostasis and fibrinolysis, assays, and clinical applications. *Advances in Clinical Chemistry, 69,* 1–46. doi:10.1016/bs.acc.2014.12.001

Park, C.K., Jung, W.-H., & Koo, J.S. (2016). Pathologic evaluation of breast cancer after neoadjuvant therapy. *Journal of Pathology and Translational Medicine, 50,* 173–180. doi:10.4132/jptm.2016.02.02

Patterson, P. (2013). Why are there so many unneeded preop tests? *OR Manager, 29*(3), 20.

Peled, A.W., Foster, R.D., Stover, A.C., Itakura, K., Ewing, C.A., Alvarado, M., … Esserman, L.J. (2012). Outcomes after total skin-sparing mastectomy and immediate reconstruction in 657 breasts. *Annals of Surgical Oncology, 19,* 3402–3409. doi:10.1245/s10434-012-2362-y

Peled, A.W., Wang, F., Foster, R.D., Alvarado, M., Ewing, C.A., Sbitany, H., & Esserman, L.J. (2016). Expanding the indications for total skin-sparing mastectomy: Is it safe for patients with locally advanced disease? *Annals of Surgical Oncology, 23,* 87–91. doi:10.1245/s10434-015-4734-6

Petty, L., & Lester, J. (2014). Distress screening in chronic disease: Essential for cancer survivors. *Journal of the Advanced Practitioner in Oncology, 5,* 107–114.

Piper, M., Peled, A.W., & Sbitany, H. (2015). Oncoplastic breast surgery: Current strategies. *Gland Surgery, 4,* 154–163. doi:10.3978/j.issn.2227-684X.2015.03.01

Quinn, T.T., Miller, G.S., Rostek, M., Cabalag, M.S., Rozen, W.M., & Hunter-Smith, D.J. (2016). Prosthetic breast reconstruction: Indications and update. *Gland Surgery, 5,* 174–186. doi:10.3978/j.issn.2227-684X.2015.07.01

Rarick, J., Kimler, B.F., & Tawfik, O. (2016). Comparison of margin status and lesional size between radioactive seed localized vs conventional wire localized breast lumpectomy specimens. *Annals of Diagnostic Pathology, 21,* 47–52. doi:10.1016/j.anndiagpath.2016.01.003

Reeder-Hayes, K.E., Wheeler, S.B., & Mayer, D.K. (2015). Health disparities across the breast cancer continuum. *Seminars in Oncology Nursing, 31,* 170–177. doi:10.1016/j.soncn.2015.02.005

Reintgen, M., Kerivan, L., Reintgen, E., Swaninathan, S., & Reintgen, D. (2016). Breast lymphatic mapping and sentinel lymph node biopsy: State of the art: 2015. *Clinical Breast Cancer, 16,* 155–165. doi:10.1016/j.clbc.2016.02.014

Rezai, M., Kraemer, S., Kimmig, R., & Kern, P. (2015). Breast conservative surgery and local recurrence. *Breast, 24*(Suppl. 2), S100–S107. doi:10.1016/j.breast.2015.07.024

Robinson, T.N., Wu, D.S., Pointer, L., Dunn, C.L., Cleveland, J.S., Jr., & Moss, M. (2013). Simple frailty score predicts postoperative complications across surgical specialties. *American Journal of Surgery, 206,* 544–550. doi:10.1016/j.amjsurg.2013.03.012

Rominger, M.B., Steinmetz, C., Westerman, R., Ramaswamy, A., & Albert, U.-S. (2015). Microcalcification-associated breast cancer: Presentation, successful first excision, long-term recurrence and survival rate. *Breast Care, 10,* 380–385. doi:10.1159/000440794

Rudolph, R. (2015). Avoiding tension of wound closure in reduction mammaplasty and mastopexy in previously irradiated breasts. *Aesthetic Surgery Journal, 35,* NP11–NP12. doi:10.1093/asj/sju101

Saha, A., Mukhopadhyay, M., Das, C., Sarkar, K., Saha, A.K., & Sarkar, D.K.R. (2016). FNAC versus core needle biopsy: A comparative study in evaluation of palpable breast lump. *Journal of Clinical and Diagnostic Research, 10,* EC05–EC08. doi:10.7860/JCDR/2016/15889.7185

Schroeder, S.M. (2014). Perioperative management of the patient with diabetes mellitus: Update and overview. *Clinics in Podiatric Medicine and Surgery, 31,* 1–10. doi:10.1016/j.cpm.2013.10.002

Schuster, F., Johannsen, S., Schneiderbanger, D., & Roewer, N. (2013). Evaluation of suspected malignant hyperthermia events during anesthesia. *BMC Anesthesiology, 13,* 24. doi:10.1186/1471-2253-13-24

Shen, Y., & Cai, T. (2016). Identifying predictive markers for personalized treatment selection. *Biometrics, 72,* 1017–1025. doi:10.1111/biom.12511

Sisco, M., Johnson, D.B., Wang, C., Rasinski, K., Rundell, V.L., & Yao, K.A. (2015). The quality-of-life benefits of breast reconstruction do not diminish with age. *Journal of Surgical Oncology, 111,* 663–668. doi:10.1002/jso.23864

Sofocleous, C.T., Sideras, P., & Petre, E.N. (2013). "How we do it"—A practical approach to hepatic metastases ablation techniques. *Techniques in Vascular and Interventional Radiology, 16,* 219–229. doi:10.1053/j.tvir.2013.08.005

Sun, S., Hennessey, H., Nakch, I.K., Alsharif, S., Meterissian, S., & Mesurolle, B. (2014). Compression-refractory breast hematoma secondary to pseudoaneurysm after stereotactically guided vacuum-assisted biopsy: The critical role of urgent surgical evacuation. *Journal of Clinical Ultrasound, 42,* 492–494. doi:10.1002/jcu.22202

Tadayyon, H., Sannachi, L., Gangeh, M., Sadeghi-Naini, A., Tran, W., Trudeau, M.E., ... Czarnota, G.J. (2016). Quantitative ultrasound assessment of breast tumor response to chemotherapy using a multi-parameter approach. *Oncotarget, 7,* 45094–45111. doi:10.18632/oncotarget.8862

Tallet, A., Lambaudie, E., Cohen, M., Minsat, M., Bannier, M., Resbeut, M., & Houvenaeghel, G. (2016). Locoregional treatment of early breast cancer with isolated tumor cells or micrometastases on sentinel lymph node biopsy. *World Journal of Clinical Oncology, 7,* 243–252. doi:10.5306/wjco.v7.i2.243

Toi, M., Winer, E.P., Benson, J.R., Inamoto, T., Forbes, J.F., von Minckwitz, G., ... Klimberg, V.S. (2015). Personalization of loco-regional care for primary breast cancer patients (part 1). *Future Oncology, 11,* 1297–1300. doi:10.2217/fon.15.65

U.S. Department of Labor. (2014, September). *Your rights after a mastectomy.* Retrieved from https://www.dol.gov/ebsa/pdf/whcra.pdf

Verheuvel, N.C., Ooms, H.W.A., Tjan-Heijnen, V.C.G., Roumen, R.M.H., & Voogd, A.C. (2016). Predictors for extensive nodal involvement in breast cancer patients with axillary lymph node metastases. *Breast, 27,* 175–181. doi:10.1016/j.breast.2016.02.006

Wallace, A.M., Han, L.K., Povoski, S.P., Deck, K., Schneebaum, S., Hall, N.C., ... Vera, D.R. (2013). Comparative evaluation of [^{99m}Tc]Tilmanocept for sentinel lymph node mapping in breast cancer patients: Results of two phase 3 trials. *Annals of Surgical Oncology, 20,* 2590–2599. doi:10.1245/s10434-013-2887-8

Zervoudis, S., Iatrakis, G., Mares, P., Boileau, L., Grammatikakis, I., Evangelinakis, N., ... Navrozoglou, I. (2014). Breast conserving surgery in multicentric breast cancer: Preliminary data of our experience. *European Journal of Gynaecological Oncology, 35,* 530–534.

CHAPTER 6

Radiation Therapy

Janet Cogswell, RN, MSN, ACNS-BC, AOCN®, Kristen McGarry, RN, BSN, OCN®, and Elfrida Bauer, BA, RN, OCN®, CBCN®

Introduction

For more than a century, radiation therapy (RT) has been used in the treatment of breast cancer. In 1896, one year after Wilhelm Röntgen defined x-rays, radiation was used to treat breast cancer (Currey, Bergom, Kelly, & Wilson, 2015). In the present day, many women diagnosed with early-stage breast cancer will receive the standard of care of breast-conserving surgery followed by whole breast radiation therapy (WBRT). Oncology nurses need to be able to provide support and education to individuals with breast cancer receiving RT as an adjuvant treatment or palliative measure.

Treatment Planning

Simulation is a critical treatment planning process that maps out the site to be irradiated through patient positioning and is a necessary first step to designing the treatment plan. This often is done with a computed tomography (CT) scan that can help visualize the target tissue. Simulation is the foundation for complex treatment planning and treatment delivery, involving treatment modalities, beam arrangements and sizes, and the production of blocks (Iwamoto, Haas, & Gosselin, 2012) (see Figure 6-1). A mold (immobilization device) may be made of the upper body so that the position is reproducible during each daily treatment (if the patient is supine). For prone treatments, a specialized prone table may be used (see Figure 6-2).

Patient data are acquired through CT, magnetic resonance imaging (MRI), or positron-emission tomography (PET). Tattoo markings (average of five to seven) are placed to ensure accurate repositioning daily. The radiation oncologist, in collaboration with the dosimetrist, selects an isocenter, determines beam placement design, contours critical structures, and transfers the data to a treatment planning system for dose calculation (Mutic, Coffey, Purdy, Michalski, & Perez, 2012). The treatment plan includes the total dose, number of fractions, dose per fraction, and energy selected. It also will include maximum tolerated doses to nearby organs or avoidance structures.

Figure 6-1. Radiation Markings Using Laser to Confirm Alignment

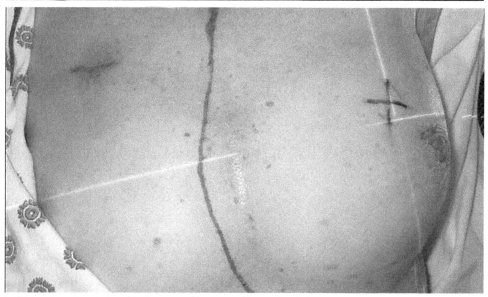

Left breast treatment planning; laser used here to guide markers' alignment.

Note. Figure courtesy of The University of Texas MD Anderson Cancer Center. Used with permission.

Figure 6-2. Molding on Breast Board as Immobilization Unit

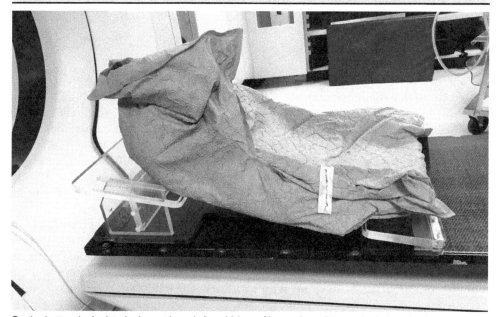

On the bottom is depicted a breast board. A mold (top of breast board) is made during simulation to reproduce the patient's position during daily treatment.

Note. Figure courtesy of The University of Texas MD Anderson Cancer Center. Used with permission.

Whole Breast Radiation Therapy

Types of WBRT include external beam radiation therapy (EBRT), three-dimensional conformal radiation therapy (3DCRT), intensity-modulated radiation therapy (IMRT), and hypofractionated WBRT.

EBRT delivers a daily fractionated (single dose of ionizing radiation) dose to a defined target. Standard RT is typically daily radiation (Monday through Friday) for six to seven weeks. The approximate dose delivered is 50 gray (Gy) in 25 fractions with a 16 Gy boost (five to eight fractions to the lumpectomy cavity) (Michalski et al., 2014) (see Figure 6-3). An additional five to seven focus treatments (referred to as a boost; see Figure 6-4) to the lumpectomy bed usually are given to reduce local recurrence (Poortmans et al., 2008). Overall, the boost offers improvement of local control (Currey et al., 2015). The results of the European Organisation for Research and Treatment of Cancer 22881-10882 trial proved that a boost dose of 16 Gy reduced the local recurrence rate for patients after a complete lumpectomy. At 10 years, the cumulative incidence of local recurrence was 6.2% for the 16 Gy boost group versus 10.2% in those who did not receive a boost dose (Poortmans et al., 2008).

Figure 6-3. Boost Treatment Shown With Boost Paddle

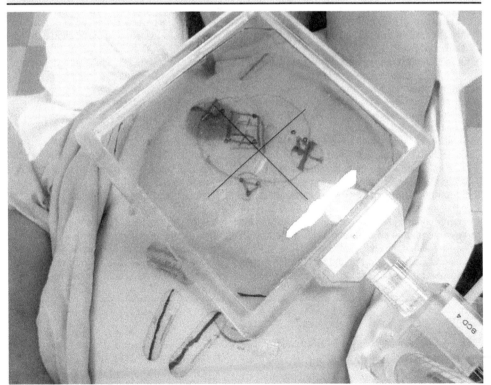

In this picture, a compression paddle is used to boost treatment focusing on the lumpectomy site. The paddle compresses the skin that will be treated during boost (the last five fractions of treatment are aimed at the tumor site using electron energy).

Note. Figure courtesy of The University of Texas MD Anderson Cancer Center. Used with permission.

Figure 6-4. Glossary

---

boost—A boost radiation dose is given to increase the amount of radiation therapy given to the area at highest risk for breast cancer recurrence.

brachytherapy—Radioactive seeds or sources are placed in or near the tumor itself, giving a high radiation dose to the tumor while reducing radiation exposure in the surrounding healthy tissues.

dermatitis—Inflammation of the skin.

electron radiation—Particle radiation that is produced by a linear accelerator. Electrons are negatively charged parts of atoms. They have a low energy level and do not penetrate deeply into the body, so this type of radiation is used most often to treat the skin, as well as tumors and lymph nodes that are close to the surface of the body.

fraction—The total radiation dose is usually divided into several fractions. Each fraction contains a small amount of radiation that gradually accumulates to form the total dose.

fractionated dosing—This technique allows the cancerous cells to be treated effectively, therefore leading to less damage to normal tissues.

Gy (gray)—A derived unit of ionizing radiation dose in the International System of Units (SI).

inframammary fold—The feature of human anatomy that is a natural boundary of a breast from below the place where the breast and the chest meet.

intensity-modulated radiation therapy (IMRT)—IMRT allows for the radiation dose to conform more precisely to the three-dimensional shape of the tumor by controlling the intensity of the radiation beam in multiple small volumes. IMRT also allows higher radiation doses to be focused to regions within the tumor while minimizing the dose to surrounding normal critical structures.

ipsilateral—On the same side.

isocenter—The point in space through which the central beam of radiation passes. Ideally, the isocenter should be placed in the center of the target volume, usually a tumor.

multileaf collimator—A device made up of individual "leaves" of a high-atomic-numbered material, usually tungsten, that can move independently in and out of the path of a particle beam in order to block it. Multileaf collimators are used on linear accelerators to provide conformal shaping of radiation treatment beams.

photon radiation (x-rays and gamma rays)—Photon beams of energy affect the cells along their path as they go through the body to get to the cancer, pass through the cancer, and then exit the body.

radiation pneumonitis—Noninfectious inflammation of the lungs.

respiratory gating—A process for continuously monitoring the movement of tumors during normal breathing. Radiation is delivered only when the tumor is exactly in the right place, and the treatment beam automatically turns off when the tumor moves outside of the target field.

simulation—The planning session; a radiation oncologist maps out the area that needs treatment. The oncologist and radiation therapist use a special machine called a CT-simulator. The patient will be fitted for an immobilization device, scanned, and tattooed. This session typically lasts an hour because it is so important to plan the position of the angles of radiation accurately.

subcutaneous fibrosis—The development of excess fibrous connective tissue in an organ under the dermis layer of the skin.

tangential beam—Direction of these beams reduces the dose-volume to the ipsilateral lung and heart.

three-dimensional conformal radiation therapy (3DCRT)—Technique where the beams of radiation used in treatment are shaped to match the tumor. Conformal radiation therapy uses the targeting information to focus precisely on the tumor while avoiding the healthy surrounding tissue. This exact targeting allows for use of higher levels of radiation in treatment, which are more effective in shrinking and killing tumors.

The 3DCRT technique is the traditional whole breast treatment that improves local control by using a multileaf collimator and electron beam boost that treats the tumor bed and avoids organs such as the heart and lung (see Figure 6-5). Use of 3DCRT planning reduces toxicity while treating breast tissue at risk for recurrence (Currey et al., 2015).

IMRT optimizes dose distribution by using smaller beam segments. IMRT has improved dose homogeneity and reduces doses to the heart, lung, and contralat-

Figure 6-5. Breath-Hold Technique: Coronal View

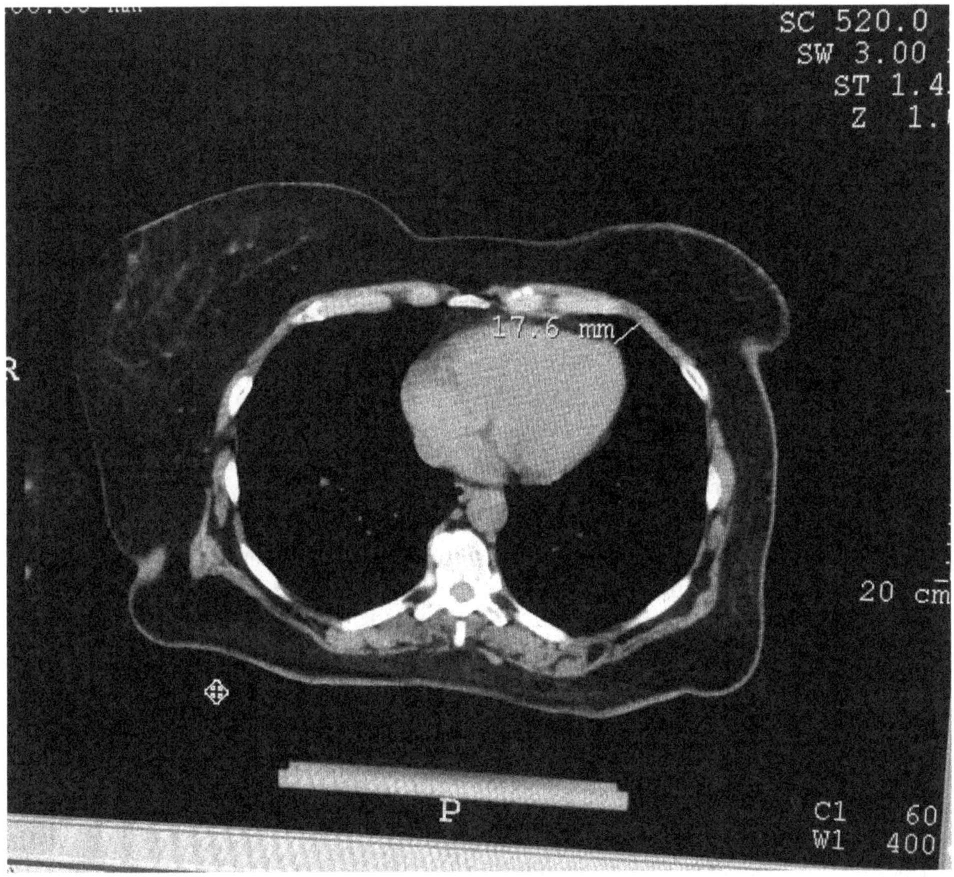

In the breath-hold technique, note the distance of the heart from the rib cage as the patient "inhales." This technique is used to minimize treatment to the heart.

Note. Figure courtesy of The University of Texas MD Anderson Cancer Center. Used with permission.

eral breast (Michalski et al., 2014). IMRT can reduce grade 3 moist desquamation and thus improve a patient's quality of life (Pignol et al., 2008). By reducing skin toxicity, it leads to better cosmesis (Currey et al., 2015). WBRT is generally well tolerated by patients with few serious side effects (Murphy & Sacchini, 2013). The treatment course is not favored by some women because of the time investment.

Hypofractionation delivers fewer fractions of radiation, meaning that the daily dose is higher. It treats all the ipsilateral breast tissue, as does WBRT, making use of the same technology. Hypofractionated WBRT is considered equivalent to standard WBRT, with 5–10 years of collected data in United Kingdom and Canadian studies (Murphy & Sacchini, 2013). A dose delivery of 4,000 cGy in 15 fractions offered rates of local-regional control and late adverse effects as favorable as standard WBRT fractionation of 5,000 cGy in 25 fractions (START Trialists' Group, 2008). A dose delivery of 4,240 cGy in 16 fractions was shown to be equivalent in terms of five-year local relapse rates and late-onset side effects when compared to 5,000 cGy in 25 fractions (Whelan et al., 2002).

Side effects such as lung fibrosis, cardiac morbidity, and impaired shoulder function were no different between hypofractionation versus standard WBRT in three published studies from the United Kingdom (Owen et al., 2006). Additionally, the cost of treatment is reduced with this schedule, which is attractive to some patients (Currey et al., 2015).

Accelerated Partial Breast Irradiation

The efficacy of APBI following breast-conserving surgery when compared to mastectomy is not yet established (Smith et al., 2009). Randomized clinical trials are underway. After completion, the data must mature for 5–15 years. Also, multiple techniques are used to deliver APBI, making analysis more difficult.

The American Society for Radiation Oncology (ASTRO) established a task force to address the use of APBI outside of clinical trials because widespread use of APBI in community and academic settings preceded the outcomes of randomized clinical trials (Smith et al., 2009). The Groupe Européen de Curiethérapie and the European Society for Radiotherapy and Oncology (GEC-ESTRO) Breast Cancer Working Group also developed guidelines for the use of APBI (Moser & Vrieling, 2012). Both associations divided patients into three groups: suitable or low risk, cautionary or intermediate risk, and unsuitable or high risk.
- **Suitable or low risk:** APBI is an acceptable treatment option. Patients who are 50–60 years old, with a tumor less than 3 cm, and with unifocal tumor characteristics would be in this low risk category.
- **Cautionary or intermediate risk:** APBI should be offered only in a clinical trial. Some of the characteristics of the cautionary group include age 40–50 years, less than 2 mm surgical margins, and limited lymphovascular invasion.
- **Unsuitable or high risk:** APBI should not be considered. The characteristics of some of these groups are younger than age 40–50 years and tumor size greater than 3 cm with any nodal involvement.

The patient characteristics in the two sets of recommendations vary slightly. One of these differences centers on estrogen receptor (ER) status. ASTRO takes ER status into consideration, whereas GEC-ESTRO does not. GEC-ESTRO recommendations also do not include *BRCA* mutation status. Furthermore, ASTRO's age threshold for low risk is 60 years and older, whereas GEC-ESTRO's is older than 50 years (Moser & Vrieling, 2012).

Four types of APBI are used: interstitial brachytherapy, intracavitary single-entry brachytherapy, intraoperative radiation therapy (IORT), and EBRT. With each type, all other breast tissue is spared, therefore causing fewer side effects than WBRT (Murphy & Sacchini, 2013).

Interstitial brachytherapy delivers a dose to the tumor bed and the immediate surrounding tissues. This type of therapy involves inserting up to 20 catheters into the breast tissue surrounding the tumor cavity. Radioactive sources are placed into the catheters to irradiate the cavity as well as a 1–2 cm margin. The most common schedule is 3,400 cGy in 10 fractions (twice daily) over five days (Moser & Vrieling, 2012). A higher dose of radiation is delivered next to the lumpectomy cavity, which is where most cases of ipsilateral breast tumor recurrences occur (Veronesi et al., 2002).

Intracavitary single-entry brachytherapy uses the MammoSite® device, in which a balloon catheter is placed into the lumpectomy cavity and the source is connected (Murphy & Sacchini, 2013) (see Figure 6-6). Another approach is the use of a silicone applicator, in which multiple catheters are connected to an afterloading system using a source of iridium-192 (Murphy & Sacchini, 2013).

All brachytherapy types require the insertion of a foreign device into the breast and thus pose a risk of possible breast infections. Therefore, prophylactic antibiotics are routinely prescribed.

IORT is radiation delivered in one treatment during surgery either by brachytherapy or mobile linear accelerators. Only the tumor bed is irradiated to a dose of 2,000 cGy (Moser & Vrieling, 2012). The short duration of therapy is attractive for some patients and helps to cut healthcare spending, but no long-term quality evidence of effectiveness exists. In 2013, the approximate cost for WBRT (using the intensity-modulated approach) was $31,172, versus $15,560 for single-channel brachytherapy (Smith et al., 2015). Radiation-induced fatigue may be lessened overall with decreased treatment time (Albuquerque et al., 2012).

Figure 6-6. Computed Tomography Cross-Section of the Multicatheter SAVI Applicator

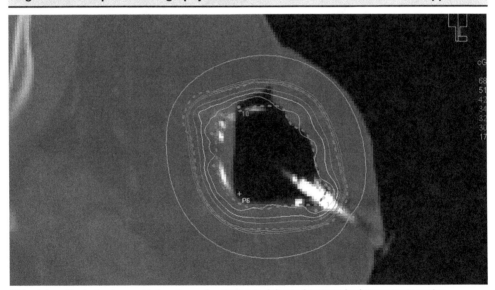

This picture illustrates how a higher dose of radiation is delivered next to the lumpectomy cavity.

SAVI—strut-adjusted volume implant

Note. Figure courtesy of The University of Texas MD Anderson Cancer Center. Used with permission.

Treatment Positions

Supine is the standard method for administering WBRT (see Figure 6-7). Women with larger breasts or high body mass index (BMI) are at increased risk for skin-

Figure 6-7. Supine Position

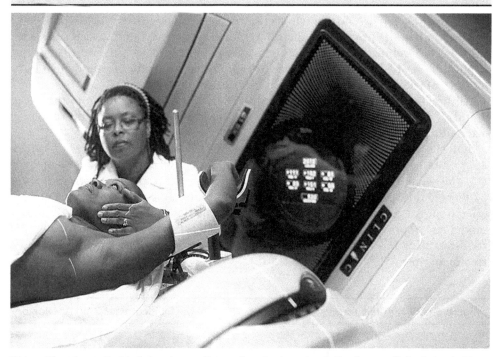

Pictured here is a patient in the supine position undergoing breast radiation therapy. Patients treated in the supine position lie on their back with the affected side arm above their head. The angle of the supine breast board flattens the chest wall and allows for more accurate planning of tangential beams. Tangential beams reduce the dose-volume to the ipsilateral lung and heart.

Note. Figure courtesy of National Cancer Institute. Photography by Rhoda Baer. Retrieved from https://visualsonline .cancer.gov/details.cfm?imageid=4485.

folds and dose inhomogeneity, leading to worse acute skin toxicities (for example, the inframammary fold). They may also get an increased dose to their heart or lungs while being treated in the supine position.

Patients treated in the supine position lie on their back with the affected side arm above their head. This allows skin to breathe rather than be occluded by a mold. Some patients find this position more comfortable than prone positioning. The disadvantage of this position is increased exposure to the lung and, if left-sided, the heart.

Prone positioning is another option. This method helps to lessen skinfolds and improve dose homogeneity (Currey et al., 2015). In randomized trials, prone positioning has proved to have fewer acute and late skin toxicities in women with large breasts or high BMI when compared with similar patients treated in the supine position (Mulliez et al., 2013). Treatment in a prone position depends on tumor location and the patient's body. Prone positioning drops the breast away from the chest wall. However, it also drops the heart toward the chest wall. Evidence exists that with proper positioning and dosimetry, the prone position may reduce radiation exposure to the heart and lung (Lymberis et al., 2012). Although some have concerns that the prone position can be difficult to reproduce on a daily basis (Shah et al., 2014), others have been able to demonstrate good reproducibility (Lymberis et al., 2012). More studies are needed to better understand the reproducibility of the prone position. While in the prone position, a woman's breast tissue gets pulled away from her chest wall, lessening the dose given to her heart and lungs. Reducing radiation exposure to the heart and lungs reduces the long-term complications of RT.

Another technique is the deep inspiration breath-hold. A person's heart may move during inspiration and expiration. When a patient is treated for left breast cancer using the deep inspiration breath-hold technique, her breast or chest wall is moved anteriorly away from her heart; the heart moves posterior and inferior to the targeted area (see Figures 6-8 and 6-9). For patients lying in the supine position, there is an increased risk of dose to the heart and lungs.

Figure 6-8. Patient Inhaling

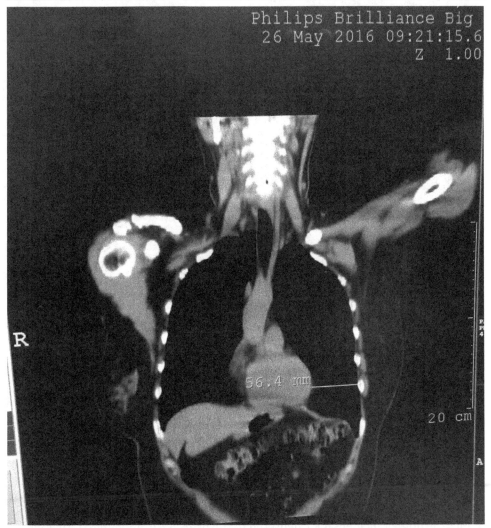

Using the breath-hold technique, the patient inhales when the radiation beam targets the left breast. The breath-hold technique provides for a greater distance between the chest wall and the heart during treatment.

Note. Figure courtesy of The University of Texas MD Anderson Cancer Center. Used with permission.

Figure 6-9. Patient Exhaling

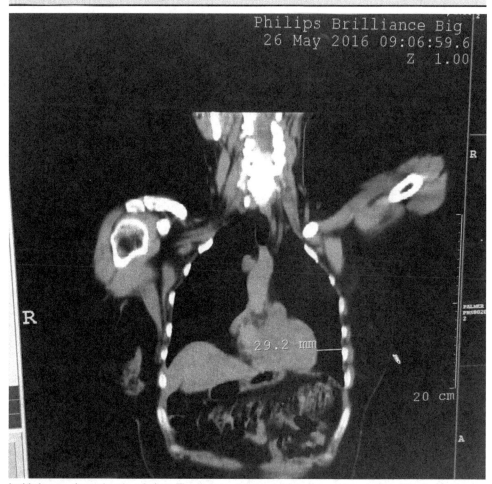

In this image, the patient is exhaling. The distance between the heart and the chest wall is closer when the patient exhales.

Note. Figure courtesy of The University of Texas MD Anderson Cancer Center. Used with permission.

An advantage of the deep inspiration breath-hold technique is that it can reduce radiation dose to the heart with the patient holding her breath for 20 seconds, especially for women receiving treatment to the left breast (Bartlett et al., 2013).

Side Effects of Radiation Therapy

End-organ toxicity from RT is dependent on the location of the field, which determines the dose of incidental RT delivered to the heart, skin, and lungs. Other factors, such as comorbid conditions of the patient, also influence the development of symptoms. Patient education on potential side effects and management strategies has been identified as an unmet need in RT (O'Gorman, Sasiadek, Denieffe, & Gooney, 2014).

There are no clear thresholds of radiation that correspond to toxicity. However, in general, the more dose (Gy) delivered, the greater the risk of toxicity. Side effects are cumulative and can be expected to increase over time. They usually manifest in the second to third week of treatment and peak at the end of treatment (Poirier, 2011).

Acute side effects include fatigue, dermatitis, and edema. Long-term effects are cosmetic and possible damage to the lung and heart. Cosmetic effects include hyperpigmentation, telangiectasia, fibrosis, and nipple retraction. End-organ damage can result in lymphedema, pneumonitis, and, though rarely since the late 1990s, cardiac toxicity (Gordils-Perez, Rawlins-Duell, & Kelvin, 2003). Concurrent systemic therapy with chemotherapy, immune therapy, or hormonal therapy could increase the potential for toxicity (Poirier, 2011).

To prevent incidental exposure to radiation, healthcare providers can use various techniques, such as patient positioning. Treatment planning should incorporate tissue dose limitations to minimize side effects while delivering the required dose to the tumor (Hogle & Pourarian, 2003).

Methods of optimizing radiation doses to tumor while sparing normal tissue include individualizing treatment plans. The use of blocks, immobilizers, and weekly imaging to verify the consistency of daily treatment is recommended. Respiratory control also is used to limit the exposure of heart and lung tissue (National Comprehensive Cancer Network®, 2017). Patients are taught to take a deep breath and hold to lift the chest wall away from these organs. It is recommended that patients be taught this technique and demonstrate it on cue prior to actual treatment.

Innovations in radiation techniques and treatment planning were developed in the late 1980s and refined in the 1990s (Emami, 2013). Techniques such as IMRT, image-guided radiation, therapy and 3DCRT allow for more precise dose delivery. CT simulation can also be used with PET or MRI to achieve more precise control of tissue exposure. Treatment teams are interprofessional with a medical oncologist, medical physicist, and dosimetrist.

When examining data on radiation-induced toxicity, it is important to attribute it to the radiation technique and era in which it was utilized. It also is important to identify the outcome defined as toxicity. Potential cardiac toxicities include pericarditis, pericardial effusion, and myocardial ischemia. A review by the group of physicians and researchers known as Quantitative Analysis of Normal Tissue Effects in the Clinic (QUANTEC), however, reported on pericarditis and long-term cardiac mortality, reflecting the current focus on survivorship (Emami, 2013). The median onset of cardiovascular disease is 13 years (Jones & Ribeiro, 1989).

Long-term cardiac mortality depends on dose and other risk factors (Taylor & Kirby, 2015). For patients without cardiac risk factors receiving a mean heart dose of 2 Gy, there is no difference in the 20-year risk of ischemic death. For patients without cardiac risk factors receiving a mean heart dose of 10 Gy, the risk is 0.8% with RT compared to 0.5% for patients not receiving RT. Patients with existing cardiac risk factors are at greater risk at both dosage levels. For patients with cardiac risk factors receiving a mean heart dose of 2 Gy, the 20-year risk of death from ischemic heart disease is 1.1% with RT versus 0.9% for patients treated without RT. At a mean heart dose of 10 Gy, the risk increases to 1.6% with RT versus 0.9% without RT (Taylor & Kirby, 2015).

Patient factors affecting incidental exposure need to be incorporated into the treatment plan. Although comorbidities such as age, smoking history, prior treatment, or chemotherapy exposure affect the response of normal tissue to therapeutic radiation, no simple method exists to predict patient toxicity. Incorporating these factors into the treatment plan continues to rely on the clinical judgment of the multimodality team (Emami, 2013).

BMI contributes to radiation-induced dermatitis. Although total dose is the greatest risk factor, three studies from Germany are investigating BMI and dermatitis. Twardella et al. (2003) reviewed the records of 478 patients. A BMI of 25.1 kg/m^2 or greater was correlated with grade 3 and 4 dermatitis. Ambrosone et al. (2006) reviewed the records of 446 patients. A BMI greater than 30 kg/m^2 was associated with 28% incidence of dermatitis, whereas a BMI less than 24.9 kg/m^2 was associated with a 10% incidence of dermatitis. Kraus-Tiefenbacher et al. (2012) found a correlation between the volumes of breast irradiated, not BMI. However, in this study, the average BMI was 23.9 kg/m^2, which was less than in the other studies.

A Radiation Therapy Oncology Group (RTOG) study reviewing the outcome of 80 patients receiving RT after lumpectomy correlated the risk of subcutaneous fibrosis with the volume of the breast irradiated (Leonard et al., 2013).

Radiation-Induced Cardiotoxicity

Although RT provides long-term benefit, it comes with the risk of cardiotoxicity. The mean dose of radiation to the heart is a better predictor of radiation-induced heart disease than any other cardiac dose measures, including mean left anterior descending coronary artery dose (Taylor & Kirby, 2015). Current methods using conformal, fused simulation techniques and free-breathing gating hopefully will continue to decrease the overall incidence. Free-breathing gating syncopates radiation with the patient's breathing.

Risk Factors

Dosing corresponds with increased risk. Incidence of pericarditis was less than 15% when the heart received less than 26 Gy. Cardiac toxicity manifests after a patient receives a dose of 4–7 Gy (Emami et al., 1991); the maximum dose is 22 Gy to prevent grade 3 pericarditis (Emami, 2013). It is estimated that each Gy a patient receives increases cardiac toxicity by 7.4% (Taylor & Kirby, 2015). EPAC1 or cAMP modulates intracellular activity in response to extracellular stimuli. This pathway is known to control aspects of cardiac function. Alterations in function are suspected to contribute to cardiac hypertrophy following RT (Monceau et al., 2014). Inflammation from fibrosis leads to acute-onset symptoms of pericarditis. This is manifested as vessel fibrosis at a younger age, arrhythmias, and cardiac blocks (Kuhnt et al., 2007).

Evaluation of the risks and benefits of potential cardiac exposure to radiation requires a holistic approach. Each patient needs to be individually evaluated for risks. Risk factors can be the result of either the patient's own health and lifestyle or can result from medical treatments. A patient's smoking history, BMI, exercise patterns, and abnormal lipid panels all contribute to risk of cardiotoxicity. For male patients with breast cancer, this includes gender (i.e., being of the male sex).

Therapies also contribute to risk factors. The addition of cardiotoxic adjuvant therapy can increase risk. The cardiotoxicity of RT is magnified by the cardiotoxicity of the other adjuvant therapies with anthracyclines and the HER2 inhibitors trastuzumab and pertuzumab. The cardiac toxicity varies. Anthracyclines appear to result in cell death, while damage from HER2 inhibitors may be reversible (Bird & Swain, 2008).

Cardiotoxicity is observed more commonly in patients receiving RT to the left breast. Patients receiving RT after left-sided mastectomy are at the highest risk, which increases as the field moves closer to the chest wall and heart (Violet & Harmer, 2004). Detailed evaluation of breast cancer survivors in the Netherlands indicated that radiation of internal mammary lymph nodes more accurately predicted the emergence of cardiac disease in survivors than left or right breast radiation (Bird & Swain, 2008). Smoking was identified as an exacerbating factor in cardiotoxicity and radiation (Bird & Swain, 2008).

Management

Techniques exist to reduce cardiac exposure to RT. Three-dimensional conformal radiation techniques are important for patients with early-stage breast cancer who are not receiving nodal radiation. Helical tomotherapy and volumetric-modulated arc therapy offer more cardiac protection for patients older than 40 years who need nodal radiation (Qi et al., 2014). Treatment planning that uses tangential fields reduces cardiac exposure. Where available, proton therapy has been proposed as a cardiac-sparing technique. However, this therapy is costlier and has limited data on its effectiveness in reducing cardiac events (Shah et al., 2014). Multileaf collimator shielding also more closely conforms the delivered dose to the intended target and away from normal tissue (Taylor & Kirby, 2015). Blocks can also be used to shield the heart. It is estimated that 2%–5% of the energy still penetrates traditional blocks or multileaf collimator shielding (Hogle, 2003). On deep inspiration, the heart is pulled away from the chest wall, which reduces cardiac exposure by 50% (Taylor & Kirby, 2015). This can be accomplished through patient education on breath holding or with electronic gated breathing technology, which delivers RT only on inspiration (see Figures 6-8 and 6-9).

Radiation Dermatitis

Radiation dermatitis is the most common and expected side effect of radiation. Depending on the study, 74%–100% of patients will experience some degree of dermatitis (Schnur, Ouellette, DiLorenzo, Green, & Montgomery, 2011). As radiation dermatitis is based on a physiologic response of normal tissue to radiation, it is questionable whether it can be prevented. The goal is to utilize radiation techniques to minimize the exposure of skin to radiation; however, often the skin remains part of the at-risk organ and must be included in the treatment field. Other treatment measures are meant to delay the onset and reduce the severity.

Pathophysiology

Basal cells are damaged by RT at a rate faster than they can be replaced. An inflammatory response to this insult also occurs, which results in erythema, edema, and pruritus from histamine. Hyperpigmentation occurs when the melanocytes move to the cell surface (McQuestion, 2006).

Radiation dermatitis is dose related. Grade 2 and higher reactions are expected between the second and third week of treatment. The following treatment factors increase the risk of radiation dermatitis: use of combined-modality treatment, including concurrent chemotherapy or following surgery where the incision is newly healed; location of the treatment, with skin in the axilla being thinner and more susceptible to irritation (Dendaas, 2012); and treatment with low-energy photon and electron beams, which deposit more energy in the skin and result in more radiation dermatitis.

Patient factors that increase the risk of radiation dermatitis and potential for skin toxicity include comorbidities of diabetes and renal failure and patient habits of smoking or poor nutrition. Older age is also a factor. The skin thins over time, making it more fragile. Postmenopausal status increases risk because it is associated with older age. BMI greater than 25 kg/m^2 increases the self-bolus of radiation through skinfolds (Dendaas, 2012). Being of the African American race increases the incidence and severity of moist desquamation (Wright et al., 2014). A German study of 211 patients receiving 3DCRT after breast-conserving surgery identified through multivariate regression analysis that large breasts and smoking are predictors of increased skin toxicity (Kraus-Tiefenbacher et al., 2012).

Assessment

The first step in management of skin toxicity is an accurate assessment and definition of the degree of the toxicity. The toxicity grading tools most often used are the National Cancer Institute Cancer Therapy Evaluation Program's (2010) Common Terminology Criteria for Adverse Events and RTOG's (n.d.) grading criteria for dermatitis. Grading also exists for pigmentation. When evaluating clinical trials, make note of the toxicity grading tool that was used. It may not be possible to directly compare trials that used different tools.

Patient Education

A grade 1 skin reaction may be more distressful to a woman than a grade 3 reaction in another. Focus on cooling imagery and vocabulary rather than burning symbolization (Schnur et al., 2011).

Improved adherence to a skin care plan is dependent on the patient's preferred learning mode (Bauer, Laszewski, & Magnan, 2015). As an example, 86 patients receiving RT were recruited in a study on adherence. They selected their preferred learning method from a video, written instructions, and demonstrations. These methods could be combined. Of the participants, 95% self-reported adherence to the skin plan to prevent, delay the onset, and decrease the severity of skin toxicity. Overall, skin toxicity was lower in the treatment arm receiving patient-preferred education compared to patients receiving standard patient health education (Bauer et al., 2015). Based on studies, patient adherence is highest when their preferred learning method is engaged.

Prevention

Delaying the onset and reducing the severity of radiation dermatitis is based more on expert opinion and institutional policy than evidence. Little evidence exists for the use of any product in reducing patient-reported symptoms, delaying onset, or decreasing healing time. Patient preferences in product, product application, and product cost should therefore be considered (McQuestion, 2006).

Washing the treatment area with soap and water or water alone reduces the severity of radiation dermatitis. In a study by Roy, Fortin, and Larochelle (2001), 99 patients with breast cancer receiving RT were randomized to washing with soap and water or no washing. The incidence of grade 2 or higher skin toxicity and moist desquamation was greater in the non-washing cohort. The evidence for the prevention and management of radiation dermatitis is summarized in the Oncology Nursing Society Putting Evidence Into Practice resource (Gosselin et al., 2017).

Two topical agents have shown effectiveness in delaying the onset and decreasing the severity of radiation dermatitis: calendula and hyaluronic acid cream.

Calendula has been shown to significantly reduce grade 2 or higher radiation dermatitis. Pommier et al. (2004) randomized 254 women with breast cancer to use either calendula or trolamine (Biafine®). Of those studied, 30% of the patients reported that the calendula cream was difficult to apply (McQuestion, 2006). This highlights the importance of selecting a skin care product that incorporates the patient's personal preferences. In addition to reduced toxicity, patients reported less pain and redness.

In a randomized placebo-controlled trial, Liguori, Guillonin, Pesce, Mirinanoff, and Bernier (1997) studied the use of hyaluronic acid cream in a diverse group of 134 patients receiving RT, which included patients with breast cancer. The placebo group had a significantly higher incidence of grade 2 radiation dermatitis compared to patients who used hyaluronic acid cream. The effect was highest in patients with head and neck cancer.

Use of deodorant does not increase skin toxicity in the axilla. In a randomized noninferiority study of 200 patients, the incidence of grade 2 skin toxicity was the same in both arms. It also maintained patients' quality of life by permitting usual and normal personal hygiene (Théberge, Harel, & Dagnault, 2009). The timing of the application of lotion or antiperspirant is based on expert recommendation rather than evidence. Generally, patients are advised to avoid the use of these agents for four hours prior to RT to avoid synergistic increase in toxicity or to avoid limiting the achievement of the full therapeutic dose (Bieck & Phillips, 2010). In a randomized trial comparing Aquaphor®, Biafine, or RadiaCare™ to a placebo of a sterile water mist, no product was superior to placebo (Gosselin, Schneider, Plambeck, & Rowe, 2010).

Treatment

Treatment of radiation dermatitis is also mostly based on expert opinion and institutional policy. Little evidence exists for the use of any product in reducing patient-reported symptoms or decreasing healing time (McQuestion, 2006).

Based on expert recommendation, gentian violet should be avoided, as it created additional toxicity in clinical trials (Feight, Baney, Bruce, & McQuestion, 2011; McQuestion, 2006). Expert opinion recommendations include wearing loose-fitting clothing made of a soft fabric to avoid friction, including avoiding underwire bras; avoiding cosmetics or perfume, which may further irritate skin; avoiding swimming in pools or hot tubs, which have disinfecting chemicals that may further irritate skin; avoiding exposure to potential infectious agents in areas such as lakes or oceans; and not using tape or adhesives on treatment areas.

Fatigue

Fatigue is a side effect experienced by up to 93% of patients receiving RT for breast cancer after the third week of treatment (Hogle, 2007). Other studies report that 65%–100% of patients identify fatigue as a distressing side effect. Traditional management strategies of energy conservation and prioritization of activities have been supplemented with moderate exercise practices. Strategies for the prevention and management of fatigue are summarized in the Oncology Nursing Society Putting Evidence Into Practice resource on fatigue (Mitchell et al., 2017).

Fatigue plays a role in undermining primary functional roles related to activities of daily living, as well as secondary roles centered on task accomplishment related to employment and household chores. Tertiary roles involving socialization, hobbies, and volunteer activities are also affected. Research is mixed regarding fatigue's effect on secondary and tertiary roles. However, studies have consistently shown that fatigue does not affect primary functional roles; patients can be offered reassurance that they are likely to continue their primary functional roles (Poirier, 2011).

Nurses should incorporate education and support into patient health education. Patients should be taught the potential impact of fatigue on their functional roles. In addition, patients need support in the discordant nature of fatigue. Patients may not be able to clean, cook, or work full time but can still participate in social and voluntary activities. They need to understand that this is not uncommon or unusual. A structured exercise program has been shown to improve fatigue in breast cancer survivors (Hsieh et al., 2008).

Survivorship Issues After Radiation Therapy

Side effects of RT can persist for years. In an underpowered study of patients receiving RT for localized prostate and breast cancer by Walker, Nail, Larsen, Magill, and Schwartz (1996), findings were inconclusive, but the unexpected finding for researchers was the persistence of symptoms over time. Cardiac and pulmonary toxicities have late-onset manifestation of symptoms. Sarcomas develop on average 8–11 years after RT (Emami, 2013).

Patients must understand the possibility of long-term persistence of treatment side effects. Survivorship care plans are necessary for long-term follow-up of potential sequelae and management of ongoing symptoms. Survivorship care plans are important because of the change in radiation techniques and the increased longevity of survivors. Survivors should know the details of their treatment plans many decades after completion of RT.

Cardiac Complications

Survivors of nonconformal (i.e., "older") radiation techniques have an increased reported rate of cardiac mortality 20 years after treatment (Mrozek & Shapiro, 2005). Survivors of new conformal radiation techniques have no increased risk of cardiac mortality at 10 years. While the hope is that this decreased risk continues over time, there has not yet been sufficient maturation of the data to support this assumption (Mrozek & Shapiro, 2005). Long-term side effects of fibrosis result in higher incidence of coronary artery disease, arrhythmias, and reduced cardiac wall compliance. Symptomatic patients have shown benefit from angiotensin-converting-enzyme inhibitors and beta-blockers. Currently, no evidence exists that these agents will prevent asymptomatic patients from developing cardiac decline (Bird & Swain, 2008).

Patient education on cardiac complications in survivors should focus on controllable factors, including not smoking, regular exercise, weight control, and diet. In a study of breast cancer survivors receiving a six-month exercise program by Hsieh et al. (2008), those who had chemotherapy and RT following surgery benefited the most from an exercise intervention. Cardiopulmonary function, as measured by predicted time and maximal oxygen consumption while using a treadmill, improved significantly.

Radiation-Induced Lung Disease

Pneumonitis is a common toxicity exhibited in patients receiving radiation for breast cancer. Radiation-induced lung disease (RILD) can have an acute onset or present as a long-term toxicity (Graves, Siddiqui, Anscher, & Movsas, 2010). Utilizing conformal techniques, the volume of lung irradiated is the key factor. However, even acute onset of radiation pneumonitis usually occurs after the end of RT. Pulmonary toxicity manifests after 2 Gy, if the entire lung is targeted. When treating a smaller volume of the lung, radiation of 6–7 Gy can be delivered. For a volume of 1,500 ml, the maximum dose is 7 Gy to avoid grade 3 lung dysfunction. Up to 7.4 Gy can be administered to 1,000 ml of the lung while avoiding grade 3 pneumonitis (Emami, 2013).

Acute-onset radiation pneumonitis occurs one to three months after completion of RT. The presenting symptoms are dyspnea ranging from mild to severe and nonproductive cough. Late-onset pulmonary fibrosis is seen at 6–24 months post-RT and is dependent on multiple factors, such as volume of lung irradiated, RT technique, and patient factors (Graves et al., 2010). In a study of 540 patients receiving thoracic RT, a mean lung dose of 15 Gy or less resulted in a 0% rate of radiation pneumonitis. A mean lung dose of 27.5 Gy or greater had a radiation pneumonitis rate of 43% (Kwa et al., 1998). In a study of 99 patients, total lung volume receiving greater than 20 Gy predicted the onset of RILD (Graham et al., 1999). Although the presenting symptom was dyspnea, many patients were asymptomatic, suggesting it may have been a radiographic finding only.

Radiation pneumonitis on x-ray is seen as a hazy confluence in the treatment field. Pulmonary fibrosis is seen as a density on CT. Pulmonary function tests (PFTs) are often used, but their correlation with RILD is weak. Forced expiratory volume in one second and diffusing capacity of the lung for carbon monoxide may improve in the setting of RILD because RT has decreased airway obstruction by the tumor. Patients do not have to experience radiation pneumonitis to develop pulmonary fibrosis.

Pathophysiology

No clear model exists to explain radiation fibrosis, including that in the lung. Radiation fibrosis is initiated by oxidative damage caused by RT. The loss of elasticity results in reduced pulmonary tissue compliance (Yarnold & Brotons, 2010).

Treatment factors that increase the risk of RILD include the dose of RT and the volume of the lung irradiated (Graves et al., 2010). Specific treatment of breast cancer also can increase the risk of RILD, with inclusion of the internal mammary lymph node chain or the supraclavicular axillary apex in the treatment field increasing the risk (Mrozek & Shapiro, 2005). Concurrent anthracycline chemotherapy increases the risk and therefore is avoided (Taghian et al., 2001).

Prevention

The goal in prevention is to reduce the exposure of normal lung tissue to radiation. Technical planning using 3DCRT and CT simulation by a multimodality team has decreased the incidental exposure of lung tissue and reduced the rate of radiation pneumonitis. A study followed 64 women treated for breast cancer longitudinally for seven months with PFTs. The incidence of symptomatic radiation pneumonitis was 1% compared to 10% in a previous study not using conformal techniques. Other variables were controlled. Women in both studies had received neoadjuvant chemotherapy. The most common regimen was cyclophosphamide, 5-fluorouracil, and methotrexate. No conclusive evidence supports that tamoxifen increases the risk of pulmonary fibrosis. The original trial, which did not use conformal techniques, showed a correlation between tamoxifen and decreased vital capacity on PFTs following RT. The current study using conformal techniques showed no correlation (Goldman, Anderson, Wennberg, & Lind, 2014).

Treatment

Radiation pneumonitis is treated with glucocorticosteroids without any evidence. Glucocorticosteroids are not recommended for the treatment of pulmonary fibrosis. Treatment for all RILD includes symptomatic support (Graves et al., 2010).

Second Primary Malignancies

Cancer in the contralateral breast is a risk of RT for breast cancer. The goal in treatment is to use multimodality treatment planning with CT simulation to spare the contralateral breast from incidental radiation that can result in breast cancer for patients younger than age 40 (Qi et al., 2014). This can occur 10 years after treatment. The risk of lung cancer following RT for breast cancer depends on the incidental exposure of lung tissue. Many of the long-term meta-analyses still include data from older nonconformal techniques. The Early Breast Cancer Trialists Collaborative Group data showed 2%–3% increased risk of lung cancer at 10 years. The National Surgical Adjuvant Breast and Bowel Project data showed a 2.1% greater risk of lung cancer in patients receiving RT following mastectomy compared to women who had surgery alone. No difference was found in the risk for lung cancer in women who had RT following breast-conserving surgery compared to women who had surgery alone (Mrozek & Shapiro, 2005).

Increased risk of breast sarcoma is a long-term complication of RT for breast cancer. Radiation-induced sarcoma occurs in the treatment field. The latency period between the end of RT and the development of a sarcoma can range from 4–24 years. The overall risk is small—0.2% at 10 years and 0.43% at 20 years—but the risk *is* real (Taghian et al., 1991). The most common sarcoma following radiation for breast cancer is angiosarcoma, based on an analysis of 274,572 women with breast cancer in the Surveillance, Epidemiology, and End Results Cancer Incidence Public-Use Database for 1973–1997. The rate of angiosarcoma of the breast following RT is 13.7%. The rate of primary angiosarcoma of the breast is 2.1% (Yap et al., 2002).

Radiation Skin Toxicity

Skin toxicity, especially pigmentation changes, have long-term implications for survivors (Schnur et al., 2011). Hyperpigmentation in breast skin experienced by African American women correlates with increased distress. Younger women and women who were not in a committed relationship were more likely to be distressed by breast skin changes (Schnur et al., 2011). It is important to identify women who are at increased risk for distress. They should be allowed to express their distress and develop management strategies without judgment.

Another skin toxicity is telangiectasia, which is the dilation of superficial capillaries and venules. In a study of 390 patients receiving RT following breast-conserving therapy between 1998 and 2001, 0.26% reported grade 3 telangiectasias, 29.9% reported grade 2 telangiectasias, and 18.81% reported grade 1 telangiectasias (Kuptsova et al., 2008). Total dose alone does not predict occurrence. Current research is investigating the role of genetic variation in oxidative stress-related enzymes. Specific genetic predictors have yet to be identified. Laser treatment is an established standard of care for vascular lesions. In a retrospective study of 11 patients, pulsed dye laser treatment provided superior results in improving appearance in four treatments (Rossi, Nehal, & Lee, 2014). Body image alterations can be seen in patients with poor outcomes, which can lead to sexual dysfunction (Hogle, 2007). This all contributes to a decreased quality of life following RT.

Radiation fibrosis of the skin can lead to undesirable cosmetic and physical outcomes through reduced elasticity of skin and connective tissue. Onset is 4–12 months following the end of treatment and may manifest without acute symptoms. Symptoms can include induration, retraction, restricted movement, and pain. Prevention centers on delivering the optimal treatment dose but no more; 3DCRT results in less radiation fibrosis. No evidence exists that pentoxifylline and vitamin E can prevent or reverse chronic fibrosis. Case studies support the use of pentoxifylline, but randomized trials failed to support them. Passive movement in the abduction of the shoulder was seen in the placebo cohort but not the pentoxifylline arm (Magnusson et al., 2009). In a randomized, double-blind, placebo-controlled trial of 68 women, pentoxifylline and vitamin E failed to prevent radiation fibrosis. Treatment is directed by the symptom compromising the quality of life of the patient (Gothard et al., 2004).

Summary

RT has added to the survival, disease-free progression, and palliation of patients with breast cancer. Thus, although it comes with significant risks, it has positively added to the treatment of patients with breast cancer. Many of the toxic side effects are an inevitable result of the beneficial effects of ionizing radiation. Modern treatment has focused on improvement of the technical delivery of the optimal dose to the target tissue. An optimal dose delivers the correct amount of radiation to the tumor and not the surrounding healthy tissue. CT-aided simulation, 3DCRT, and the inclusion of a multimodality treatment team has pushed this concept into realization. Although control of symptoms initially appears to be largely a matter of the technical delivery of radiation, clinical research has shown that this is not the case. Patients must understand the importance of the technical plan in sparing healthy tissue and replicating the treatment plan daily. It is of utmost importance that patients understand the inevitable side effects that are based on biology and physics and know that they have control over the other aspects. With their intrinsic holistic approach to patient care, radiation oncology nurses are the bridge between technology and the human experience. They understand the technology and guide patients in managing the toxicities to reach a mutually determined goal. Nurses teach, counsel, and support patients. They have one foot in technology and one foot in the life of their patients.

References

Albuquerque, K., Tell, D., Lobo, P., Millbrandt, L., Mathews, H.L., & Janusek, L.W. (2012). Impact of partial versus whole breast radiation therapy on fatigue, perceived stress, quality of life and natural killer cell activity in women with breast cancer. *BMC Cancer, 12,* 251. doi:10.1186/1471-2407 -12-251

Ambrosone, C.B., Tian, C., Ahn, J., Kropp, S., Helmbold, I., von Fournier, D., … Chang-Claude, J. (2006). Genetic predictors of acute toxicities related to radiation therapy following lumpectomy for breast cancer: A case-series study. *Breast Cancer Research, 8*(4), R40. doi:10.1186/bcr1526

Bartlett, F.R., Colgan, R.M., Carr, K., Donovan, E.M., McNair, H.A., Locke, I., … Kirby, A.M. (2013). The UK HeartSpare Study: Randomised evaluation of voluntary deep-inspiratory breath-hold in women undergoing breast radiotherapy. *Radiotherapy and Oncology, 108,* 242–247. doi:10.1016/j.radonc.2013.04.021

Bauer, C., Laszewski, P., & Magnan, M. (2015). Promoting adherence to skin care practices among patients receiving radiation therapy. *Clinical Journal of Oncology Nursing, 19,* 196–203. doi:10.1188/15.CJON.196-203

Bieck, T., & Phillips, S. (2010). Appraising the evidence for avoiding lotions or topical agents prior to radiation therapy. *Clinical Journal of Oncology Nursing, 14,* 103–105. doi:10.1188/10.CJON.103-105

Bird, B.R.J.H., & Swain, S.M. (2008). Cardiac toxicity in breast cancer survivors: Review of potential cardiac problems. *Clinical Cancer Research, 14,* 14–24. doi:10.1158/1078-0432.CCR-07-1033

Currey, A.D., Bergom, C., Kelly, T.R., & Wilson, J.F. (2015). Reducing the human burden of breast cancer: Advanced radiation therapy yields improved treatment outcomes. *Breast Journal, 21,* 610–620. doi:10.1111/tbj.12495

Dendaas, N. (2012). Toward evidence and theory-based skin care in radiation oncology. *Clinical Journal of Oncology Nursing, 16,* 520–525. doi:10.1188/12.CJON.520-525

Emami, B. (2013). Tolerance of normal tissue to therapeutic radiation. *Reports of Radiotherapy and Oncology, 1*(1), 35–48. Retrieved from http://journals.sbmu.ac.ir/rro/article/view/4316

Emami, B., Lyman, J., Brown, A., Coia, L., Goitein, M., Munzenrider, J.E., … Wesson, M. (1991). Tolerance of normal tissue to therapeutic irradiation. *International Journal of Radiation Oncology, Biology, Physics, 21,* 109–122. doi:10.1016/0360-3016(91)90171-Y

Feight, D., Baney, T., Bruce, S., & McQuestion, M. (2011). Putting evidence into practice: Evidence-based interventions for radiation dermatitis. *Clinical Journal of Oncology Nursing, 15,* 481–492. doi:10.1188/11.CJON.481-492

Goldman, U.B., Anderson, M., Wennberg, B., & Lind, P. (2014). Radiation pneumonitis and pulmonary function with lung dose–volume constraints in breast cancer irradiation. *Journal of Radiotherapy in Practice, 13,* 211–217. doi:10.1017/S1460396913000228

Gordils-Perez, J., Rawlins-Duell, R., & Kelvin, J.F. (2003). Advances in radiation treatment of patients with breast cancer. *Clinical Journal of Oncology Nursing, 7,* 629–636. doi:10.1188/03.CJON.629-636

Gosselin, T.K., Beamer, L., Ciccolini, K., Merritt, C., Omabegho, M., Shaftic, A., & Lucas, A.S. (2017, May). ONS PEP resource: Radiodermatitis. Retrieved from https://www.ons.org/practice-resources/pep/radiodermatitis

Gosselin, T.K., Schneider, S.M., Plambeck, M.A., & Rowe, K. (2010). A prospective randomized, placebo-controlled skin care study in women diagnosed with breast cancer undergoing radiation therapy. *Oncology Nursing Forum, 37,* 619–626. doi:10.1188/10.ONF.619-626

Gothard, L., Cornes, P., Earl, J., Hall, E., MacLaren, J., Mortimer, P., … Yarnold, J. (2004). Double-blind placebo-controlled randomised trial of vitamin E and pentoxifylline in patients with chronic arm lymphoedema and fibrosis after surgery and radiotherapy for breast cancer. *Radiotherapy and Oncology, 73,* 133–139. doi:10.1016/j.radonc.2004.09.013

Graham, M.V., Purdy, J.A., Emami, B., Harms, W., Bosch, W., Lockett, M.A., & Perez, C.A. (1999). Clinical dose–volume histogram analysis for pneumonitis after 3D treatment for non-small cell lung cancer (NSCLC). *International Journal of Radiation Oncology, Biology, Physics, 45,* 323–329. doi:10.1016/S0360-3016(99)00183-2

Graves, P.R., Siddiqui, F., Anscher, M.S., & Movsas, B. (2010). Radiation pulmonary toxicity: From mechanics to management. *Seminars in Radiation Oncology, 20,* 201–207. doi:10.1016/j.semradonc.2010.01.010

Hogle, W.P. (2003). Radiation therapy 101: The basics every nurse needs to know. *Clinical Journal of Oncology Nursing, 7,* 230–232. doi:10.1188/03.CJON.230-232

Hogle, W.P. (2007). Radiation therapy in the treatment of breast cancer. *Seminars in Oncology Nursing, 23,* 20–28. doi:10.1016/j.soncn.2006.11.004

Hogle, W.P., & Pourarian, R. (2003). Sparing critical organs from the effects of radiation therapy. *Clinical Journal of Oncology Nursing, 7,* 587–589. doi:10.1188/03.CJON.587-589

Hsieh, C.C., Sprod, L.K., Hydock, D.S., Carter, S.D., Hayward, R., & Schneider, C.M. (2008). Effects of a supervised exercise intervention on recovery from treatment regimens in breast cancer survivors. *Oncology Nursing Forum, 35,* 909–915. doi:10.1188/08.ONF.909-915

Iwamoto, R.R., Haas, M.L., & Gosselin, T.K. (Eds.). (2012). *Manual for radiation oncology nursing practice and education* (4th ed.). Pittsburgh, PA: Oncology Nursing Society.

Jones, J.M., & Ribeiro, G.G. (1989). Mortality patterns over 34 years of breast cancer patients in a clinical trial of post-operative radiotherapy. *Clinical Radiology, 40,* 204–208. doi:10.1016/S0009-9260(89)80099-6

Kraus-Tiefenbacher, U., Sfintizky, A., Welzel, G., Simeonova, A., Sperk, E., Siebenlist, K., ... Wenz, F. (2012). Factors of influence on acute skin toxicity of breast cancer patients treated with standard three-dimensional conformal radiotherapy (3D-CRT) after breast conversing surgery (BCS). *Radiation Oncology, 7,* 217. doi:10.1186/1748-717X-7-217

Kuhnt, T., Friese, M., Janich, M., Gerlach, R., Pelz, T., & Haensgen, G. (2007). Possibility of radiotherapy-associated cardiovascular side effects in breast cancer patients by modern radiotherapy techniques. *Breast Journal, 13,* 103–105. doi:10.1111/j.1524-4741.2006.00378.x

Kuptsova, N., Chang-Claude, J., Kropp, S., Helmbold, I., Schmezer, P., von Fournier, D., ... Ambrosone, C.B. (2008). Genetic predictors of long-term toxicities after radiation therapy for breast cancer. *International Journal of Cancer, 122,* 1333–1339. doi:10.1002/ijc.23138

Kwa, S.L., Lebesque, J.V., Theuws, J.C., Marks, L.B., Munley, M.T., Bentel, G., ... Ten Haken, R.K. (1998). Radiation pneumonitis as a function of mean lung dose: An analysis of pooled data of 540 patients. *International Journal of Radiation Oncology, Biology, Physics, 42,* 1–9. doi:10.1016/S0360-3016(98)00196-5

Leonard, K.L., Hepel, J.T., Hiatt, J.R., Dipetrillo, T.A., Price, L.L., & Wazer, D.E. (2013). The effect of dose-volume parameters and interfraction interval on cosmetic outcome and toxicity after 3-dimensional conformal accelerated partial breast irradiation. *International Journal of Radiation Oncology,* Biology, Physics, *85,* 623–629. doi:10.1016/j.ijrobp.2012.06.052

Liguori, V., Guillemin, C., Pesce, G.F., Mirimanoff, R.O., & Bernier, J. (1997). Double-blind, randomized clinical study comparing hyaluronic acid cream to placebo in patients treated with radiotherapy. *Radiotherapy and Oncology, 42,* 155–161. doi:10.1016/S0167-8140(96)01882-8

Lymberis, S.C., deWyngaert, J.K., Parhar, P., Chhabra, A.M., Fenton-Kerimian, M., Chang, J., ... Formenti, S.C. (2012). Prospective assessment of optimal individual position (prone versus supine) for breast radiotherapy: Volumetric and dosimetric correlations in 100 patients. *International Journal of Radiation Oncology, Biology, Physics, 84,* 902–909. doi:10.1016/j.ijrobp.2012.01.040

Magnusson, M., Höglund, P., Johansson, K., Jönsson, C., Killander, F., Malmström, P., ... Kjellén, E. (2009). Pentoxifylline and vitamin E treatment for prevention of radiation-induced side-effects in women with breast cancer: A phase two, double-blind, placebo-controlled randomised clinical trial (Ptx-5). *European Journal of Cancer, 45,* 2488–2495. doi:10.1016/j.ejca.2009.05.015

McQuestion, M. (2006). Evidence-based skin care management in radiation therapy. *Seminars in Oncology Nursing, 22,* 163–173. doi:10.1016/j.soncn.2006.04.004

Michalski, A., Atyeo, J., Cox, J., Rinks, M., Morgia, M., & Lamoury, B. (2014). A dosimetric comparison of 3D-CRT, IMRT, and static tomotherapy with an SIB for large and small breast volumes. *Medical Dosimetry, 39,* 163–168. doi:10.1016/j.meddos.2013.12.003

Mitchell, S.A., Albrecht, T.A., Alkaiyat, M.O., Browne, K., Clark, J.C., DeGennaro, R.M., ... Weisbrod, B.M. (2017, April). ONS PEP resource: Fatigue. Retrieved from https://www.ons.org/practice-resources/pep/fatigue

Monceau, V., Llach, A., Azria, D., Bridier, A., Petit, B., Mazevet, M., ... Vozenin, M.C. (2014). Epac contributes to cardiac hypertrophy and amyloidosis induced by radiotherapy but not fibrosis. *Radiotherapy and Oncology, 111,* 63–71. doi:10.1016/j.radonc.2014.01.025

Moser, E.C., & Vrieling, C. (2012). Accelerated partial breast irradiation: The need for well-defined patient selection criteria, improved volume definitions, close follow-up and discussion of salvage treatment. *Breast, 21,* 707–715. doi:10.1016/j.breast.2012.09.014

Mrozek, E., & Shapiro, C.L. (2005). Survivorship and complications of treatment in breast cancer. *Clinical Advances in Hematology and Oncology, 3,* 211–222, 238.

Mulliez, T., Veldeman, L., van Greveling, A., Speleers, B., Sadeghi, S., Berwouts, D., ... De Neve, W. (2013). Hypofractionated whole breast irradiation for patients with large breasts: A randomized trial comparing prone and supine positions. *Radiotherapy and Oncology, 108,* 203–208. doi:10.1016/j.radonc.2013.08.040

Murphy, J.O., & Sacchini, V.S. (2013). New innovative techniques in radiotherapy for breast cancer. *Minerva Chirurgica, 68,* 139–154.

Mutic, S., Coffey, M., Purdy, J.A., Michalski, J.M., & Perez, C.A. (2012). Simulation in the determination and definition of treatment volume and treatment planning. In S.H. Levitt, J.A. Purdy, C.A. Perez, & P. Poortmans (Eds.), *Technical basis of radiation therapy: Practical clinical applications* (5th ed., pp. 133–156). New York, NY: Springer.

National Cancer Institute Cancer Therapy Evaluation Program. (2010). *Common terminology criteria for adverse events* [v.4.03]. Retrieved from http://evs.nci.nih.gov/ftp1/CTCAE/CTCAE_4.03_2010-06-14_QuickReference_5x7.pdf

National Comprehensive Cancer Network. (2017). *NCCN Clinical Practice Guidelines in Oncology (NCCN Guidelines®): Breast cancer* [v.2.2017]. Retrieved from http://www.nccn.org/professionals/physician_gls/pdf/breast.pdf

O'Gorman, C., Sasiadek, W., Denieffe, S., & Gooney, M. (2014). Predicting radiotherapy-related clinical toxicities in cancer: A literature review [Online exclusive]. *Clinical Journal of Oncology Nursing, 18,* E37–E44. doi:10.1188/14.CJON.E37-E44

Owen, J.R., Ashton, A., Bliss, J.M., Homewood, J., Harper, C., Hanson, J., ... Yarnold, J.R. (2006). Effect of radiotherapy fraction size on tumour control in patients with early-stage breast cancer after local tumour excision: Long-term results of a randomised trial. *Lancet Oncology, 7,* 467–471. doi:10.1016/S1470-2045(06)70699-4

Pignol, J.-P., Olivotto, I., Rakovitch, E., Gardner, S., Sixel, K., Beckham, W., ... Paszat, L. (2008). A multicenter randomized trial of breast intensity-modulated radiation therapy to reduce acute radiation dermatitis. *Journal of Clinical Oncology, 26,* 2085–2092. doi:10.1200/JCO.2007.15.2488

Poirier, P. (2011). The impact of fatigue on role functioning during radiation therapy. *Oncology Nursing Forum, 38,* 457–465. doi:10.1188/11.ONF.457-465

Pommier, P., Gomez, F., Sunyach, M.P., D'Hombres, A., Carrie, C., & Montbarbon, X. (2004). Phase III randomized trial of *Calendula officinalis* compared with trolamine for the prevention of acute dermatitis during irradiation for breast cancer. *Journal of Clinical Oncology, 22,* 1447–1453. doi:10.1200/JCO.2004.07.063

Poortmans, P.M., Collette, L., Bartelink, H., Struikmans, H., Van den Bogaert, W.F., Fourquet, A., ... Horiot, J.-C. (2008). The addition of a boost dose on the primary tumour bed after lumpectomy in breast conserving treatment for breast cancer: A summary of the results of EORTC 22881-10882 "boost versus no boost" trial. *Cancer/Radiothérapie, 12,* 565–570. doi:10.1016/j.canrad.2008.07.014

Qi, X.S., Liu, T.X., Liu, A.K., Newman, F., Rabinovitch, R., Kavanagh, B., & Hu, Y.A. (2014). Left-sided breast cancer irradiation using rotational and fixed-field radiotherapy. *Medical Dosimetry, 39,* 227–234. doi:10.1016/j.meddos.2014.02.005

Radiation Therapy Oncology Group. (n.d.). Adverse event and safety information. Retrieved from https://www.rtog.org/ResearchAssociates/AdverseEventReporting.aspx

Rossi, A.M., Nehal, K.S., & Lee, E.H. (2014). Radiation-induced breast telangiectasias treated with the pulsed dye laser. *Journal of Clinical and Aesthetic Dermatology, 7,* 34–37.

Roy, I., Fortin, A., & Larochelle, M. (2001). The impact of skin washing with water and soap during breast irradiation: A randomized study. *Radiotherapy and Oncology, 58,* 333–339. doi:10.1016/s0167-8140(00)00322-4

Schnur, J.B., Ouellette, S.C., DiLorenzo, T.A., Green, S., & Montgomery, G.H. (2011). A qualitative analysis of acute skin toxicity among breast cancer radiotherapy patients. *Psycho-Oncology, 20,* 260–268. doi:10.1002/pon.1734

Shah, C., Badiyan, S., Berry, S., Khan, A.J., Goyal, S., Schulte, K., ... Vicini, F.A. (2014). Cardiac dose sparing and avoidance techniques in breast cancer radiotherapy. *Radiotherapy and Oncology, 112,* 9–16. doi:10.1016/j.radonc.2014.04.009

Smith, B.D., Arthur, D.W., Buchholz, T.A., Haffty, B.G., Hahn, C.A., Hardenbergh, P.H., ... Harris, J.R. (2009). Accelerated partial breast irradiation consensus statement from the American Society for Radiation Oncology (ASTRO). *Journal of the American College of Surgeons, 209,* 269–277. doi:10.1016/j.jamcollsurg.2009.02.066

Smith, G.L., Huo, J., Giordano, S.H., Hunt, K.K., Buchholz, T.A., & Smith, B.D. (2015). Utilization and outcomes of breast brachytherapy in younger women. *International Journal of Radiation Oncology, Biology, Physics, 93,* 91–101. doi:10.1016/j.ijrobp.2015.05.010

START Trialists' Group. (2008). The UK Standardisation of Breast Radiotherapy (START) Trial B of radiotherapy hypofractionation for treatment of early breast cancer: A randomised trial. *Lancet, 371,* 1098–1107. doi:10.1016/S0140-6736(08)60348-7

Taghian, A.G., Assaad, S.I., Niemierko, A., Kuter, I., Younger, J., Schoenthaler, R., ... Powell, S.N. (2001). Risk of pneumonitis in breast cancer patients treated with radiation therapy and combination chemotherapy with paclitaxel. *Journal of the National Cancer Institute, 93,* 1806–1811.

Taghian, A.G., de Vathaire, F., Terrier, P., Le, M., Auquier, A., Mouriesse, H., ... Tubiana, M. (1991). Long-term risk of sarcoma following radiation treatment for breast cancer. *International Journal of Radiation Oncology, Biology, Physics, 21,* 361–367.

Taylor, C.W., & Kirby, A.M. (2015). Cardiac side-effects from breast cancer radiotherapy. *Clinical Oncology, 27,* 621–629. doi:10.1016/j.clon.2015.06.007

Théberge, V., Harel, F., & Dagnault, A. (2009). Use of axillary deodorant and effect on acute skin toxicity during radiotherapy for breast cancer: A prospective randomized noninferiority trial. *International Journal of Radiation Oncology, Biology, Physics, 75,* 1048–1052. doi:10.1016/j.ijrobp.2008.12.046

Twardella, D., Popanda, O., Helmbold, I., Ebbeler, R., Benner, A., von Fournier, D., … Chang-Claude, J. (2003). Personal characteristics, therapy modalities and individual DNA repair capacity as predictive factors of acute skin toxicity in an unselected cohort of breast cancer patients receiving radiotherapy. *Radiotherapy and Oncology, 69,* 145–153. doi:10.1016/S0167-8140(03)00166-X

Veronesi, U., Cascinelli, N., Mariani, L., Greco, M., Saccozzi, R., Luini, A., … Marubini, E. (2002). Twenty-year follow-up of a randomized study comparing breast-conserving surgery with radical mastectomy for early breast cancer. *New England Journal of Medicine, 347,* 1227–1232. doi:10.1056/NEJMoa020989

Violet, J.A., & Harmer, C. (2004). Breast cancer: Improving outcome following adjuvant radiotherapy. *British Journal of Radiology, 77,* 811–820. doi:10.1259/bjr/44576710

Walker, B.L., Nail, L.M., Larsen, L., Magill, J., & Schwartz, A. (1996). Concerns, affect, and cognitive disruption following completion of radiation treatment for localized breast or prostate cancer. *Oncology Nursing Forum, 23,* 1181–1187.

Whelan, T., MacKenzie, R., Julian, J., Levine, M., Shelley, W., Grimard, L., … Szechtman, B. (2002). Randomized trial of breast irradiation schedules after lumpectomy for women with lymph node-negative breast cancer. *Journal of the National Cancer Institute, 94,* 1143–1150. doi:10.1093/jnci/94.15.1143

Wright, J.L., Takita, C., Reis, I.M., Zhao, W., Lee, E., & Hu, J.J. (2014). Racial variations in radiation-induced skin toxicity severity: Data from a prospective cohort receiving postmastectomy radiation. *International Journal of Radiation Oncology, Biology, Physics, 90,* 335–343. doi:10.1016/j.ijrobp.2014.06.042

Yap, J., Chuba, P.J., Thomas, R., Aref, A., Lucas, D., Severson, R.K., & Hamre, M. (2002). Sarcoma as a second malignancy after treatment for breast cancer. *International Journal of Radiation Oncology, Biology, Physics, 52,* 1231–1237. doi:10.1016/S0360-3016(01)02799-7

Yarnold, J., & Brotons, M.-C.V. (2010). Pathogenetic mechanisms in radiation fibrosis. *Radiotherapy and Oncology, 97,* 149–161. doi:10.1016/j.radonc.2010.09.002

CHAPTER 7

Chemotherapy and Biotherapy

Marlon G. Saria, PhD, RN, AOCNS®, FAAN, and
Tara S. Baney, CRNP, MS, ANP-BC, AOCNP®

Introduction

Chemotherapy has improved the long-term survival in people diagnosed with breast cancer. This is, in part, due to many randomized trials designed to identify the most effective regimens. More recently, targeted therapy has led to even better outcomes in appropriately selected patients. Oncology nurses need to understand the common regimens used in the treatment of breast cancer so that they can provide effective patient education and support.

Brief History

Reduction in the risk of recurrence with the addition of adjuvant therapy was documented in the 1970s (Bonadonna et al., 1976; Verrill, 2009). The combination of cyclophosphamide, methotrexate, and 5-fluorouracil (CMF) was reported to be the first effective chemotherapy regimen for breast cancer (Bonadonna et al., 1976; Verrill, 2009). This was followed by multiple trials to improve efficacy by substituting one or more of its agents. Replacing methotrexate with an anthracycline resulted in the regimens known as FAC (5-fluorouracil, doxorubicin, cyclophosphamide) and FEC (5-fluorouracil, epirubicin, cyclophosphamide) (French Adjuvant Study Group, 2001; Levine et al., 1998; Martin et al., 2003; Verrill, 2009). Instead of substituting an anthracycline for methotrexate, the National Epirubicin Adjuvant Trial added four cycles of epirubicin prior to four cycles of CMF, resulting in significantly improved efficacy (Poole et al., 2006; Verrill, 2009). The TAC regimen, wherein the 5-fluorouracil component of FAC is substituted with docetaxel, was reported to significantly improve efficacy (Martin et al., 2005; Verrill, 2009).

Clinical trials for doxorubicin and cyclophosphamide (AC), the first anthracycline-containing regimen to become a "gold standard," were first reported in the 1990s (Fisher et al., 1990; Verrill, 2009). AC followed by paclitaxel was found to be more effective than AC alone, and increasing the dose density with granulocyte–colony-stimulating factor support further increased the efficacy (Citron et al., 2003; Henderson et al., 2003; Verrill, 2009). See Figure 7-1 for current U.S. Food and Drug

---

Figure 7-1. Classification of Chemotherapy and Biotherapy Agents Used in Breast Cancer Treatment

Chemotherapy Agents
- Alkylating agents
  - Cyclophosphamide
  - Thiotepa
- Antimetabolites
  - Capecitabine
  - 5-Fluorouracil
  - Gemcitabine
  - Methotrexate
- Antitumor antibiotics (anthracyclines)
  - Doxorubicin
  - Epirubicin
- Miscellaneous
  - Eribulin
  - Ixabepilone
- Plant alkaloids (taxanes)
  - Docetaxel
  - Paclitaxel
  - Paclitaxel protein-bound particles
- Plant alkaloids (vinca alkaloids)
  - Vinblastine

Biotherapy Agents
- Monoclonal antibodies
  - Ado-trastuzumab emtansine
  - Pertuzumab
  - Trastuzumab
- Small molecule inhibitor (tyrosine-kinase inhibitor)
  - Lapatinib
- Small molecule inhibitor (cyclin-dependent kinase inhibitor)
  - Palbociclib

Note. Based on information from Polovich et al., 2014.

Administration (FDA)-approved chemotherapy and biotherapy agents for breast cancer.

Principles of Chemotherapy and Biotherapy

Adjuvant Therapy

Delivered after surgery, adjuvant systemic chemotherapy, endocrine therapy, and biologic therapy significantly reduce the risk of recurrence and improve overall survival (Anampa, Makower, & Sparano, 2015; Haddad & Goetz, 2015). The choice of regimen will depend on disease-specific factors, including tumor size, lymph node status, recurrence risk, and predicted response to chemotherapy, and patient-specific variables, including age, comorbidities, and risk tolerance (see Figure 7-2).

Neoadjuvant Therapy

Neoadjuvant therapy refers to the administration of chemotherapy, hormonal therapy, or biologic therapy in the presurgical setting (Haddad & Goetz, 2015). Women with early-stage, operable disease, those with inoperable or inflammatory disease, and those with triple-negative breast cancer have been shown to benefit from neoadjuvant therapy (Santa-Maria et al., 2015). Benefits of neoadjuvant therapy include downstaging of disease to allow breast-conserving therapy and reduction in morbidity related to axillary lymph node surgery.

Figure 7-2. Neoadjuvant and Adjuvant Therapy Regimens

HER2-Negative Breast Cancer
- Dose-dense AC followed by paclitaxel every 2 weeks*
- Dose-dense AC followed by weekly paclitaxel*
- TC*
- Dose-dense AC
- AC every 3 weeks
- CMF
- AC followed by docetaxel every 3 weeks
- AC followed by weekly paclitaxel
- EC
- FEC/CEF followed by docetaxel
- FEC/CEF followed by weekly paclitaxel
- FAC followed by weekly paclitaxel
- TAC

HER2-Positive Breast Cancer
- AC followed by paclitaxel plus trastuzumab*
- Dose-dense AC followed by paclitaxel plus trastuzumab*
- AC followed by paclitaxel plus trastuzumab + pertuzumab*
- TCH*
- TCH + pertuzumab*
- AC followed by docetaxel + trastuzumab
- AC followed by docetaxel + trastuzumab + pertuzumab
- Docetaxel + cyclophosphamide + trastuzumab
- FEC followed by docetaxel + trastuzumab + pertuzumab
- FEC followed by paclitaxel + trastuzumab + pertuzumab
- Paclitaxel + trastuzumab
- Pertuzumab + trastuzumab + docetaxel followed by FEC
- Pertuzumab + trastuzumab + paclitaxel followed by FEC

* Preferred regimens

AC—doxorubicin and cyclophosphamide; CMF—cyclophosphamide, methotrexate, 5-fluorouracil; EC—epirubicin and cyclophosphamide; FAC—5-fluorouracil, doxorubicin, cyclophosphamide; FEC/CEF—5-fluorouracil, epirubicin, cyclophosphamide; TAC—docetaxel, doxorubicin, cyclophosphamide; TC—docetaxel and cyclophosphamide; TCH—docetaxel, carboplatin, trastuzumab

Note. Based on information from National Comprehensive Cancer Network, 2017b.

Metastatic Breast Cancer

Clinical trial participation is a crucial part of current oncology practice for the treatment of metastatic breast cancer (Santa-Maria & Gradishar, 2015). Current standard of care options include the following: premenopausal women treated with ovarian ablation may receive regimens indicated for postmenopausal women; frontline therapy should be based on previous therapy received for early-stage disease; and chemotherapy may be considered at any point if a visceral crisis is suspected (see Figures 7-3 and 7-4).

Chemotherapy Agents

Capecitabine

Indications: Metastatic breast cancer in combination with docetaxel after failure of prior anthracycline-containing therapy or as monotherapy in patients resistant to both paclitaxel and an anthracycline-containing regimen (Genentech USA, Inc., 2015; Polovich, Olsen, & LeFebvre, 2014)

Mechanism of action: Inhibits DNA synthesis and cell division and interferes with RNA processing and protein synthesis

Administration: In combination with docetaxel, the recommended dose of capecitabine is 1,250 mg/m^2 twice daily for two weeks followed by a one-week rest

Figure 7-3. Chemotherapy Regimens for Recurrent or Metastatic Breast Cancer

Preferred Single Agents
- Capecitabine
- Doxorubicin
- Eribulin
- Gemcitabine
- Paclitaxel
- Pegylated liposomal doxorubicin
- Vinorelbine

Other Single Agents
- Albumin-bound paclitaxel
- Carboplatin
- Cisplatin
- Cyclophosphamide
- Docetaxel
- Epirubicin
- Ixabepilone

Combination Regimens
- Doxorubicin + cyclophosphamide
- Cyclophosphamide + methotrexate + 5-fluorouracil
- Docetaxel + capecitabine
- Epirubicin + cyclophosphamide
- 5-Fluorouracil + doxorubicin + cyclophosphamide
- 5-Fluorouracil + epirubicin + cyclophosphamide
- Gemcitabine + carboplatin
- Gemcitabine + paclitaxel
- Paclitaxel + bevacizumab

Note. Based on information from National Comprehensive Cancer Network, 2017b.

Figure 7-4. Chemotherapy Regimens for Recurrent or Metastatic HER2-Positive Breast Cancer

Preferred First-Line Agents
- Pertuzumab + trastuzumab + docetaxel
- Pertuzumab + trastuzumab + paclitaxel

Other Agents
- Ado-trastuzumab emtansine
- Trastuzumab + capecitabine
- Trastuzumab + docetaxel
- Trastuzumab + paclitaxel
- Trastuzumab + paclitaxel + carboplatin
- Trastuzumab + vinorelbine

Agents for Trastuzumab-Exposed HER2-Positive Disease
- Lapatinib + capecitabine
- Trastuzumab + capecitabine
- Trastuzumab + lapatinib

Note. Based on information from National Comprehensive Cancer Network, 2017b; Polovich et al., 2014.

period, combined with docetaxel at 75 mg/m^2 as a one-hour IV infusion every three weeks. As monotherapy, the recommended dose of capecitabine is 1,250 mg/m^2 PO twice daily (morning and evening; equivalent to 2,500 mg/m^2 total daily dose) for two weeks followed by a one-week rest period given as three-week cycles.

Side effects: Dose reduction is recommended for patients with grade 3 hand-foot syndrome (palmar-plantar erythrodysesthesia). Diarrhea and vomiting may require dose reductions, intensive antiemetic therapy, and intensive fluid management. Interactions may occur between capecitabine and warfarin, phenytoin, and antacids (Frye, 2009).

Nursing considerations: Capecitabine is an oral drug designed to deliver 5-fluorouracil directly to the tumor site. When dose reductions are needed, it is important to remember that patients may be reluctant to reduce the dose for fear of reduced efficacy. Nonadherence has been reported as a major threat to successful therapy (Frye, 2009).

Cyclophosphamide

Indications: Breast carcinoma (Baxter Healthcare Corp., 2013; Polovich et al., 2014)

Mechanism of action: Cross-links tumor cell DNA

Administration: Initial course for patients with no hematologic deficiency: 40–50 mg/kg in divided doses over two to five days. Other regimens include 10–15 mg/kg given every 7–10 days, or 3–5 mg/kg twice weekly.

Side effects: Hemorrhagic cystitis is a dose-limiting toxicity. Nausea, vomiting, alopecia, and myelosuppression are common side effects. Cardiotoxicity (myocarditis, myopericarditis, pericardial effusion including cardiac tamponade, and congestive heart failure [CHF]) and pulmonary toxicity (pneumonitis, pulmonary fibrosis, pulmonary veno-occlusive disease) have been reported. Cyclophosphamide can cause secondary malignancies (urinary tract cancer, acute leukemia, lymphoma, thyroid cancer, and sarcoma), as well as impaired male and female reproductive function and fertility.

Nursing considerations: Aggressive hydration with forced diuresis and frequent bladder emptying can reduce the frequency and severity of bladder toxicity. Administering the medication in the morning rather than later in the day will limit the exposure of the drug within the bladder, as the patient will be awake and able to void frequently. Mesna has been used to prevent severe bladder toxicity. The risk of cardiotoxicity may be increased with high doses of cyclophosphamide, in patients with advanced age, and in patients with previous radiation treatment to the cardiac region or previous or concomitant treatment with other cardiotoxic agents.

Docetaxel

Indications: Locally advanced or metastatic breast cancer after failure of prior chemotherapy and in combination with doxorubicin and cyclophosphamide for the adjuvant treatment of patients with operable node-positive breast cancer (Polovich et al., 2014; Sanofi-Aventis U.S. LLC, 2010)

Mechanism of action: Disrupts the microtubular network in cells that is essential for mitotic and interphase cellular functions

Administration: For locally advanced or metastatic breast cancer after failure of prior chemotherapy, 60–100 mg/m² IV administered over one hour every three weeks. For the adjuvant treatment of operable node-positive breast cancer, 75 mg/m² administered one hour after doxorubicin 50 mg/m² and cyclophosphamide 500 mg/m² every three weeks for six courses.

Side effects: Hypersensitivity reactions have been reported, particularly during the first and second infusions. Severe fluid retention has been reported following therapy.

Nursing considerations: On the day before treatment, patients should be premedicated with dexamethasone 8 mg PO BID for three days to decrease the incidence of a hypersensitivity reaction and fluid retention. Docetaxel is an irritant. Infusion site reactions are generally mild and include hyperpigmentation, inflammation, redness or dryness of the skin, phlebitis, extravasation, or swelling of the vein.

Doxorubicin

Indications: Used as a component of multiagent neoadjuvant or adjuvant chemotherapy for treatment of women with axillary lymph node involvement following resection of primary breast cancer and for metastatic breast cancer (Bedford Laboratories, 2014; Polovich et al., 2014)

Mechanism of action: Interacts with DNA by nucleotide base intercalation and cell membrane lipid binding

Administration: Single agent: 60–75 mg/m² IV given every 21 days. Combination therapy: 40–75 mg/m² IV given every 21–28 days.

Side effects: The black box warning includes cardiomyopathy, secondary malignancies, extravasation and tissue necrosis, and severe myelosuppression.

Nursing considerations: Do not exceed lifetime cumulative dose of 550 mg/m² (450 mg/m² for patients who have had prior chest irradiation or concomitant cyclophosphamide). Assess left ventricular ejection fraction (LVEF) before and regularly during and after treatment. Doxorubicin can increase radiation-induced toxicity to the myocardium, mucosa, skin, and liver. Radiation recall, including but not limited to cutaneous and pulmonary toxicity, can occur in patients who receive doxorubicin after prior radiation therapy.

Epirubicin

Indications: Used as a component of adjuvant therapy in patients with evidence of axillary node tumor involvement following resection of primary breast cancer (Pharmacia & Upjohn Co., 2011; Polovich et al., 2014)

Mechanism of action: Anthracycline cytotoxic agent that interferes with a number of biochemical and biologic functions within eukaryotic cells

Administration: The starting dose is 100–120 mg/m². Administer intravenously in repeated three- to four-week cycles, either total dose on day 1 of each cycle or divided equally and given on days 1 and 8 of each cycle. Dosage reductions are possible when given in certain combinations.

Side effects: Severe local tissue necrosis associated with extravasation has been reported, as well as myocardial toxicity manifested by potentially fatal CHF. Secondary acute myeloid leukemia and severe myelosuppression have been observed. Reduce dosage in patients with impaired hepatic function.

Nursing considerations: The risk of developing CHF rises rapidly with increasing total cumulative doses in excess of 900 mg/m². The risk of serious cardiac impairment may be decreased through regular monitoring of LVEF during the course of treatment. Serum creatinine should be assessed before and during therapy. Dosage adjustment is necessary in patients with serum creatinine greater than 5 mg/dl. Administration after previous radiation therapy may induce an inflammatory recall reaction at the site of the irradiation.

Eribulin

Indications: Metastatic breast cancer in patients who have previously received at least two chemotherapy regimens for the treatment of metastatic disease. Prior therapy should have included an anthracycline and a taxane in either the adjuvant or metastatic setting (Eisai Inc., 2016; Polovich et al., 2014).

Mechanism of action: Inhibits the growth phase of microtubules without affecting the shortening phase and sequesters tubulin into nonproductive aggregates, leading to G_2/M cell-cycle block, disruption of mitotic spindles, and, ultimately, apoptotic cell death after prolonged mitotic blockage

Administration: 1.4 mg/m^2 IV administered over two to five minutes on days 1 and 8 of a 21-day cycle

Side effects: The most common adverse reactions reported were neutropenia, anemia, asthenia/fatigue, alopecia, peripheral neuropathy, nausea, and constipation. Peripheral neuropathy was the most common toxicity leading to discontinuation of therapy.

Nursing considerations: If a dose has been delayed for toxicity and toxicities have recovered to a severity of grade 2 or less, resume eribulin at a reduced dose. Do not reescalate the dose after it has been reduced. Do not dilute in or administer through an IV line containing solutions with dextrose.

5-Fluorouracil

Indications: Palliative management of breast carcinoma (Gensia Sicor Pharmaceuticals, Inc., 1999; Polovich et al., 2014)

Mechanism of action: Interferes with the synthesis of DNA and to a lesser extent inhibits the formation of RNA

Administration: 12 mg/kg IV once daily for four successive days. The daily dose should not exceed 800 mg. If no toxicity is observed, 6 mg/kg are given on the 6th, 8th, 10th, and 12th days unless toxicity occurs. No therapy is given on the 5th, 7th, 9th, or 11th days. Therapy is to be discontinued at the end of the 12th day, even if no toxicity has become apparent.

Side effects: Therapy is to be discontinued promptly with any of the following toxicities: at the first visible sign of stomatitis or esophageal pharyngitis, leukopenia (white blood cell count less than 3,500/mm^3) or a rapidly falling white blood cell count, intractable vomiting, diarrhea (frequent bowel movements or watery stools), gastrointestinal ulceration and bleeding, and thrombocytopenia (platelet count less than 100,000/mm^3). Hemorrhage from any site and palmar-plantar erythrodysesthesia syndrome (also known as hand-foot syndrome) have been reported, and acute cerebellar syndrome may occur. Ophthalmic adverse events reported include lacrimal duct stenosis, visual changes, lacrimation, and photophobia.

Nursing considerations: Leucovorin is often given concurrently to enhance efficacy.

Gemcitabine

Indications: In combination with paclitaxel for first-line treatment of patients with metastatic breast cancer after failure of prior anthracycline-containing adjuvant chemotherapy, unless anthracyclines were clinically contraindicated (Eli Lilly and Co., 1996; Polovich et al., 2014)

Mechanism of action: Inhibits DNA synthesis

Administration: 1,250 mg/m^2 over 30 minutes on days 1 and 8 of each 21-day cycle

Side effects: Most common adverse events include nausea and vomiting, anemia, alanine transaminase (ALT), aspartate transaminase (AST), neutropenia, leukopenia, alkaline phosphatase, proteinuria, fever, hematuria, rash, thrombocytopenia, and dyspnea. Gemcitabine may cause severe and life-threatening radiation toxicity because of its radiation-sensitizing property.

Nursing considerations: Increased toxicity can occur with an infusion time longer than 60 minutes or dosing more frequently than once weekly.

Ixabepilone

Indications: In combination with capecitabine for the treatment of patients with metastatic or locally advanced breast cancer resistant to treatment with an anthracycline and a taxane or whose cancer is taxane resistant and for whom further anthracycline therapy is contraindicated (Bristol-Myers Squibb Co., 2016; Polovich et al., 2014)

Mechanism of action: Blocks cells in the mitotic phase of the cell division cycle, leading to cell death

Administration: 40 mg/m^2 IV administered over three hours every three weeks

Side effects: Must not be given in combination with capecitabine to patients with AST or ALT greater than 2.5 times the upper limit of normal or bilirubin greater than one times the upper limit of normal because of the increased risk of toxicity and neutropenia-related death. Most common adverse reactions include peripheral sensory neuropathy, fatigue or asthenia, myalgia or arthralgia, alopecia, nausea, vomiting, stomatitis or mucositis, diarrhea, and musculoskeletal pain.

Nursing considerations: Patients with a history of a severe hypersensitivity reaction to agents containing polyoxyl 35 castor oil or its derivatives (e.g., polyoxyethylated castor oil) should not be treated with ixabepilone. All patients must be premedicated approximately one hour before the infusion with diphenhydramine and an H$_2$ antagonist. Patients who experienced a hypersensitivity reaction require premedication with corticosteroids. Only the supplied diluent must be used for constituting ixabepilone. Mix only in lactated Ringer's and administer through a 0.2–1.2 micron in-line filter. The infusion must be prepared in a DEHP (di-[2-ethylhexyl] phthalate)-free bag.

Methotrexate

Indications: Used alone or in combination with other anticancer agents in the treatment of breast cancer (Polovich et al., 2014; Xanodyne Pharmaceuticals, Inc., 2003)

Mechanism of action: Interferes with DNA synthesis, repair, and cellular replication

Administration: Dosage varies widely from 30–40 mg/m^2/week to 100–12,000 mg/m^2 with leucovorin rescue.

Side effects: Acute (elevated transaminases) and chronic (fibrosis and cirrhosis) hepatotoxicity and renal damage that may lead to acute renal failure are dose-limiting toxicities. Nonspecific pneumonitis occurring during methotrexate therapy may be indicative of a potentially dangerous lesion and require interruption of treatment and careful investigation. Transient acute neurologic syndrome has been observed in patients treated with high-dose regimens. Most frequently reported adverse events include ulcerative stomatitis, leukopenia, nausea, and abdominal distress.

Nursing considerations: Timely administration of leucovorin and vigorous hydration must follow any high-dose methotrexate. Sodium bicarbonate should be included in IV fluid to ensure urine pH is greater than 7.0. Methotrexate levels should also be monitored. Instruct the patient to avoid supplements with folic acid because it may counteract the effects of methotrexate.

Paclitaxel

Indications: Neoadjuvant and adjuvant treatment of node-positive breast cancer administered sequentially to standard doxorubicin-containing combination chemotherapy. It also is indicated for the treatment of breast cancer after failure of combination chemotherapy for metastatic disease or relapse within six months of adjuvant chemotherapy. Prior therapy should have included an anthracycline unless clinically contraindicated (Bristol-Myers Squibb Co., 2011; Polovich et al., 2014).

Mechanism of action: Interferes with the normal breakdown of microtubules during cell division

Administration: For neoadjuvant therapy, the recommended dose is 175 mg/m^2 IV over three hours every three weeks for four cycles or 80 mg/m^2 IV over one hour weekly for 12 weeks. For the adjuvant treatment of node-positive breast cancer, the recommended regimen is paclitaxel at a dose of 175 mg/m^2 IV over three hours every three weeks for four courses administered sequentially to doxorubicin-containing combination chemotherapy. After failure of initial chemotherapy for metastatic disease or relapse within six months of adjuvant chemotherapy, paclitaxel is given at a dose of 175 mg/m^2 IV administered over three hours every three weeks.

Side effects: Severe hypersensitivity reactions, such as hypotension requiring treatment, dyspnea requiring bronchodilators, angioedema, or generalized urticaria, require immediate discontinuation of paclitaxel and aggressive symptomatic therapy. Peripheral neuropathy frequently has been reported. Severe symptoms will require a dose reduction of 20% for all subsequent courses. Injection site reactions have been observed more frequently with the 24-hour infusion than with the 3-hour infusion. Reactions were usually mild and consisted of erythema, tenderness, skin discoloration, or swelling at the injection site.

Nursing considerations: Patients with a history of severe hypersensitivity reactions to products containing polyoxyl 35 castor oil (e.g., cyclosporin for injection concentrate and teniposide for injection concentrate) should not be treated with paclitaxel. It is recommended that all patients be pretreated with corticosteroids, diphenhydramine, and H$_2$ antagonists to reduce the incidence of anaphylaxis and severe hypersensitivity; however, fatal reactions have occurred in patients despite premedication. Paclitaxel should preferably be stored in bottles (glass, polypropylene) or plastic bags (polypropylene, polyolefin) and administered through polyethylene-lined administration sets to prevent contact with plasticized polyvinyl chloride equipment or devices. Paclitaxel must be administered through an in-line filter with a microporous membrane not greater than 0.22 micron.

Paclitaxel Protein-Bound Particles

Indications: Treatment of breast cancer after failure of combination chemotherapy for metastatic disease or for relapse within six months of adjuvant chemotherapy. Prior therapy should have included an anthracycline unless clinically contraindicated (Celgene Corp., 2015; Polovich et al., 2014).

Mechanism of action: Is a microtubule inhibitor that promotes the assembly of microtubules from tubulin dimers and stabilizes microtubules by preventing depolymerization

Administration: 260 mg/m^2 IV administered over 30 minutes every three weeks

Side effects: Bone marrow suppression (primarily neutropenia) is dose dependent and a dose-limiting toxicity. Sensory neuropathy is dose and schedule dependent.

Severe events such as phlebitis, cellulitis, induration, necrosis, and fibrosis have been reported.

Nursing considerations: Premedication is not required. Patients who experience severe neutropenia or severe sensory neuropathy should have the dosage reduced to 220 mg/m^2 for subsequent courses. Recurrence of severe neutropenia or severe sensory neuropathy requires an additional dose reduction to 180 mg/m^2.

Thiotepa

Indications: Adenocarcinoma of the breast (Polovich et al., 2014; West-Ward Pharmaceuticals, 2015)

Mechanism of action: Prevents DNA replication

Administration: May be given by rapid IV administration in doses of 0.3–0.4 mg/kg. Doses should be given at one- to four-week intervals.

Side effects: Myelosuppression is a dose-limiting toxicity. Hypersensitivity reactions, fatigue, weakness, contact dermatitis, nausea, vomiting, conjunctivitis, amenorrhea, and interference with spermatogenesis have been reported.

Nursing considerations: Weekly blood and platelet counts are recommended during therapy and for at least three weeks after therapy has been discontinued. Monitor for delayed myelosuppression (14–28 days).

Vinblastine

Indications: Carcinoma of the breast that is unresponsive to appropriate endocrine surgery and hormone therapy (Bedford Laboratories, 2012; Polovich et al., 2014)

Mechanism of action: Inhibits microtubule formation in the mitotic spindle, resulting in an arrest of dividing cells at the metaphase stage

Administration: Initiate therapy for adults by administering a single IV dose of 3.7 mg/m^2, a second dose of 5.5 mg/m^2, a third dose of 7.4 mg/m^2, a fourth dose of 9.25 mg/m^2, and a fifth dose of 11.1 mg/m^2, with the maximum dose not to exceed 18.5 mg/m^2.

Side effects: Leukopenia and neurotoxicity are dose-limiting toxicities. Alopecia, constipation, paresthesias, malaise, bone pain, and jaw pain have been reported.

Nursing consideration: Fatal if given intrathecally. Syringe containing a specific dose must be labeled "FOR INTRAVENOUS USE ONLY—FATAL IF GIVEN BY OTHER ROUTES."

Extravasation during IV injection may lead to cellulitis and phlebitis. If the amount of extravasation is great, sloughing may occur.

Targeted Therapy

Ado-Trastuzumab Emtansine

Indications: As a single agent for the treatment of patients with HER2-positive, metastatic breast cancer who previously received trastuzumab and a taxane, separately or in combination. Patients should have either received prior therapy for metastatic disease or developed disease recurrence during or within six months of completing adjuvant therapy (Genentech USA, Inc., 2016b; Polovich et al., 2014).

Mechanism of action: Is an HER2-targeted antibody–drug conjugate that inhibits HER2 receptor signaling, mediates antibody-dependent cell-mediated cytotoxicity (ADCC), and inhibits shedding of the HER2 extracellular domain in human breast cancer cells that overexpress HER2

Administration: 3.6 mg/kg given as an IV infusion every three weeks (21-day cycle) until disease progression or unacceptable toxicity

Side effects: Hepatotoxicity, liver failure, and death have occurred in patients treated with ado-trastuzumab emtansine. Monitor hepatic function prior to initiation and each dose. Institute dose modifications or permanently discontinue as appropriate. May lead to reductions in left ventricular ejection fraction (LVEF). Assess LVEF prior to initiation. Monitor and withhold dosing or discontinue as appropriate. Most common adverse reactions include fatigue, nausea, musculoskeletal pain, hemorrhage, thrombocytopenia, headache, increased transaminases, constipation, and epistaxis. Management of increased serum transaminases, hyperbilirubinemia, left ventricular dysfunction, thrombocytopenia, pulmonary toxicity, or peripheral neuropathy may require temporary interruption, dose reduction, or treatment discontinuation.

Nursing considerations: Do not substitute ado-trastuzumab emtansine for or with trastuzumab. Do not administer as an IV push or bolus. Do not use dextrose (5%) solution. Use a 0.2 or 0.22 micron in-line polyethersulfone filter during infusion. Assess LVEF prior to initiation and at regular intervals. Do not reescalate the dose after a dose reduction has been made.

Reactions secondary to extravasation have been observed more frequently within 24 hours of infusion; they usually were mild and included erythema, tenderness, skin irritation, pain, or swelling at the infusion site.

Everolimus

Indications: Advanced hormone receptor–positive, HER2-negative breast cancer in combination with exemestane after failure of treatment with letrozole or anastrozole in postmenopausal women (Novartis Pharmaceuticals Corp., 2016)

Mechanism of action: Blocks the mammalian target of rapamycin pathway to slow the growth and spread of cancer cells

Administration: 10 mg PO taken consistently with or without food and at the same time every day

Side effects: Most common adverse reactions (incidence of 30% or higher) include stomatitis, infections, rash, fatigue, diarrhea, edema, abdominal pain, nausea, fever, asthenia, cough, headache, and decreased appetite.

Nursing considerations: Avoid concomitant use with cytochrome P450 3A4 (CYP3A4) inhibitors or inducers; instruct the patient to limit exposure to sunlight, wear protective clothing, use a sunscreen with a high ultraviolet protection factor (SPF 30 or greater), and avoid tanning beds or sunlamps; advise the patient to take the tablet at the same time each day. It may be taken with or without food; however, if it is taken with food, then it should always be taken with food, and if it is taken without food, then it should always be taken without food.

Lapatinib

Indications: Used in combination with capecitabine for the treatment of patients with advanced or metastatic breast cancer whose tumors overexpress HER2 and who have received prior therapy including an anthracycline, a taxane, and trastuzumab. It also is indicated in combination with letrozole for the treatment of postmenopausal women with hormone receptor–positive metastatic breast cancer that overexpresses the HER2 receptor for whom hormonal therapy is indicated (GlaxoSmithKline, 2014; Polovich et al., 2014).

Mechanism of action: Inhibits ErbB-driven tumor cell growth

Administration: For HER2-positive metastatic breast cancer, give 1,250 mg PO once daily on days 1–21 in combination with capecitabine 2,000 mg/m²/day (administered orally in two doses approximately 12 hours apart) on days 1–14 in a repeating 21-day cycle. For hormone receptor–positive, HER2-positive metastatic breast cancer, give 1,500 mg PO once daily in combination with letrozole.

Side effects: Hepatotoxicity has been observed in clinical trials and postmarketing experience. It may be severe, and deaths have been reported. Most common adverse reactions include diarrhea, palmar-plantar erythrodysesthesia, nausea, rash, vomiting, and fatigue.

Nursing considerations: Lapatinib should be taken at least one hour before or one hour after a meal. When given in combination with capecitabine, take into consideration that capecitabine should be taken with food or within 30 minutes after food.

Modify the dose for cardiac and other toxicities, severe hepatic impairment, and CYP3A4 drug interactions. Monitor liver function tests before initiation of treatment, every four to six weeks during treatment, and as clinically indicated. Confirm normal LVEF before starting therapy and continue evaluations during treatment.

Palbociclib

Indications: Hormone receptor–positive, HER2-negative advanced or metastatic breast cancer in combination with letrozole as initial endocrine-based therapy in postmenopausal women, or fulvestrant in women with disease progression following endocrine therapy (Pfizer Labs, 2016; Polovich et al., 2014)

Mechanism of action: Inhibits cyclin-dependent kinase (CDK) 4 and 6. Cyclin D1 and CDK4/6 are downstream of signaling pathways that lead to cellular proliferation.

Administration: 125 mg capsule PO once daily for 21 consecutive days followed by 7 days off treatment to form a complete cycle of 28 days

Side effects: Pulmonary embolism was reported at a higher rate in patients treated with palbociclib. Common adverse reactions include neutropenia, leukopenia, infections, fatigue, nausea, anemia, stomatitis, headache, diarrhea, thrombocytopenia, constipation, alopecia, vomiting, rash, and decreased appetite.

Nursing considerations: Monitor complete blood count prior to the start of therapy and at the beginning of each cycle, as well as on day 14 of the first two cycles, and as clinically indicated. Monitor patients for signs and symptoms of pulmonary embolism and treat as medically appropriate. Encourage patients to take their dose at approximately the same time each day.

Pertuzumab

Indications: Used in combination with trastuzumab and docetaxel for the treatment of patients with HER2-positive metastatic breast cancer who have not received prior anti-HER2 therapy or chemotherapy for metastatic disease. Also used in combination with trastuzumab and docetaxel in neoadjuvant treatment in patients with HER2-positive, locally advanced, inflammatory, or early-stage breast cancer (either greater than 2 cm in diameter or node positive) (Genentech USA, Inc., 2016c; Polovich et al., 2014).

Mechanism of action: Targets the extracellular dimerization domain (subdomain II) of the HER2 protein and thereby blocks ligand-dependent heterodimerization of HER2 with other HER family members, including EGFR, HER3, and HER4. Inhibition of these signaling pathways can result in cell growth arrest and apoptosis. Pertuzumab also mediates ADCC.

Administration: Initial dose is 840 mg IV infused over 60 minutes, followed every three weeks by a dose of 420 mg IV infused over 30–60 minutes. For neoadjuvant treatment, administer every three weeks for three to six cycles as part of one of the following treatment regimens for early-stage breast cancer:

- Four preoperative cycles of pertuzumab in combination with trastuzumab and docetaxel followed by three postoperative cycles of FEC
- Three preoperative cycles of FEC alone followed by three preoperative cycles of pertuzumab in combination with docetaxel and trastuzumab
- Six preoperative cycles of pertuzumab in combination with docetaxel, carboplatin, and trastuzumab (escalation of docetaxel greater than 75 mg/m^2 is not recommended)

Side effects: Subclinical and clinical cardiac failure manifesting as decreased LVEF and CHF can occur. Most common adverse reactions include fatigue, alopecia, diarrhea, nausea, vomiting, and neutropenia.

Nursing considerations: Evaluate cardiac function prior to and during treatment. Discontinue pertuzumab for a confirmed clinically significant decrease in left ventricular function. Pertuzumab should be discontinued if trastuzumab treatment is discontinued. Dilute with 0.9% sodium chloride injection only. Do not use dextrose (5%) solution.

Trastuzumab

Indications: Adjuvant treatment of HER2-overexpressing, node-positive or node-negative (estrogen receptor or progesterone receptor negative or with one high-risk feature) breast cancer as part of a treatment regimen comprising doxorubicin, cyclophosphamide, and either paclitaxel or docetaxel; in a regimen with docetaxel and carboplatin; or as a single agent following multimodality anthracycline-based therapy. For metastatic breast cancer, it is used in combination with paclitaxel for first-line treatment of HER2-overexpressing metastatic breast cancer or as a single agent for treatment of HER2-overexpressing breast cancer in patients who have received one or more chemotherapy regimens for metastatic disease (Genentech USA, Inc., 2016a; Polovich et al., 2014).

Mechanism of action: Mediates ADCC. Trastuzumab-mediated ADCC has been shown to be preferentially exerted on HER2-overexpressing cancer cells compared with cancer cells that do not overexpress HER2.

Administration: Trastuzumab is administered according to the following doses and schedules:

- Adjuvant treatment during and following paclitaxel, docetaxel, or docetaxel/carboplatin (total of 52 weeks of trastuzumab therapy):
  - Initial dose of 4 mg/kg as an IV infusion over 90 minutes, then 2 mg/kg as an IV infusion over 30 minutes weekly during chemotherapy for the first 12 weeks (paclitaxel or docetaxel) or 18 weeks (docetaxel/carboplatin)

– One week following the last weekly dose of trastuzumab, administer trastuzumab 6 mg/kg as an IV infusion over 30–90 minutes every three weeks.
• Adjuvant treatment as a single agent within three weeks following completion of a multimodality, anthracycline-based chemotherapy regimen (total of 52 weeks of trastuzumab therapy):
  – Initial dose of 8 mg/kg as an IV infusion over 90 minutes
  – Subsequent doses of 6 mg/kg as an IV infusion over 30–90 minutes every three weeks
• For metastatic breast cancer, administer trastuzumab at an initial dose of 8 mg/kg as a 90-minute IV infusion followed by subsequent doses of 6 mg/kg as an IV infusion over 30–90 minutes every three weeks until disease progression.

Side effects: Treatment can result in subclinical and clinical cardiac failure manifesting as CHF and decreased LVEF, with greatest risk when administered concurrently with anthracyclines. Discontinue treatment for anaphylaxis, angioedema, interstitial pneumonitis, or acute respiratory distress syndrome. Trastuzumab can result in serious and fatal pulmonary toxicity. Pulmonary toxicity includes dyspnea, interstitial pneumonitis, pulmonary infiltrates, pleural effusions, noncardiogenic pulmonary edema, pulmonary insufficiency and hypoxia, acute respiratory distress syndrome, and pulmonary fibrosis.

Nursing considerations: Do not substitute trastuzumab for or with ado-trastuzumab emtansine. Do not use dextrose solution for dilution. Evaluate LVEF prior to and during treatment.

Toxicities

Cardiotoxicities

Definition

Cardiotoxicity is a well-recognized adverse event associated with certain chemotherapy and biotherapy agents (Viale & Yamamoto, 2008). Cardiotoxicity can be manifested as myocardial infarction, myocarditis or pericarditis, cardiomyopathy, arrhythmias or changes in cardiac conduction, and hypertension.

Risk Factors

Various chemotherapy and biotherapy agents are risk factors for cardiotoxicity (Thomy & Theobald, 2015). See Table 7-1 for details on treatment-induced cardiotoxicity and the reversibility of the effects. Radiation therapy is also a risk factor. Mediastinal irradiation is widely used for breast cancer, and cardiotoxicity is a critical dose-limiting aspect of radiation therapy. Risk increases with the use of anthracycline-based chemotherapy. Finally, lifestyle factors can create risk, including body mass index, smoking, physical inactivity, alcohol intake, poor diet, hypertension, and diabetes. Nonmodifiable factors include older age at treatment and genetic predisposition for heart disease.

Identification

Early identification and prompt treatment can help reduce the complications from cardiotoxicity (Curigliano et al., 2016; Thomy & Theobald, 2015). Echocardiography (two-dimensional imaging, two-dimensional echocardiogram) is the most widely used technique to monitor cardiac function during and after chemotherapy. LVEF

Table 7-1. Chemotherapy and Biotherapy Agents Associated With Cardiotoxicity

Drug Class	Drug Name	Treatment-Induced Cardiotoxicity	Reversibility
Chemotherapy Agents			
Alkylating agents	Cyclophosphamide	Cardiac decompensation Cardiomyopathy	Irreversible
Antimetabolites	Capecitabine 5-Fluorouracil Gemcitabine	Angina pectoris Arrhythmias Left ventricular dysfunction Myocardial infarction	Reversible
Antitumor antibiotics (anthracyclines)	Doxorubicin Epirubicin	Cardiomyopathy Congestive heart failure	Irreversible
Plant alkaloids (taxanes)	Docetaxel Paclitaxel	Atrioventricular block Heart failure Ischemia Sinus bradycardia Ventricular tachycardia	Reversible
Biotherapy Agents			
Monoclonal antibodies	Ado-trastuzumab emtansine Pertuzumab Trastuzumab	Left ventricular ejection fraction decrease or asymptomatic heart failure	Reversible
Small molecule inhibitors	Lapatinib	Heart failure Hypertension Left ventricular dysfunction Myocardial ischemia	Reversible

Note. From "Cardiotoxicity Related to Anti-Cancer Drug Treatment: A Literature Review," by L.B. Thomy and K. Theobald, 2015, *Australian Journal of Cancer Nursing, 16*(2), p. 5. Copyright 2015 by Cambridge Publishing. Adapted with permission.

is the most commonly accepted parameter of cardiac function. Multigated acquisition scans also can determine LVEF. Known disadvantages include radiation exposure and limited information on cardiac structure and diastolic function. Cardiac biomarkers are reported to be more sensitive and specific for early identification of therapy-induced cardiotoxicity. Troponins are the most cardiac-specific biomarkers of cardiac injury. Brain natriuretic peptide, also called B-type natriuretic peptide, is useful in the diagnosis of heart failure.

Management

Prevention: Cardioprotective agents are used as a preventive measure (Curigliano et al., 2016; Thomy & Theobald, 2015). Dexrazoxane is the preferred agent to reduce anthracycline-related cardiotoxicity. It is recommended for use in patients with metastatic breast cancer who have already received more than 300 mg/m² of doxorubicin. Beta-blockers and angiotensin-converting enzyme inhibitors have been used as cardioprotective agents during therapy with anthracyclines.

Treatment: Beta-blockers and angiotensin-converting enzyme inhibitors have been shown to improve cardiac function in patients with anthracycline-induced left ventricular dysfunction. Periodic monitoring with electrocardiograms and electrolyte panels during treatment should be considered for patients with a history of QT interval prolongation, including those who are taking antiarrhythmics or who have bradycardia or thyroid dysfunction. Monitor and manage hypertension in collaboration with the patient's primary healthcare provider and cardiologist. Consider prophylactic use of low-molecular-weight heparin in patients receiving chemotherapy or antiangiogenic agents.

Cutaneous Toxicities

Definition

Cutaneous toxicities are some of the most frequently reported adverse effects associated with chemotherapy and biotherapy (see Table 7-2). The rapidly dividing cells of the skin are more susceptible to the effects of chemotherapy. Unlike conventional chemotherapy drugs, biotherapy drugs cause cutaneous toxicities because of their direct effect on target molecules present in the skin.

Alopecia

Alopecia occurs with many of the regimens and agents used to treat breast cancer, including cyclophosphamide, anthracyclines, 5-fluorouracil, methotrexate, and tax-

Table 7-2. Chemotherapy and Biotherapy Agents Associated With Cutaneous Toxicities

Drug Class	Drug Name	Treatment-Induced Cutaneous Toxicities
Chemotherapy Agents		
Alkylating agents	Cyclophosphamide Thiotepa	Hyperpigmentation, alopecia, urticarial hypersensitivity, neutrophilic eccrine hidradenitis, porphyria cutanea tarda, and radiation recall
Antimetabolites	Gemcitabine	Maculopapular or bullous reactions
	Capecitabine 5-Fluorouracil	Hand-foot syndrome, photosensitivity, hyperpigmentation, alopecia, stomatitis, inflammation of actinic keratosis, cutaneous lupus, pyogenic granuloma, and granulomatous septal panniculitis
Antitumor antibiotics (anthracyclines)	Doxorubicin	Hand-foot syndrome, follicular rash, intertrigo-like eruption melanotic macules, and radiation recall
Plant alkaloids (taxanes)	Docetaxel Paclitaxel	Taxane-induced hand-foot syndrome, nail changes, alopecia, hypersensitivity, and edema
Plant alkaloids (vinca alkaloids)	Vinblastine	Alopecia, maculopapular rash, erythema multiforme–like lesions, and hand-foot syndrome
Biotherapy Agents		
Small molecule inhibitors (dual kinase inhibitors of EGFR and HER2)	Lapatinib	Papulopustular eruption, xerosis, hair changes, mucositis, and paronychia

Note. Based on information from Macdonald et al., 2015; Reyes-Habito & Roh, 2014.

anes. It can begin as early as seven days after the first chemotherapy dose. Hair loss usually starts on the scalp and progresses to whole body alopecia with continued treatment (Sanborn & Sauer, 2008). Some experts recommend cutting long hair before treatment to minimize the psychological trauma associated with hair loss. Encourage patients to wear head covers, including wigs, hats, or scarves. Hair regrowth happens approximately six weeks after treatment. Biotherapy-associated alopecia is often mild and may cause trichomegaly (curly, thick, long eyelashes), whereas chemotherapy may cause the loss of eyelashes (Peuvrel & Dréno, 2014).

Palmar-Plantar Erythrodysesthesia

Palmar-plantar erythrodysesthesia or acral erythema, more commonly known as hand-foot syndrome, is the development of swelling and formation of erythematous macules on the palms of the hands and the soles of the feet. Blistering and desquamation may be seen and often occurs in areas of pressure or friction and can be painful.

To manage this syndrome, the patient's hands and feet should be keep well moisturized (Sanborn & Sauer, 2008). Instruct the patient to apply emollient before bed and wear cotton gloves and socks to retain moisture. Comfortable, well-fitting shoes are also helpful. If necessary, steroid cream can be applied to affected areas to decrease inflammation (Peuvrel & Dréno, 2014). In severe cases, dose reduction or discontinuation of the causative agent may be necessary.

Paronychia

Paronychia is an infection in the skin causing pain or discharge at the junction of the nail and the lateral subungual fold. This is not as common as skin changes but occurs in approximately 10%–30% of patients (Peuvrel & Dréno, 2014).

Primary treatment is the use of emollient and topical steroids. If this is not effective, semisynthetic tetracyclines can be added. If a suprainfection occurs, a bacterial swab should be completed and appropriate antibiotics should be administered based on culture and sensitivity. To prevent infection, keep nails short, avoid skin trauma, and wear gloves when handling irritants (Peuvrel & Dréno, 2014).

Rash

Acneform rash generally occurs on the face, trunk, and extremities. Skin care is important when agents that cause cutaneous toxicities are being used. Advise patients to limit sun exposure and use sun protection. Avoid skin products containing alcohol, exfoliating agents, and face masks, as they can be irritating.

If an acneform rash occurs, a semisynthetic tetracycline such as doxycycline or minocycline can be started along with a topical steroid cream or clindamycin cream applied to affected areas. If the rash does not respond, oral steroids can be attempted along with a topical agent. If still no response, the dose may need to be modified or the agent may need to be discontinued (Peuvrel & Dréno, 2014).

Gastrointestinal Toxicities

Diarrhea

Diarrhea can occur with the use of chemotherapy and biotherapy agents. Agents that increase the risk for treatment-related diarrhea include capecitabine, eribulin, 5-fluorouracil, and lapatinib. When on capecitabine, 40% of patients reported all grades of diarrhea and 10% reported grade 3–4 diarrhea. Diarrhea is less common in patients using eribulin, with 14%–18% reporting low-grade diarrhea (grades 1–2) (Doherty & Morris, 2015). A 5-fluorouracil–induced diarrhea is dose and schedule dependent and particularly seen with bolus administration. Approximately 1%–2% of the population has a genetic mutation causing dihydropyrimidine dehydrogenase deficiency. This reduces the clearance of fluoropyrimidines, resulting in longer exposure to the agent and increased toxicity (Andreyev et al., 2014). When lapatinib was given in combination with either capecitabine or paclitaxel, 65% of patients reported all grades of diarrhea and 14% reported grade 3–4 diarrhea (Metzger Filho, Saini, Azim, & Awada, 2012).

Management of diarrhea ranges from simple lifestyle changes to medication and, in some cases, hospitalization. According to the latest recommendations from the Oncology Nursing Society (ONS) Putting Evidence Into Practice (PEP) resources, loperamide and octreotide are the two interventions reported as likely be effective (Thorpe et al., 2017). Grade 1–2 diarrhea can be controlled with simple changes in diet. Patients should avoid lactose-containing products and increase fluids to at least 8–10 large glasses of clear fluid. Small, frequent meals are better tolerated than a large volume being put into the gastrointestinal tract. Grade 2 diarrhea requires interruption of all chemotherapy. Loperamide should be administered and continued until the patient is diarrhea-free for 12 hours. Consider hospital admission, octreotide, and IV fluids for grade 3–4 diarrhea. Prophylactic antibiotics may be necessary if diarrhea persists beyond 24 hours or if fever or neutropenia is present (Andreyev et al., 2014).

Mucositis

Mucositis is a common adverse event with the use of conventional chemotherapy and biotherapy agents. Approximately 4% of patients receiving commonly used agents will develop grade 3–4 toxicity (Seiler, Kosse, Loibl, & Jackisch, 2014). Weekly doxorubicin and cyclophosphamide has the highest rate of grade 3–4 toxicity (Seiler et al., 2014). Other chemotherapy agents known to cause oral mucositis include 5-fluorouracil, anthracyclines, and taxanes. Biotherapy agents used in metastatic breast cancer that are known to cause mucositis include lapatinib and palbociclib. Oral mucositis was only noted when lapatinib was used with capecitabine (Metzger Filho et al., 2012). The incidence and severity vary based on treatment- and patient-related factors. Currently, there is no way to predict the occurrence and severity of mucositis.

Based on the ONS PEP resources, interventions that are recommended for the prevention and treatment of mucositis that have strong evidence of efficacy include cryotherapy prior to, during, and after rapid infusions of mucotoxic agents with short half-life, low-level laser therapy in patients receiving stem cell transplantation conditioning or radiation therapy to the oral cavity area, an oral care protocol, palifermin, and sodium bicarbonate (Eilers et al., 2017). A dental examination before treatment and preventive care during cancer therapy are indicated. Mouthwashes with alcohol, peroxide, iodine, and thyme should be avoided, as they will most likely aggravate the symptom. Good mouth care with a soft-bristle toothbrush and floss is encouraged. Chlorhexidine rinse may also be beneficial in the prevention of oral mucositis but not the treatment (Eilers, Harris, Henry, & Johnson, 2014). Patients should avoid smoking, alcohol, spicy foods, acidic foods, or very hot foods. Despite lack of evidence, different oral topical agents such as lidocaine, magic mouthwash, Gelclair™, or Caphosol™ may be effective in reducing pain. Oral intake should also be monitored, as weight loss and dehydration can occur if intake is decreased or restricted because of pain. Soft foods and nutritional supplements may help to ensure adequate calorie consumption. Nystatin can be used with fungal infections, as oral antifungals such as fluconazole may interact with anticancer therapies (Eilers et al., 2014).

Chemotherapy-Induced Nausea and Vomiting

Chemotherapy-induced nausea and vomiting (CINV) is a common adverse event, occurring in 38%–60% of patients receiving chemotherapy. Often, agents may only have low or moderate emetogenic potential as a single agent but, when given in combination with other agents, result in a higher emetogenic potential. Well-known risk factors include female gender, high body mass index, drug dosage, number of cycles, and light alcohol consumption. Risk is higher in patients with a history of motion sickness or nausea during pregnancy. Frequency of emesis is associated with the emetogenicity of agents, with highly emetogenic regimens causing acute emesis in more than 90% of the patients who do not receive effective prophylaxis (National Comprehensive Cancer Network®, 2017a).

Interventions recommended for the prevention and management of CINV include cannabis/cannabinoids, netupitant–palonosetron combination, neurokinin 1 (NK_1) receptor antagonists, serotonin ($5\text{-}HT_3$) receptor antagonists, transdermal granisetron, and a triple-drug regimen consisting of a steroid (dexamethasone), a $5\text{-}HT_3$ receptor antagonist, and an NK_1 receptor antagonist (Lee et al., 2017). Other interventions considered likely to be effective include gabapentin, hypnosis for anticipatory CINV, olanzapine for breakthrough CINV, oral palonosetron, progestins, progressive muscle relaxation and guided imagery, single-agent dexamethasone, and sustained-release granisetron (Lee et al., 2017).

Hepatotoxicity

Definition

As the major site of drug metabolism and detoxification, the liver is vulnerable to the toxic effects of chemotherapy agents. Drug-induced hepatotoxicity is one of the major dose-limiting adverse effects of certain agents. An increased incidence of hepatotoxicity has been reported with the use of combination therapy (Dai et al., 2015).

Risk Factors

Two of the HER2-targeted therapies, ado-trastuzumab emtansine and lapatinib, have been shown to cause hepatotoxicity and include black box warnings for this side effect. In patients treated with ado-trastuzumab emtansine, 28% developed an elevation in the aminotransferase, while 14% developed grade 3 or 4 toxicity (Amiri-Kordestani et al., 2014). Lapatinib had a 37%–53% incidence of elevated ALT and AST, with 2%–6% being grade 3 or 4.

Identification

Obtain baseline hepatic function panel prior to initiation of treatment and monitor liver enzymes during treatment.

Management

In grade 1 or 2 hepatotoxicity, dose modifications may be necessary. Grade 3 or 4 hepatotoxicity warrants treatment interruption until liver function has returned to normal.

Chemotherapy-Related Cognitive Impairment
Definition

Many patients with breast cancer have reported cognitive issues such as attention deficit, memory loss, and executive function impairment after chemotherapy. Studies indicate that 30%–60% of patients with breast cancer will experience cognitive impairment (Player, Mackenzie, Willis, & Loh, 2014). *Chemo brain* and *chemo fog* are terms used by cancer survivors to describe cognitive changes after chemotherapy. Cognitive impairment has been reported in some breast cancer survivors many years after treatment. The pathophysiology is not clear, but cognitive impairment may be due to damage to myelin (Staat & Segatore, 2005).

Risk Factors

No single chemotherapy agent or regimen is known to cause cognitive impairment; however, all agents and regimens have the potential. Several studies have noted that cognitive changes are more prevalent with an increase in the number of chemotherapy cycles (Staat & Segatore, 2005).

Often, patients experience fatigue, psychological stress, and anxiety that can complicate cognitive functioning. In one study, a strong correlation existed between self-perceived cognition loss and objective scores by neuropsychological testing (Schagen & Wefel, 2013).

Identification

Baseline neuropsychological testing becomes increasingly important as patients with cancer live longer. The majority of neuropsychological studies have demonstrated cognitive decline in patients who received chemotherapy compared to non-cancer controls (Schagen & Wefel, 2013).

Management

Cognitive training provided to individuals in a group setting is the only intervention listed as likely to be effective on the ONS PEP resource page (Jansen, Von Ah, Allen, Merriman, & Myers, 2017). A review of the literature shows that medicinal treatments are ineffective; restorative and exercise treatments have mixed results; and cognitive therapy has had success in various cognitive areas. Another study looked at different methods to assist with cognitive changes, which included taking notes using a diary, smartphone, or calendar; participating in regular exercise and relaxation sessions; allowing another person to assist with appointment scheduling; recognizing limitations on a daily basis; completing Sudoku puzzles; and participating in artistic activities (Morean, O'Dwyer, & Cherney, 2015). Getting enough sleep can also help with cognitive function. Acupuncture may also be beneficial because it dilates cerebral blood vessels, improving circulation and oxygenation to the brain. Computerized cognitive training may prove effective in the treatment of cognitive changes due to chemotherapy (Staat & Segatore, 2005).

Pulmonary Toxicities

Definition

Pulmonary toxicity is a rare complication of chemotherapy and biotherapy and includes interstitial pneumonitis, infectious pneumonia, diffuse alveolar hemorrhage, and respiratory failure requiring ventilatory support.

Risk Factors

Pulmonary toxicities can be seen in approximately 10% of patients receiving chemotherapy and often are associated with high-dose regimens (Chi et al., 2012). Dyspnea was apparent in 25% of patients treated with gemcitabine; however, serious pulmonary toxicity is much less common (Chi et al., 2012). Docetaxel can cause pulmonary toxicity, which is thought to be a delayed hypersensitivity reaction. Paclitaxel has been associated with interstitial pneumonitis. Weekly doses may increase the risk of interstitial pneumonitis when compared to every-three-weeks dosing schedules (Omarini, Thanopoulou, & Johnston, 2014). Although rare (1%), pulmonary toxicities, specifically acute interstitial pneumonitis and fibrotic lung disease, have been noted with the use of cyclophosphamide (Omarini et al., 2014). Anthracyclines can cause pulmonary toxicities when given with other chemotherapy agents. Vinorelbine is associated with pneumonitis and interstitial pneumonia when given with other chemotherapy agents. Acute respiratory infusion reactions are the most common trastuzumab-related pulmonary toxicity. This is rare complication (0.3%) that usually occurs during or shortly after the first infusion (Omarini et al., 2014). Interstitial pneumonitis has also been reported, yet most cases occurred after taxane administration with trastuzumab so it is difficult to discern if trastuzumab is the real offending agent. Even when lapatinib is given in combination with capecitabine, lapatinib-induced pulmonary toxicity occurs in less than 1% of the time (Omarini et al., 2014). Preexisting pulmonary disease predisposes an individual to the development of pulmonary complications during treatment.

Identification

The diagnosis of chemotherapy-induced pulmonary toxicity can be difficult to confirm. The mode of onset and timing of clinical manifestations are highly variable—they may occur during the initial treatment, after subsequent cycles, or years after treatment. High-resolution computed tomography may reveal ground-glass opacities, usually bilateral. Bronchoscopic or surgical lung biopsy usually does not provide specific findings (Ryu, 2010).

Management

Management of chemotherapy-induced pulmonary toxicity usually includes discontinuing the offending drug and administering corticosteroid therapy either orally or intravenously (Ryu, 2010).

Summary

Recent advances have led to more personalization of systemic therapy for breast cancer. Systemic therapy can be given in multiple settings, including neoadjuvant, adjuvant, and palliative care settings. Research continues to improve existing therapies and identify better treatment options with fewer side effects. Nurses must remain current in their knowledge of these agents, exercise caution with their administration, be proactive in managing their side effects, and provide the necessary patient education. Multiple combinations of agents are possible, and patients diagnosed with breast cancer need individualized education on the purpose of the agents, the potential side effects, and the management of side effects.

References

Amiri-Kordestani, L., Blumenthal, G.M., Xu, Q.C., Zhang, L., Tang, S.W., Ha, L., ... Cortazar, P. (2014). FDA approval: Ado-trastuzumab emtansine for the treatment of patients with HER2-positive metastatic breast cancer. *Clinical Cancer Research, 20,* 4436–4441. doi:10.1158/1078-0432.CCR-14-0012

Anampa, J., Makower, D., & Sparano, J.A. (2015). Progress in adjuvant chemotherapy for breast cancer: An overview. *BMC Medicine, 13,* 195. doi:10.1186/s12916-015-0439-8

Andreyev, J., Ross, P., Donnellan, C., Lennan, E., Leonard, P., Waters, C., ... Ferry, D. (2014). Guidance on the management of diarrhoea during cancer chemotherapy. *Lancet Oncology, 15,* e447–e460. doi:10.1016/S1470-2045(14)70006-3

Baxter Healthcare Corp. (2013). *Cyclophosphamide* [Package insert]. Deerfield, IL: Author.

Bedford Laboratories. (2012). *Vinblastine sulfate* [Package insert]. Bedford, OH: Author.

Bedford Laboratories. (2014). *Adriamycin® (doxorubicin)* [Package insert]. Bedford, OH: Author.

Bonadonna, G., Brusamolino, E., Valagussa, P., Rossi, A., Brugnatelli, L., Brambilla, C., ... Veronesi, U. (1976). Combination chemotherapy as an adjuvant treatment in operable breast cancer. *New England Journal of Medicine, 294,* 405–410. doi:10.1056/NEJM197602192940801

Bristol-Myers Squibb Co. (2011). *Taxol® (paclitaxel)* [Package insert]. Princeton, NJ: Author.

Bristol-Myers Squibb Co. (2016). *Ixempra® (ixabepilone)* [Package insert]. Princeton, NJ: Author.

Celgene Corp. (2015). *Abraxane (paclitaxel protein-bound)* [Package insert]. Summit, NJ: Author.

Chi, D.-C., Brogan, F., Turenne, I., Zelonis, S., Schwartz, L., & Saif, M.W. (2012). Gemcitabine-induced pulmonary toxicity. *Anticancer Research, 32,* 4147–4149. Retrieved from http://ar.iiarjournals.org/content/32/9/4147.long

Citron, M.L., Berry, D.A., Cirrincione, C., Hudis, C., Winer, E.P., Gradishar, W.J., ... Norton, L. (2003). Randomized trial of dose-dense versus conventionally scheduled and sequential versus concurrent combination chemotherapy as postoperative adjuvant treatment of node-positive primary breast cancer: First report of Intergroup Trial C9741/Cancer and Leukemia Group B Trial 9741. *Journal of Clinical Oncology, 21,* 1431–1439. doi:10.1200/JCO.2003.09.081

Curigliano, G., Cardinale, D., Dent, S., Criscitiello, C., Aseyev, O., Lenihan, D., & Cipolla, C.M. (2016). Cardiotoxicity of anticancer treatments: Epidemiology, detection, and management. *CA: A Cancer Journal for Clinicians, 66,* 309–325. doi:10.3322/caac.21341

Dai, C., Ma, S., Wang, F., Zhao, H., Wu, X., Huang, Z., ... Fu, L. (2015). Lapatinib promotes the incidence of hepatotoxicity by increasing chemotherapeutic agent accumulation in hepatocytes. *Oncotarget, 6,* 17738–17752. doi:10.18632/oncotarget.3921

Doherty, M.K., & Morris, P.G. (2015). Eribulin for the treatment of metastatic breast cancer: An update on its safety and efficacy. *International Journal of Women's Health, 7,* 47–58. doi:10.2147/IJWH.S74462

Eilers, J.G., Asakura, Y., Blecher, C.S., Burgoon, D., Chiffelle, R., Ciccolini, K., ... Valinski, S. (2017, May 10). ONS PEP resource: Mucositis. Retrieved from https://www.ons.org/practice-resources/pep/mucositis

Eilers, J.G., Harris, D., Henry, K., & Johnson, L.A. (2014). Evidence-based interventions for cancer treatment-related mucositis: Putting evidence into practice. *Clinical Journal of Oncology Nursing, 18*(6, Suppl. 3), 80–96. doi:10.1188/14.CJON.S3.80-96

Eisai Inc. (2016). *Halaven® (eribulin mesylate)* [Package insert]. Woodcliff Lake, NJ: Author.

Eli Lilly and Co. (1996). *Gemzar® (gemcitabine for injection)* [Package insert]. Indianapolis, IN: Author.

Fisher, B., Brown, A.M., Dimitrov, N.V., Poisson, R., Redmond, C., Margolese, R.G., ... Kardinal, C.G. (1990). Two months of doxorubicin-cyclophosphamide with and without interval reinduction therapy compared with 6 months of cyclophosphamide, methotrexate, and fluorouracil in positive-node breast cancer patients with tamoxifen-nonresponsive tumors: Results from the National Surgical Adjuvant Breast and Bowel Project B-15. *Journal of Clinical Oncology, 8,* 1483–1496. doi:10.1200/JCO.1990.8.9.1483

French Adjuvant Study Group. (2001). Benefit of a high-dose epirubicin regimen in adjuvant chemotherapy for node-positive breast cancer patients with poor prognostic factors: 5-year follow-up results of French Adjuvant Study Group 05 randomized trial. *Journal of Clinical Oncology, 19,* 602–611. doi:10.1200/JCO.2001.19.3.602

Frye, D.K. (2009). Capecitabine-based combination therapy for breast cancer: Implications for nurses. *Oncology Nursing Forum, 36,* 105–113. doi:10.1188/09.ONF.105-113

Genentech USA, Inc. (2015). *Xeloda® (capecitabine)* [Package insert]. South San Francisco, CA: Author.

Genentech USA, Inc. (2016a). *Herceptin® (trastuzumab)* [Package insert]. South San Francisco, CA: Author.

Genentech USA, Inc. (2016b). *Kadcyla® (ado-trastuzumab emtansine)* [Package insert]. South San Francisco, CA: Author.

Genentech USA, Inc. (2016c). *Perjeta® (pertuzumab)* [Package insert]. South San Francisco, CA: Author.

Gensia Sicor Pharmaceuticals, Inc. (1999). *Fluorouracil* [Package insert]. Irvine, CA: Author.

GlaxoSmithKline. (2014). *Tykerb® (lapatinib)* [Package insert]. Research Triangle Park, NC: Author.

Haddad, T.C., & Goetz, M.P. (2015). Landscape of neoadjuvant therapy for breast cancer. *Annals of Surgical Oncology, 22,* 1408–1415. doi:10.1245/s10434-015-4405-7

Henderson, I.C., Berry, D.A., Demetri, G.D., Cirrincione, C.T., Goldstein, L.J., Martino, S., … Norton, L. (2003). Improved outcomes from adding sequential paclitaxel but not from escalating doxorubicin dose in an adjuvant chemotherapy regimen for patients with node-positive primary breast cancer. *Journal of Clinical Oncology, 21,* 976–983. doi:10.1200/JCO.2003.02.063

Jansen, C.E., Von Ah, D., Allen, D.H., Merriman, J.D., & Myers, J.S. (2017, April 3). ONS PEP resource: Cognitive impairment. Retrieved from https://www.ons.org/practice-resources/pep/cognitive-impairment

Lee, J., Cherwin, C., Czaplewski, L.M., Dabbour, R., Doumit, M., Lewis, C., … Whiteside, S. (2017, April 14). ONS PEP resource: Chemotherapy-induced nausea and vomiting—Adult. Retrieved from https://www.ons.org/practice-resources/pep/chemotherapy-induced-nausea-and-vomiting/chemotherapy-induced-nausea-and

Levine, M.N., Bramwell, V.H., Pritchard, K.I., Norris, B.D., Shepherd, L.E., Abu-Zahra, H., … Tu, D. (1998). Randomized trial of intensive cyclophosphamide, epirubicin, and fluorouracil chemotherapy compared with cyclophosphamide, methotrexate, and fluorouracil in premenopausal women with node-positive breast cancer. National Cancer Institute of Canada Clinical Trials Group. *Journal of Clinical Oncology, 16,* 2651–2658. doi:10.1200/JCO.1998.16.8.2651

Macdonald, J.B., Macdonald, B., Golitz, L.E., LoRusso, P., & Sekulic, A. (2015). Cutaneous adverse effects of targeted therapies: Part I: Inhibitors of the cellular membrane. *Journal of the American Academy of Dermatology, 72,* 203–218. doi:10.1016/j.jaad.2014.07.032

Martin, M., Pienkowski, T., Mackey, J., Pawlicki, M., Guastalla, J.-P., Weaver, C., … Vogel, C. (2005). Adjuvant docetaxel for node-positive breast cancer. *New England Journal of Medicine, 352,* 2302–2313. doi:10.1056/NEJMoa043681

Martin, M., Villar, A., Sole-Calvo, A., Gonzalez, R., Massuti, B., Lizon, J., … Diaz-Rubio, E. (2003). Doxorubicin in combination with fluorouracil and cyclophosphamide (I.V. FAC regimen, day 1, 21) versus methotrexate in combination with fluorouracil and cyclophosphamide (I.V. CMF regimen, day 1, 21) as adjuvant chemotherapy for operable breast cancer: A study by the GEICAM group. *Annals of Oncology, 14,* 833–842. doi:10.1093/annonc/mdg260

Metzger Filho, O., Saini, K.S., Azim, H.A., Jr., & Awada, A. (2012). Prevention and management of major side effects of targeted agents in breast cancer. *Critical Reviews in Oncology/Hematology, 84*(Suppl. 1), e79–e85. doi:10.1016/j.critrevonc.2010.07.014

Morean, D.F., O'Dwyer, L., & Cherney, L.R. (2015). Therapies for cognitive deficits associated with chemotherapy for breast cancer: A systematic review of objective outcomes. *Archives of Physical Medicine and Rehabilitation, 96,* 1880–1897. doi:10.1016/j.apmr.2015.05.012

National Comprehensive Cancer Network. (2017a). *NCCN Clinical Practice Guidelines in Oncology (NCCN®): Antiemesis* [v.2.2017]. Retrieved from http://www.nccn.org/professionals/physician_gls/pdf/antiemesis.pdf

National Comprehensive Cancer Network. (2017b). *NCCN Clinical Practice Guidelines in Oncology (NCCN®): Breast cancer* [v.2.2017]. Retrieved from https://www.nccn.org/professionals/physician_gls/pdf/breast.pdf

Novartis Pharmaceuticals Corp. (2016). *Afinitor® (everolimus)* [Package insert]. East Hanover, NJ: Author.

Omarini, C., Thanopoulou, E., & Johnston, S.R. (2014). Pneumonitis and pulmonary fibrosis associated with breast cancer treatments. *Breast Cancer Research and Treatment, 146,* 245–258. doi:10.1007/s10549-014-3016-5

Peuvrel, L., & Dréno, B. (2014). Dermatological toxicity associated with targeted therapies in cancer: Optimal management. *American Journal of Clinical Dermatology, 15,* 425–444. doi:10.1007/s40257-014-0088-2

Pfizer Labs. (2016). *Ibrance® (palbociclib)* [Package insert]. New York, NY: Author.

Pharmacia & Upjohn Co. (2011). *Ellence® (epirubicin hydrochloride injection)* [Package insert]. New York, NY: Author.

Player, L., Mackenzie, L., Willis, K., & Loh, S.Y. (2014). Women's experiences of cognitive changes or 'chemobrain' following treatment for breast cancer: A role for occupational therapy? *Australian Occupational Therapy Journal, 61,* 230–240. doi:10.1111/1440-1630.12113

Polovich, M., Olsen, M., & LeFebvre, K.B. (Eds.). (2014). *Chemotherapy and biotherapy guidelines and recommendations for practice* (4th ed.). Pittsburgh, PA: Oncology Nursing Society.

Poole, C.J., Earl, H.M., Hiller, L., Dunn, J.A., Bathers, S., Grieve, R.J., ... Twelves, C.J. (2006). Epirubicin and cyclophosphamide, methotrexate, and fluorouracil as adjuvant therapy for early breast cancer. *New England Journal of Medicine, 355,* 1851–1862. doi:10.1056/NEJMoa052084

Reyes-Habito, C.M., & Roh, E.K. (2014). Cutaneous reactions to chemotherapeutic drugs and targeted therapies for cancer: Part I. Conventional chemotherapeutic drugs. *Journal of the American Academy of Dermatology, 71,* 203.e1–203.e12. doi:10.1016/j.jaad.2014.04.014

Ryu, J.H. (2010). Chemotherapy-induced pulmonary toxicity in lung cancer patients. *Journal of Thoracic Oncology, 5,* 1313–1314. doi:10.1097/JTO.0b013e3181e9dbb9

Sanborn, R.E., & Sauer, D.A. (2008). Cutaneous reactions to chemotherapy: Commonly seen, less described, little understood. *Dermatologic Clinics, 26,* 103–119. doi:10.1016/j.det.2007.08.006

Sanofi-Aventis U.S. LLC. (2010). *Taxotere® (docetaxel)* [Package insert]. Bridgewater, NJ: Author.

Santa-Maria, C.A., Camp, M., Cimino-Mathews, A., Harvey, S., Wright, J., & Stearns, V. (2015). Neoadjuvant therapy for early-stage breast cancer: Current practice, controversies, and future directions. *Oncology, 29,* 828–838.

Santa-Maria, C.A., & Gradishar, W.J. (2015). Changing treatment paradigms in metastatic breast cancer: Lessons learned. *JAMA Oncology, 1,* 528–534. doi:10.1001/jamaoncol.2015.1198

Schagen, S.B., & Wefel, J.S. (2013). Chemotherapy-related changes in cognitive functioning. *EJC Supplements, 11,* 225–232. doi:10.1016/j.ejcsup.2013.07.007

Seiler, S., Kosse, J., Loibl, S., & Jackisch, C. (2014). Adverse event management of oral mucositis in patients with breast cancer. *Breast Care, 9,* 232–237. doi:10.1159/000366246

Staat, K., & Segatore, M. (2005). The phenomenon of chemo brain. *Clinical Journal of Oncology Nursing, 9,* 713–721. doi:10.1188/05.CJON.713-721

Thomy, L.B., & Theobald, K. (2015). Cardiotoxicity related to anti-cancer drug treatment: A literature review. *Australian Journal of Cancer Nursing, 16*(2), 4–10.

Thorpe, D.M., Byar, K.L., Conley, S., Drapek, L., Held-Warmkessel, J., Ramsdell, M.J., ... Wolles, B. (2017, February 27). ONS PEP resource: Chemotherapy-induced diarrhea. Retrieved from https://www.ons.org/practice-resources/pep/diarrhea/chemotherapy-induced-diarrhea

Verrill, M. (2009). Chemotherapy for early-stage breast cancer: A brief history. *British Journal of Cancer, 101*(Suppl. 1), S2–S5. doi:10.1038/sj.bjc.6605268

Viale, P.H., & Yamamoto, D.S. (2008). Cardiovascular toxicity associated with cancer treatment. *Clinical Journal of Oncology Nursing, 12,* 627–638. doi:10.1188/08.CJON.627-638

West-Ward Pharmaceuticals. (2015). *Thiotepa* [Package insert]. Eatontown, NJ: Author.

Xanodyne Pharmaceuticals, Inc. (2003). *Methotrexate sodium* [Package insert]. Florence, KY: Author.

CHAPTER 8

Endocrine Therapy

Patricia Gordon, MSN, CRNP, NP-C, Susan Beikman, MSN, CRNP, AOCNP®,
and Mary Ann Zalewski, MSN, CRNP, AOCNP®

Introduction

Approximately 75%–80% of all breast cancers are hormone sensitive, meaning the tumor is responsive to estrogen and/or progesterone produced by the body (in both males and females) (Williams & Harris, 2014). This is an important prognostic factor for survival and recurrence of breast cancer (Bender et al., 2014). Hormone-sensitive breast cancers have a better prognosis than hormone-negative breast cancers, with lower mortality rates. For hormone-positive breast cancers, the patient is eligible for endocrine therapy to suppress the growth of the cancer or prevent development of a second breast cancer. The goal of endocrine therapy is to reduce the availability of estrogen to the estrogen receptor (ER)-positive breast cancer cell. This is achieved by the blocking of ERs on breast cancer cells, suppression of estrogen synthesis, or ovarian ablation or suppression. These therapies have evolved over time but remain an important part of treatment of any hormone-positive breast cancer. Table 8-1 illustrates the types of endocrine therapies, specific drugs, and common side effects. The general classes include selective estrogen receptor modulators (SERMs), selective estrogen receptor downregulators, and aromatase inhibitors (AIs).

Classes of Antiestrogen Hormone Therapy

Selective Estrogen Receptor Modulators

Raloxifene

Indications: Prevention only in postmenopausal women (not studied in premenopausal women); never studied for use in patients with breast cancer (Visvanathan et al., 2013)

Mechanism of action: Raloxifene is a benzothiophene derivative that binds to the ER, similar to tamoxifen (Vogel & Bevers, 2003). This binding results in activation of estrogenic pathways in some tissues (agonism) and blockade of estrogenic pathways in others (antagonism). Its agonistic activity at some receptors and antagonistic activ-

---

Table 8-1. Endocrine Therapies Used in Breast Cancer Treatment

Types of Endocrine Therapies	Drugs	Common Side Effects
Selective estrogen receptor modulator	Tamoxifen (Nolvadex®, various generic) Toremifene (Fareston®) Raloxifene (Evista®, various generic)	Hot flashes, vaginal discharge, endometrial changes, menstrual irregularities, thromboembolic events
Selective estrogen receptor downregulator	Fulvestrant (Faslodex®)	Hot flashes, arthralgias, injection site pain
Aromatase inhibitor	Anastrozole (Arimidex®, various generic) Letrozole (Femara®, various generic) Exemestane (Aromasin®)	Hot flashes, arthralgias, bone loss, vaginal dryness

Note. Based on information from Burstein et al., 2016; National Cancer Institute, 2017; Reinbolt et al., 2015; Rydén et al., 2016; Vogel & Bevers, 2003; Vogel et al., 2006; Williams & Harris, 2014.

---

ity at others makes it a SERM (see Figure 8-1). Raloxifene works by blocking estrogen in the breast tissue of women at increased risk by preventing the development of tumors that require estrogen to grow. Raloxifene appears to act as an estrogen agonist in bone.

Administration: 60 mg PO per day

Side effects: Hot flashes, leg cramps, and deep vein thrombosis

Nursing considerations: Contraindicated in patients with prior clotting event or high risk for a clotting event, a history of coronary artery disease, atrial fibrillation, factor V Leiden, lupus anticoagulant, or known sensitivity, and women who are pregnant or considering pregnancy

History: The Multiple Outcomes of Raloxifene Evaluation (MORE) trial demonstrated effectiveness in 1998, but raloxifene was not approved by the U.S. Food and Drug Administration (FDA) until following the Study of Tamoxifen and Raloxifene (STAR) trial in 2005. It is used in women who meet criteria to be considered high risk based on family history or high-risk pathology (atypia, lobular neoplasia, Gail score higher than 1.66% for five-year risk) (Vogel et al., 2006).

Tamoxifen

Indications: Prevention, neoadjuvant and adjuvant therapy, and treatment of metastatic breast cancer in premenopausal or postmenopausal women

Mechanism of action: Triphenylethylene has been shown to be tissue specific and disease specific and binds to ERs (Vogel & Bevers, 2003). Tamoxifen (a derivative of this chemical) was then developed. Breast tissue has ERs, and tamoxifen blocks the receptors, so estrogen cannot be introduced into the tissue (see Figure 8-2).

Administration: 20 mg PO per day or 10 mg PO twice per day. Initial use of 5 years, with 10 years recommended in premenopausal women with invasive breast cancer or a combination of tamoxifen and an AI (if postmenopausal) for a total of 10 years (Burstein et al., 2014).

Figure 8-1. Selective Estrogen Receptor Modulators (SERMs)

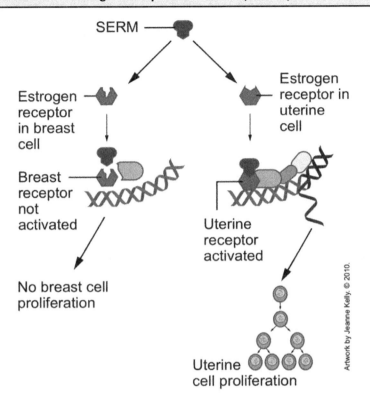

In working on the development of antiestrogens, scientists have made a somewhat surprising discovery. Some drugs that block the action of estrogen in certain tissues actually can mimic the action of estrogen in other tissues. Such selectivity is made possible by the fact that the estrogen receptors of different target tissues vary in chemical structure. These differences allow estrogen-like drugs to interact in different ways with the estrogen receptors of different tissues. Such drugs are called selective estrogen receptor modulators, or SERMs, because they selectively stimulate or inhibit the estrogen receptors of different target tissues. For example, a SERM might inhibit the estrogen receptor found in breast cells but activate the estrogen receptor present in uterine endometrial cells. A SERM of this type would inhibit cell proliferation in breast cells, but stimulate the proliferation of uterine endometrial cells.

Note. Figure courtesy of National Cancer Institute. Illustration created by Jeanne Kelly.

Side effects: Hot flashes, increased risk of endometrial cancer (see Table 8-1), cataracts, vaginal discharge, and thromboembolic events, including stroke, deep vein thrombosis, transient ischemic attack, and pulmonary embolism

Nursing considerations: Contraindicated in patients with known thromboembolic events or high risk for thromboembolic events, patients currently using hormonal contraception or hormone replacement, and women who are pregnant or considering pregnancy. Tamoxifen is effective in the prevention of breast cancer in women at high risk for the disease. This includes women with a family history of breast cancer or high-risk pathology including atypical hyperplasia or lobular neoplasia (lobular carcinoma in situ) (Visvanathan et al., 2013). Prevention trials in the 1990s, the National Surgical Adjuvant Breast and Bowel Project P-1 trial (Fisher et

Figure 8-2. Tamoxifen and Cancer

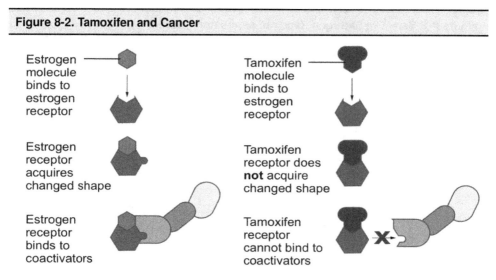

Estrogen molecule binds to estrogen receptor

Estrogen receptor acquires changed shape

Estrogen receptor binds to coactivators

Tamoxifen molecule binds to estrogen receptor

Tamoxifen receptor does **not** acquire changed shape

Tamoxifen receptor cannot bind to coactivators

The first selective estrogen receptor modulator to be investigated extensively for its anticancer properties was a drug called tamoxifen. Tamoxifen blocks the action of estrogen in breast tissue by binding to the estrogen receptors of breast cells, thereby preventing estrogen molecules from binding to these receptors. But unlike what occurs when estrogen binds to its receptor, tamoxifen binds but does not change the receptor's shape, so coactivators are unable to bind. As a result, the genes that stimulate cell proliferation cannot be activated. By interfering with estrogen receptors in this way, tamoxifen blocks the ability of estrogen to stimulate the proliferation of breast cells.

Note. Figure courtesy of National Cancer Institute. Illustration created by Jeanne Kelly.

al., 1998) as well as the STAR trials, showed its role in prevention. Overall risk reduction was approximately 50%. Women aged 35 years and older and with a five-year Gail model score of 1.67% or greater are eligible for tamoxifen.

History: Tamoxifen has been used since the 1970s to block estrogen in ER-positive breast cancer. Recent research (the Adjuvant Tamoxifen: Longer Against Shorter [ATLAS] and Adjuvant Tamoxifen—To Offer More? [aTTom] trials) has shown 10 years of adjuvant therapy to be superior to 5 years of therapy (Williams & Harris, 2014).

Toremifene

Indications: Treatment of metastatic breast cancer in postmenopausal women (Kyowa Kirin, Inc., n.d.)

Mechanism of action: Binds to the ER (see Figure 8-2) as a nonsteroidal antiestrogen triphenylethylene derivative (Gerken, 2004)

Administration: 60 mg PO per day

Side effects: QT prolongation and other arrhythmias, cataracts, dry eyes, and elevated liver function tests

Nursing considerations: Contraindicated in patients with prior clotting events or increased risk of a clotting event, history of coronary artery disease, atrial fibrillations, factor V Leiden, lupus anticoagulant, QT prolongation, known sensitivity to the drug or its components, impaired renal or liver function, or endometrial hyperplasia, and in women who are considering pregnancy (Gerken, 2004)

History: Toremifene was approved in the 1990s (Vogel, Johnston, Capers, & Braccia, 2014). Three older clinical studies demonstrated efficacy and safety comparable to that of tamoxifen in postmenopausal women with ER-positive or ER-unknown metastatic breast cancer (Gershanovich et al., 1997; Hayes et al., 1995; Hertz, McLeod, & Irvin, 2012).

Selective Estrogen Receptor Downregulator

Fulvestrant

Indications: Treatment of locally advanced or metastatic breast cancer in postmenopausal women after AI therapy

Mechanism of action: Fulvestrant is a pure ER antagonist that works by downregulating the ER, causing antiproliferative activity and apoptosis. *Downregulating* means the drug is actually decreasing the number of ERs. The drug binds, blocks, and increases degradation (Robertson, 2007).

Administration: 250 mg intramuscularly in each buttock (500 mg total) on days 0, 14, and 28 and monthly thereafter. This dosing is based on the Comparison of Faslodex in Recurrent or Metastatic Breast Cancer (CONFIRM) trial, which revealed that the 500 mg dose significantly improved time to progression and overall survival compared to the 250 mg monthly dose. Overall, a 20% relative risk reduction was seen. It also is used in combination with exemestane (AstraZeneca Pharmaceuticals, 2016).

Side effects: Injection site pain, nausea, and bone pain

Nursing considerations: Contraindicated in patients with liver problems, blood clotting disorder, or decreased platelets, and women who are pregnant or breastfeeding

History: In the Fulvestrant First-Line Study Comparing Endocrine Treatments (FIRST) clinical trial, fulvestrant was found to have overall survival benefit and time to progression over anastrozole (Williams & Harris, 2014). In the North American study, Osborne et al. (2002) concluded that fulvestrant was at least as effective as anastrozole, with efficacy endpoints slightly favoring fulvestrant. Fulvestrant represents an additional treatment option for postmenopausal women with advanced breast cancer whose disease has progressed on tamoxifen therapy.

Aromatase Inhibitors

Aromatase is the enzyme that synthesizes estrogen. Because breast and ovarian cancers require estrogen to grow, AIs are used to either block the production of estrogen or to block the action of estrogen on receptors. The primary source of estrogen is the ovaries in premenopausal women and the peripheral tissues in postmenopausal women. AIs block the aromatase enzyme, which catalyzes the final step in estrogen production from the adrenal androgen, and aromatization is suppressed by 98%. AIs are used in postmenopausal women (natural menopause or ovarian suppression). They have been found to be superior to tamoxifen in postmenopausal women (Rydén, Arnlind, Vitols, Höistad, & Ahlgren, 2016). Three AIs are commonly prescribed: anastrozole, exemestane, and letrozole. The two types of AIs are nonsteroidal and steroidal. Nonsteroidal AIs bind noncovalently and reversibly to the aromatase protein. Steroidal AIs bind covalently (molecular bond) and irreversibly.

Anastrozole

Indications: Neoadjuvant therapy (first-line treatment of breast cancer, prior to surgery or chemotherapy), adjuvant therapy (following primary treatment with chemotherapy and/or surgery), and metastatic breast cancer (even if prior AI used during primary breast cancer treatment)

Mechanism of action: Acts as a nonsteroidal AI

Administration: 1 mg per day for 5–10 years

Side effects: Arthralgias, bone loss, hot flashes, myalgias, vaginal dryness, decreased libido, hair thinning, depression, mood swings, hyperlipidemia, hypertension, and carpal tunnel syndrome

Nursing considerations: Contraindicated in patients who are pregnant, premenopausal women, and patients with hypersensitivity, ischemic heart disease, osteopenia, or osteoporosis

History: Anastrozole received FDA approval in 1996 for postmenopausal breast cancer after progression on tamoxifen. The Arimidex, Tamoxifen, Alone or in Combination (ATAC) trial showed superiority of anastrozole versus tamoxifen in the adjuvant setting for postmenopausal women. Disease-free survival for anastrozole was 89.4% compared to 87.4% with tamoxifen (National Comprehensive Cancer Network® [NCCN®], 2017).

Exemestane

Indications: Neoadjuvant and adjuvant therapy, metastatic breast cancer, and prevention (in women never diagnosed with breast cancer but defined as high risk based on family and personal history)

Mechanism of action: Exemestane is a steroidal aromatase inactivator. Steroidal AIs also inactivate the aromatase enzyme, but they bind irreversibly, as opposed to the nonsteroidal agents, whose activity is reversible. However, both classes are very active in suppressing the enzymatic activity of aromatase by 97%–99%.

Administration: 25 mg PO daily

Side effects: Hot flashes, bone loss, arthralgias and myalgias, and vaginal dryness

Nursing considerations: Contraindicated in patients with known hypersensitivity to the drug or its components, premenopausal women, pregnant women, and patients with osteoporosis

History: Exemestane received FDA approval in October 2005 for adjuvant endocrine therapy in postmenopausal, ER-positive breast cancer after completion of two to three years of tamoxifen. The National Cancer Institute of Canada Clinical Trials Group Mammary Prevention (MAP.3) trial showed prevention benefit in postmenopausal high-risk women (Williams & Harris, 2014). The relative risk reduction was approximately 65%.

Letrozole

Indications: Neoadjuvant and adjuvant therapy, metastatic breast cancer

Mechanism of action: Acts as a nonsteroidal AI

Administration: 2.5 mg PO daily

Side effects: Hot flashes, bone loss, arthralgias and myalgias, vaginal dryness, decreased libido, hair thinning, carpal tunnel syndrome, hypertension, hypercholesterolemia, depression, and mood swings

Nursing considerations: Contraindicated in patients with severe liver disease, increased cardiovascular event risk, osteoporosis, or abnormal liver function tests, and in women who are pregnant, breast-feeding, or premenopausal

History: Letrozole received FDA approval in December 2005 for ER-positive early-stage breast cancer in postmenopausal women. The Breast International Group 1-98 (BIG 1-98) trial showed letrozole to be superior to tamoxifen alone. Disease-free survival was 84% with letrozole compared to 81.4% with tamoxifen (NCCN, 2017).

Ovarian Ablation and Suppression Therapies

Ablation can either be permanent, through surgical oophorectomy or ovarian irradiation, or temporary, through the use of medications. Patients with higher-risk breast cancer should receive ovarian suppression (Burstein et al., 2016). Higher-risk women are defined as premenopausal women younger than age 35, women who have received chemotherapy, women with larger tumors, and women with positive lymph nodes.

Goserelin

Indications: Ovarian suppression for premenopausal, ER-positive females with breast cancer (adjuvant, neoadjuvant) with endocrine therapy

Mechanism of action: Goserelin is a luteinizing hormone–releasing hormone (LHRH) agonist that suppresses luteinizing hormone. Luteinizing hormone is associated with ovarian stimulation in women and testosterone production in men. In women with breast cancer, goserelin works by telling the brain to stop the production of both luteinizing hormone and follicle-stimulating hormone, thereby stopping the ovaries from making estrogen. Ovarian function may resume once the medication is stopped.

Administration: 3.6 mg every 4 weeks or 10.8 mg every 12 weeks by injection of a subcutaneous cylinder in the abdomen. The biodegradable cylinder by which the medication is delivered was developed to allow for a continuous release of goserelin, resulting in a suppression of the luteinizing hormone (or testosterone) over 4 or 12 weeks. It is recommended as monthly injections to reliably suppress estrogen levels (NCCN, 2017).

Side effects: Hot flashes, night sweats, bone loss, vaginal dryness, headache, nausea, decreased libido, and erectile dysfunction in men

Nursing considerations: Contraindicated in women who are pregnant or considering pregnancy and those with hypersensitivity, undiagnosed vaginal bleeding, or QT prolongation

History: The Tamoxifen and Exemestane Trial (TEXT) and the Suppression of Ovarian Function Trial (SOFT) showed benefit of ovarian suppression with an AI versus tamoxifen alone or tamoxifen with ovarian suppression (Reinbolt et al., 2015). Five-year disease-free survival was 67.7% with tamoxifen alone, 78.9% with tamoxifen and ovarian suppression, and 83.4% with exemestane and ovarian suppression.

Leuprolide

Indications: Ovarian suppression for premenopausal, ER-positive females with breast cancer

Mechanism of action: Leuprolide is an LHRH agonist that signals the pituitary gland to begin producing luteinizing hormone, which then signals the ovaries to produce estrogen. Normally, LHRH is sent in pulses. Leuprolide confuses this signal by sending LHRH in a prolonged surge (LHRH agonist), which tricks the pituitary into thinking that no pulses are being sent (NCCN, 2017).

Administration: 7.5 mg every 4 weeks or 22.5 mg every 12 weeks by intramuscular injection

Side effects: Decreased libido, bone loss

Nursing considerations: Contraindicated in women who are pregnant or considering pregnancy, women who are breast-feeding, and patients with hypersensitivity, undiagnosed vaginal bleeding, or history of convulsions

History: Leuprolide was first approved by FDA to treat advanced prostate cancer in April 1985. Since then, it has been approved for the treatment of some breast cancers, endometriosis, and fibroids (National Cancer Institute, 2017).

Progestin Therapy

Megestrol

Indications: Treatment of metastatic disease if progression occurs on standard medications; used more commonly for appetite stimulation

Mechanism of action: Megestrol is a synthetic derivative of naturally occurring progesterone ("Megestrol Acetate," n.d.). Progestins suppress the effects of estrogen on cancer cells. The exact mechanism of action is unknown, but they are thought to have activity as agonists to exogenous estrogen.

Administration: 160 mg, with higher doses for appetite stimulation

Side effects: Weight gain, deep vein thrombosis, and other thromboembolic diseases

Nursing considerations: Contraindicated in patients who are pregnant or considering pregnancy and those with hypersensitivity, heart failure, high blood pressure, diabetes, increased blood sugar, adrenal gland dysfunction, history of a clotting event, or renal impairment

History: Megestrol originally was used as a contraceptive in 1963 and, in 1967, was used in the treatment of breast cancer (Argilés, Anguera, & Stemmler, 2013). In 1993, it was approved for the treatment of anorexia-cachexia in people with AIDS. It has not been used recently in breast cancer treatment but may be a reasonable option for postmenopausal women who have progressed on an AI or in cost-sensitive environments (Bines et al., 2014).

Adherence

Although all these therapies have shown great promise in treating or preventing breast cancer, one of the challenges noted in the literature is patient adherence (Wuensch et al., 2015). Healthcare providers are well aware of the benefits of these medications but, unless the patient is taking the medication, the disease can recur or progress. When most therapies were recommended for five years of time, only about 50% of the patients met this goal (Chlebowski, Kim, & Haque, 2014).

Studies have shown a direct correlation between the length of treatment and recurrence rates (Bender et al., 2014). Healthcare providers play an integral part in identifying reasons for nonadherence (see Table 8-2). One study showed that patients felt inadequately prepared to take endocrine therapies and felt inadequate in the management of side effects (van Londen et al., 2014). Another study showed that patients value direct communication about the medication and management of possible side

Table 8-2. Nursing Interventions for Increased Endocrine Therapy Adherence

Area of Intervention	Strategies and Teaching Points
Education	Explain the importance of the medication. Emphasize that it is as important as other areas of treatment (e.g., surgery, chemotherapy, radiation). Discuss possible side effects. Explain that most women complete therapy. Stress the importance of communication with the provider regarding any problems (e.g., side effects, cost, other concerns).
Follow-up	At *every* appointment (surgery, radiation, medical oncology, gynecology, primary care provider), ask the patient about adherence in a nonjudgmental manner. Listen to any and all concerns from the patient and discuss with the provider. Ascertain whether the patient is able to obtain prescription (many pharmaceutical companies have options available). Compliance tends to decrease with patient age and length of therapy; continue to monitor the patient.
Management of side effects	Based on provider recommendations, can have patient stop medication briefly (2 weeks) to see if side effect is related to the endocrine therapy. Try another medication if possible or restart the same medication. Look for other methods of treating the side effects (e.g., hot flashes may be managed with acupuncture, antidepressants, or other methods).

Note. Based on information from Chlebowski et al., 2014; Gerken, 2004; Hadji et al., 2013; Murphy et al., 2012; Vogel & Bevers, 2003; Ziller et al., 2013.

effects (Wuensch et al., 2015). These factors should be considered when educating patients about the importance of and how to take endocrine therapy for the treatment of breast cancer.

Summary

Endocrine therapy has progressed over the years and will continue to change as new studies show more about the precise amount of therapy needed, as well as other targets are identified. Previous use of androgen therapy is recently being re-studied to see what role it will play. This therapy may be beneficial in women with hormone receptor negative disease (Williams & Harris, 2014).

Oncology nurses have a large responsibility to assure adherence to endocrine therapy, which ultimately influences the long-term survival of breast cancer. This education includes how to take the medication, the importance of the medication, and potential side effects. Nurses need to monitor for side effects and, whenever possible, suggest evidence-based management strategies.

References

Argilés, J.M., Anguera, A., & Stemmler, B. (2013). A new look at an old drug for the treatment of cancer cachexia: Megestrol acetate. *Clinical Nutrition, 32,* 319–324. doi:10.1016/j.clnu.2013.01.004

AstraZeneca Pharmaceuticals. (2016). *Faslodex® (fulvestrant) injection* [Package insert]. Wilmington, DE: Author.

Bender, C.M., Gentry, A.L., Brufsky, A.M., Casillo, F.E., Cohen, S.M., Dailey, M.M., ... Sereika, S.M. (2014). Influence of patient and treatment factors on adherence to adjuvant endocrine therapy in breast cancer. *Oncology Nursing Forum, 41,* 274–285. doi:10.1188/14.ONF.274-285

Bines, J., Dienstmann, R., Obadia, R.M., Branco, L.G.P., Quintella, D.C., Castro, T.M., ... Costa, M.E.F. (2014). Activity of megestrol acetate in postmenopausal women with advanced breast cancer after nonsteroidal aromatase inhibitor failure: A phase II trial. *Annals of Oncology, 25,* 831–836. doi:10.1093/annonc/mdu015

Burstein, H.J., Lacchetti, C., Anderson, H., Buchholz, T.A., Davidson, N.E., Gelmon, K.E., ... Griggs, J.J. (2016). Adjuvant endocrine therapy for women with hormone receptor-positive breast cancer: American Society of Clinical Oncology clinical practice guideline update on ovarian suppression. *Journal of Clinical Oncology, 34,* 1689–1701. doi:10.1200/JCO.2015.65.9573

Burstein, H.J., Temin, S., Anderson, H., Buchholz, T.A., Davidson, N.E., Gelmon, K.E., ... Griggs, J.J. (2014). Adjuvant endocrine therapy for women with hormone receptor–positive breast cancer: American Society of Clinical Oncology clinical practice guideline focused update. *Journal of Clinical Oncology, 32,* 2255–2269. doi:10.1200/JCO.2013.54.2258

Chlebowski, R.T., Kim, J., & Haque, R. (2014). Adherence to endocrine therapy in breast cancer adjuvant and prevention settings. *Cancer Prevention Research, 7,* 378–387. doi:10.1158/1940-6207.CAPR-13-0389

Fisher, B., Costantino, J.P., Wickerham, D.L., Redmond, C.K., Kavanah, M., Cronin, W.M., ... Wolmark, N. (1998). Tamoxifen for prevention of breast cancer: Report of the National Surgical Adjuvant Breast and Bowel Project P-1 study. *Journal of the National Cancer Institute, 90,* 1371–1388. doi:10.1093/jnci/90.18.1371

Gerken, P. (2004). Toremifene citrate (Fareston®). *Clinical Journal of Oncology Nursing, 8,* 529–530. doi:10.1188/04.CJON.529-530

Gershanovich, M., Garin, A., Baltina, D., Kurvet, A., Kangas, L., & Ellmén, J. (1997). A phase III comparison of two toremifene doses to tamoxifen in postmenopausal women with advanced breast cancer. Eastern European Study Group. *Breast Cancer Research and Treatment, 45,* 251–262. doi:10.1023/A:1005891506092

Hadji, P., Blettner, M., Harbeck, N., Jackisch, C., Lück, H.-J., Windemuth-Kieselbach, C., ... Kreienberg, R. (2013). The Patient's Anastrozole Compliance to Therapy (PACT) Program: A randomized, in-practice study on the impact of a standardized information program on persistence and compliance to adjuvant endocrine therapy in postmenopausal women with early breast cancer. *Annals of Oncology, 24,* 1505–1512. doi:10.1093/annonc/mds653

Hayes, D.F., Van Zyl, J.A., Hacking, A., Goedhals, L., Bezwoda, W.R., Mailliard, J.A., ... Shemano, I. (1995). Randomized comparison of tamoxifen and two separate doses of toremifene in postmenopausal patients with metastatic breast cancer. *Journal of Clinical Oncology, 13,* 2556–2566. doi:10.1200/JCO.1995.13.10.2556

Hertz, D.L., McLeod, H.L., & Irvin, W.J., Jr. (2012). Tamoxifen and CYP2D6: A contradiction of data. *Oncologist, 17,* 620–630. doi:10.1634/theoncologist.2011-0418

Kyowa Kirin, Inc. (n.d.). Fareston® 60 mg (toremifene citrate) tablets. Retrieved from http://fareston.com/hcp/index.html

Megestrol acetate. (n.d.). In *NCI drug dictionary.* Retrieved from https://www.cancer.gov/publications/dictionaries/cancer-drug?CdrID=43435

Murphy, C.C., Bartholomew, L.K., Carpentier, M.Y., Bluethmann, S.M., & Vernon, S.W. (2012). Adherence to adjuvant hormonal therapy among breast cancer survivors in clinical practice: A systematic review. *Breast Cancer Research and Treatment, 134,* 459–478. doi:10.1007/s10549-012-2114-5

National Cancer Institute. (2017). Hormone therapy for breast cancer. Retrieved from https://www.cancer.gov/types/breast/breast-hormone-therapy-fact-sheet

National Comprehensive Cancer Network. (2017). *NCCN Clinical Practice Guidelines in Oncology (NCCN Guidelines®): Breast cancer* [v.2.2017]. Retrieved from http://www.nccn.org/professionals/physician_gls/pdf/breast.pdf

Osborne, C.K., Pippen, J., Jones, S.E., Parker, L.M., Ellis, M., Come, S., ... Buzdar, E.A. (2002). Double-blind, randomized trial comparing the efficacy and tolerability of fulvestrant versus anastrozole in postmenopausal women with advanced breast cancer progressing on prior endocrine therapy: Results of a North American trial. *Journal of Clinical Oncology, 20,* 3386–3395. doi:10.1200/jco.2002.10.058

Reinbolt, R.E., Mangini, N., Hill, J.L., Levine, L.B., Dempsey, J.L., Singaravelu, J., ... Lustberg, M.B. (2015). Endocrine therapy in breast cancer: The neoadjuvant, adjuvant, and metastatic approach. *Seminars in Oncology Nursing, 31,* 146–155. doi:10.1016/j.soncn.2015.02.002

Robertson, J.F.R. (2007). Fulvestrant (Faslodex®)—How to make a good drug better. *Oncologist, 12,* 774–784. doi:10.1634/theoncologist.12-7-774

Rydén, L., Arnlind, M.H., Vitols, S., Höistad, M., & Ahlgren, J. (2016). Aromatase inhibitors alone or sequentially combined with tamoxifen in postmenopausal early breast cancer compared with tamoxifen or placebo—Meta-analyses on efficacy and adverse events based on randomized clinical trials. *Breast, 26,* 106–114. doi:10.1016/j.breast.2016.01.006

van Londen, G.J., Donovan, H.S., Beckjord, E.B., Cardy, A.L., Bovbjerg, D.H., Davidson, N.E., ... Dew, M.A. (2014). Perspectives of postmenopausal breast cancer survivors on adjuvant endocrine therapy-related symptoms. *Oncology Nursing Forum, 41,* 660–668. doi:10.1188/14.ONF.660-668

Visvanathan, K., Hurley, P., Bantug, E., Brown, P., Col, N.F., Cuzick, J., ... Lippman, S.M. (2013). Use of pharmacologic interventions for breast cancer risk reduction: American Society of Clinical Oncology clinical practice guideline. *Journal of Clinical Oncology, 31,* 2942–2962. doi:10.1200/JCO.2013.49.3122

Vogel, C.L., Johnston, M.A., Capers, C., & Braccia, D. (2014). Toremifene for breast cancer: A review of 20 years of data. *Clinical Breast Cancer, 14,* 1–9. doi:10.1016/j.clbc.2013.10.014

Vogel, V.G., & Bevers, T. (Eds.). (2003). *Handbook of breast cancer risk-assessment: Evidence-based guidelines for evaluation, prevention, counseling, and treatment.* Burlington, MA: Jones & Bartlett Learning.

Vogel, V.G., Costantino, J.P., Wickerham, D.L., Cronin, W.M., Cecchini, R.S., Atkins, J.N., ... Wolmark, N. (2006). Effects of tamoxifen vs raloxifene on the risk of developing invasive breast cancer and other disease outcomes. The NSAP Study of Tamoxifen and Raloxifene (STAR) P-2 Trial. *JAMA, 295,* 2727–2741. doi:10.1001/jama.295.23.joc60074

Williams, N., & Harris, L.N. (2014). The renaissance of endocrine therapy in breast cancer. *Current Opinion in Obstetrics and Gynecology, 26,* 41–47. doi:10.1097/GCO.0000000000000039

Wuensch, P., Hahne, A., Haidinger, R., Meißler, K., Tenter, B., Stoll, C., ... Huebner, J. (2015). Discontinuation and non-adherence to endocrine therapy in breast cancer patients: Is lack of communication the decisive factor? *Journal of Cancer Research and Clinical Oncology, 141,* 55–60. doi:10.1007/s00432-014-1779-z

Ziller, V., Kyvernitakis, I., Knöll, D., Storch, A., Hars, O., & Hadji, P. (2013). Influence of a patient information program on adherence and persistence with an aromatase inhibitor in breast cancer treatment—The COMPAS study. *BMC Cancer, 13,* 407. doi:10.1186/1471-2407-13-407

CHAPTER 9

Side Effect Management

Marcelle Kaplan, MS, RN, CBCN®

Introduction

Multiple treatment options exist for women diagnosed with breast cancer, each of which can cause side effects that can be physically and psychologically life altering. The side effects may appear early or late and be temporary or long-lasting, reversible, or permanent. This chapter will review the most common side effects specific to breast cancer treatment and present evidence-based management strategies.

Lymphedema

Overview

Breast cancer–related lymphedema (BCRL) is a greatly feared complication of breast cancer therapy because of its physical, psychological, social, and financial consequences. BCRL typically presents within 12 months of breast surgery (Hayes et al., 2012), but the risk for occurrence is lifelong (Helyer, Varnic, Le, Leong, & McCready, 2010; Ostby et al., 2014). BCRL results from impaired lymphatic drainage that leads to tissue swelling due to accumulation of protein-rich fluid in the interstitial spaces (Hayes et al., 2012; Helyer et al., 2010). The arm, hand, breast, and torso on the affected side can be involved with lymphedema (Hayes et al., 2012).

Utilization of healthcare resources and medical costs are greatly increased when BCRL is present. A review of medical insurance claims showed that costs were twice as high for women with BCRL compared to unaffected women, mostly due to recurrent arm infections, labor-intensive physical therapy, and compression pumps, supplies, and other costs for advanced care (Shih et al., 2009). A review of hospital charges within two years of breast cancer surgery found that costs for all-cause hospital admissions were seven times greater for women with BCRL than for unaffected women (Basta et al., 2016). The presence of BCRL has been reported to be prognostic for decreased length of survival compared to breast cancer survivors without lymphedema (Hayes et al., 2012).

Incidence

Reports of BCRL vary widely. However, based on the results of a meta-analysis of prospective cohort studies, arm lymphedema has been reported in 21% of worldwide survivors of unilateral breast cancer (DiSipio, Rye, Newman, & Hayes, 2013). The incidence was four times greater in women who had axillary lymph node dissection compared with those who had sentinel lymph node biopsy (DiSipio et al., 2013). (See Chapter 5 for descriptions of these procedures.) Incidence of arm lymphedema may increase for two years or longer after breast cancer diagnosis or surgery (DiSipio et al., 2013). Lymphedema involving the breast only (rather than the arm) has been reported to occur in 30% of women who had breast-conserving surgery plus an axillary procedure; the incidence in women whose surgery did not include axillary surgery was 0% (Boughey et al., 2014). BCRL severity increased over a five-year period in one-third of women treated for breast cancer, especially those who were older than 65 years at the time of diagnosis (Bar Ad et al., 2012).

Pathophysiology

Lymphatic fluid is composed of plasma proteins, extravascular blood cells, excess water, and cellular waste products that are too large for uptake by the veins. The lymphatic system returns these elements from the interstitial spaces to the venous system (International Society of Lymphology [ISL], 2013; National Cancer Institute [NCI], 2015). Lymphedema develops when the amount of lymphatic fluid drainage exceeds the transport capacity of the lymphatic system so that protein-rich fluid accumulates in the interstitial spaces (NCI, 2015).

Lymphedema can be classified as primary or secondary. Primary lymphedema is a congenital disorder caused by an underdeveloped or malformed lymphatic system that is insufficient to transport the volume of lymph fluid (ISL, 2013). Secondary lymphedema results from acquired damage to lymphatic vessels or lymph nodes that obliterates or obstructs the lymphatic transport system (ISL, 2013). Conditions that disrupt the lymphatic system (e.g., surgical removal of axillary lymph nodes or lymph vessels, tissue scarring) reduce the carrying capacity of the system and lead to secondary lymphedema (Ridner, 2013). Radiation therapy can cause lymphedema secondary to radiation-induced tissue damage and the resulting inflammatory response and fibrosis and scarring of lymph nodes that obstructs lymphatic drainage (Ridner, 2013). As lymphedema progresses, the lymphedematous tissue transforms from mostly fluid to fibrosis, fat, and protein (Bernas, 2013; Penha et al., 2013), and risks for infection (cellulitis) and poor wound healing increase greatly (Boughey et al., 2014).

Risk Factors

The two factors most strongly associated with increased risk for BCRL are (a) surgical removal of axillary lymph nodes and (b) obesity at the time of diagnosis (Bar Ad et al., 2012; Boughey et al., 2014; Dominick, Madlensky, Natarajan, & Pierce, 2013). Any type of axillary surgery can lead to BCRL. Having a sentinel lymph node biopsy alone, rather than an axillary lymph node dissection, can diminish risk; however, both procedures have been shown to result in BCRL (Helyer et al., 2010). Breast reconstruction, whether immediate or postponed, does not appear to add to lymphedema risk (Basta et al., 2016). Obese women were reported to have twice the risk for BCRL as normal weight women (Dominick et al., 2013). The odds of BCRL were two to three times higher in women with a body mass index (BMI) of 30–34 kg/m^2 (obesity) or 35 kg/m^2 or greater (morbid obesity) compared to those with a BMI less than 25 kg/m^2 (healthy weight) (Bar Ad et al., 2012; Boughey et al., 2014).

Reports about the risks for BCRL posed by adjuvant radiation therapy following breast-conserving surgery or mastectomy are conflicting. Several studies have reported increased risk, especially when axillary or regional lymph nodes were irradiated (Bar Ad et al., 2012; Dominick et al., 2013; Hayes et al., 2012; Warren et al., 2014). Other investigators reported that breast radiation therapy did not contribute to lymphedema because of advances in the planning and delivery of radiation treatments (Brown, Mutter, & Halyard, 2015; Shah, Arthur, Riutta, Whitworth, & Vicini, 2012).

Postoperative seroma (fluid collection in the axilla) formation and infection on the side of surgery have been reported to increase BCRL risk (Kwan et al., 2010; Ridner, 2013). Other factors that have not shown a consistent association with BRCL risk include older age at diagnosis, tumor size, disease stage, number of axillary lymph nodes removed, menopausal status, and type of adjuvant therapy other than radiation (Hayes et al., 2012; Helyer et al., 2010; Paskett, Dean, Oliveri, & Harrop, 2012).

Signs and Symptoms

Signs of lymphedema include swelling (leading to pain, decreased function in the arm, and arm disfigurement), redness, firmness, and changes in skin texture (Boughey et al., 2014; DiSipio et al., 2013). Dry skin may increase infection risk (Bernas, 2013; Fu, Deng, & Armer, 2014). Symptoms include patient reports of aching, discomfort, heaviness, and tightness in arm (Fu et al., 2014).

Stages of Lymphedema

No standardized method exists for staging lymphedema. The ISL (2013) Consensus Document describes criteria for staging lymphedema based on the characteristics of the edema and the skin. Functional limitations and quality-of-life indicators are not considered in this staging system (ISL, 2013). For the stages of lymphedema, see Table 9-1.

Table 9-1. Stages of Lymphedema

Stages	Physical Characteristics
0 Latency stage	Underlying changes in lymphatic system are not clinically evident. Patients are asymptomatic but may report feeling of heaviness in the limb. May exist for months to years before progressing.
I (mild) Reversible lymphedema	Skin is very soft. Fluid with high protein content is accumulating. Pitting edema is present, but swelling resolves with prolonged elevation of the limb.
II (moderate) Spontaneously irreversible lymphedema	Tissue fibrosis is present. Skin is firm and does not "pit" easily. Swelling is constant and does not resolve with limb elevation. Excess fat and fibrosis cause increased arm volume. The limb is more prone to skin infections.
III (severe) Lymphostatic elephantiasis	Skin is fibrotic, hard, and nonpitting. Arm volume increases greatly with adipose subcutaneous fat deposition. Skin changes and warty growths occur. Bacterial and fungal infections of the skin and nails are common and recurrent.

Note. Based on information from Bernas, 2013; International Society of Lymphology, 2013; Lawenda et al., 2009.

Diagnosis

The diagnosis of lymphedema can be obtained through reviewing the patient's history and conducting a physical examination and imaging procedures. A review of the patient's breast cancer history, including types of breast surgical and axillary lymph node procedures and adjuvant therapies, comorbid conditions, and results of the physical examination, are generally sufficient to establish the presence of lymphedema (Bernas, 2013; ISL, 2013). Soft tissue imaging such as magnetic resonance imaging (MRI), computed tomography (CT), and ultrasound examinations are essential to rule out recurrent cancer and can detect the presence of increased interstitial fluid and fluid accumulations (Armer et al., 2013; Bernas, 2013). Lymphatic system imaging tests include lymphangioscintigraphy and noninvasive duplex-Doppler studies. Lymphangioscintigraphy is the current "gold standard." A radioactive tracer is injected into the hand (either intradermally or subcutaneously) to visualize lymphatic flow. It provides images of peripheral lymph channels and lymph nodes and reveals abnormalities and sites of blockage (Bernas, 2013; Ostby et al., 2014). Noninvasive duplex-Doppler studies are used to examine the deep venous system and complement evaluation of limb edema (ISL, 2013).

Objective Assessment of Arm Volume

Objective measures are used to quantify the presence and severity of lymphedema and to follow response to treatment. Tape measurements are commonly used in clinical practice because of convenience. Measurements of arm circumference are taken at defined intervals along both arms from the hand to the axilla for comparison and to assess treatment efficacy over time (Phillips, 2014). Lymphedema exists when there is a difference of at least 2 cm between the arms at one anatomic point (Bernas, 2013; Ostby et al., 2014; Phillips, 2014). See Figure 9-1 for hand and arm measurement techniques for patients with breast cancer and lymphedema. Figure 9-2 lists the severity categories of lymphedema based on limb volumes.

Perometry is a validated measure of arm volume using an infrared optical electronic scanner and computer software to calculate overall arm volume (O'Toole et al., 2013).

Water displacement is the "gold standard" for measuring arm volume. The arm is immersed in a cylinder filled with water, and the volume of water displaced is measured. This method is rarely used because of inconvenience and hygienic precautions (Bernas, 2013; Ostby et al., 2014).

Figure 9-1. Breast Cancer Lymphedema Hand and Arm Measurement Technique

1. Measure using the centimeter side of a flexible tape measure. Note all measurements.
2. Start with the unaffected arm. Place a measuring tape above the thumb (under the index finger), and measure around the hand.
3. Measure the wrist circumference.
4. Continue to measure every 4 cm, starting from the wrist and advancing upward to the shoulder.
5. Next, measure the affected arm, making note of all measurements.
6. Compare the measurements for both arms.
7. If the difference between the arms is 2 cm or more, the findings are clinically significant and the patient should be referred to a lymphedema specialist.

Note. From "Breast Cancer Lymphedema Hand/Arm Measurements," by J. Phillips, 2014, *Lymphedema Management Special Interest Group Newsletter, 25*(2). Retrieved from http://onsopcontent.ons.org/Publications/SIGNewsletters/lym/lym25.2.html#story2. Copyright 2014 by Oncology Nursing Society. Adapted with permission.

Figure 9-2. Severity Categories of Lymphedema Based on Limb Volumes*

- Minimal: Measured limb volume is < 20% greater.
- Moderate: Measured limb volume is 20%–40% greater.
- Severe: Measured limb volume is > 40% greater.

*Compared to volume of the unaffected limb

Note. Based on information from Bernas, 2013; International Society of Lymphology, 2013.

Bioimpedance spectroscopy provides a reliable measure of extracellular fluid content (DiSipio et al., 2013). An electrical current is passed through each arm, and the impedance (resistance to the current) is measured and compared. The higher the fluid content in the arm, the lower the impedance. Bioimpedance spectroscopy is very sensitive and can detect changes in the arm before clinical presentation (Armer et al., 2013; Hayes et al., 2012).

Interprofessional Management

Effective management of the patient at risk for or with existing BCRL incorporates the expertise of members of an interprofessional team, including breast surgery, radiation therapy, medical oncology, oncology nursing, rehabilitation medicine and physical therapy, and psychology, as appropriate (Patricolo, Armstrong, Riutta, & Lanni, 2015). Goals of therapy are to reduce swelling by moving fluid from the affected area to functional areas of the lymphatic system, alleviate symptoms, prevent infection, improve functional status, and enhance quality of life (Hayes et al., 2012; Ridner, 2013).

Complete decongestive therapy (CDT) is the standard of care treatment regimen (Fu et al., 2014; ISL, 2013; Lasinski, 2013). CDT consists of two phases (see Table 9-2). Phase I is intensive treatment by trained lymphedema therapists to reduce arm volume. Phase II is lifelong self-management to conserve arm volume reduction.

Intermittent pneumatic compression therapy is self-care therapy for select patients. A pneumatic compression pump with a segmented sleeve is programmed to intermit-

Table 9-2. Complete Decongestive Therapy

Phase	Goals	Time Frame
Phase I: Reductive phase—performed by lymphedema therapist	Reduce the size of the affected area through: • Manual lymphatic drainage • Compression bandages • Exercise program Educate the patient about proper skin care.	5 days/week for 3–8 weeks
Phase II: Maintenance phase—self-care performed by patient	Self-care strategies: • Wear compression sleeves and garments. • Maintain proper skin care to minimize risk for infection. • Continue exercise program. • Perform self–manual lymphatic drainage massage as needed.	Years or lifelong

Note. Based on information from Fu et al., 2014; International Society of Lymphology, 2013; Lasinski, 2013.

tently inflate and deflate sequentially along the length of the patient's arm to move lymph fluid from the arm toward the heart. A systemic review of the evidence-based literature has ranked ICP as "effectiveness not established" and noted that adverse events, including increased swelling in the arm and torso, have been reported (Fu et al., 2014). However, use of intermittent pneumatic compression as an adjunct to CDT has been reported as safe (Chang & Cormier, 2013; Feldman et al., 2012) and has been shown to reduce episodes of cellulitis and costs of care for cancer- and noncancer-related lymphedema (Karaca-Mandic, Hirsch, Rockson, & Ridner, 2015).

Exercise Interventions

Exercise recommendations for patients at risk for BCRL or who have existing lymphedema have been conflicting because of arm safety concerns. Systematic reviews of the evidence suggest that a slowly progressive program of resistance exercises (e.g., weight lifting with free weights or machines, use of elastic bands, water-based exercises), supervised by an experienced trainer, is safe to start at any point following breast cancer surgery and does not increase the risk for or exacerbate BCRL (Fu et al., 2014; Kwan, Cohn, Armer, Stewart, & Cormier, 2011; Stuiver et al., 2015). Evidence to support the use of compression garments (i.e., sleeves) during exercise was insufficient to make a practice recommendation (Kwan et al., 2011). However, the National Lymphedema Network (2013) supports the use of compression garments during exercise in patients with existing lymphedema.

Surgical Interventions

Axillary reverse mapping is a BCRL risk reduction technique that spares uninvolved lymph vessels from damage during surgical excision of sentinel or axillary lymph nodes. Dye is injected prior to surgery to help identify and avoid injury to these lymph vessels (Bernas, 2013; Dayan, Dayan, & Smith, 2015). Surgical treatment of existing BCRL generally is reserved for patients with chronic, advanced lymphedema who have not responded to conservative first-line therapies (Chang & Cormier, 2013; Hayes et al., 2012). Goals of surgical treatment of BCRL are to reduce the volume of the arm, improve lymphatic function, relieve symptoms and disability related to BCRL, and allow conservative therapies (e.g., use of compression sleeves) to be discontinued (Basta, Gao, & Wu, 2014; Penha et al., 2013).

Surgical approaches are selected based on individual patient factors and include, in order of frequency: (a) excision of lymphedematous tissue, (b) microsurgical reconstruction of lymphatic pathways, and (c) tissue transfer techniques (Chang & Cormier, 2013; Cormier, Rourke, Crosby, Chang, & Armer, 2012; Hayes et al., 2012).

Excisional procedures involve debulking of the affected arm by removing excess subcutaneous fat and skin using liposuction (Cormier et al., 2012; Hayes et al., 2012). In reconstruction of lymphatic pathways (lymphovenous shunt), microsurgical techniques are employed to shunt lymphatic fluid around obstructed areas by anastomosing lymph vessels or lymph nodes to veins (ISL, 2013; Ridner, 2013). In the third surgical option, tissue transfer, normal superficial lymph nodes and their vascular supply are removed from an unaffected extremity (e.g., the groin) and transplanted to involved sites (e.g., the axilla) to enhance lymph return from the arm (Basta et al., 2014; ISL, 2013).

Quantitative improvements, such as reduction in arm circumference, have been reported postoperatively. Although no complications were reported, evidence is lacking to recommend a particular procedure (Basta et al., 2014; Penha et al., 2013). The greatest subjective improvement was reported by patients undergoing lymph node transplantation procedures; they were most likely to be able to discontinue the use of compression garments (Basta et al., 2014; Penha et al., 2013).

Other Treatment Approaches

Oral benzopyrones, selenium, and diuretics have been investigated as drug therapy for managing BCRL, but the evidence does not support their use in clinical practice (Fu et al., 2014; ISL, 2013; NCI, 2015).

Weight loss, low-level laser therapy, electronic devices, aqua lymphatic therapy, and complementary and alternative approaches (e.g., massage, acupuncture, yoga, meditation, nutritional supplements) do not have sufficient evidence to support their use in clinical practice, and some may have adverse side effects (Fu et al., 2014; Ostby et al., 2014; Rodrick et al., 2014).

Psychosocial Impact

Breast cancer survivors with chronic BCRL experience tremendous psychosocial and emotional distress in all aspects of life related to the visual appearance of the lymphedematous arm, which serves as a persistent reminder of their disease, and the associated physical symptoms, which require daily complex self-management (DiSipio et al., 2013; Ostby et al., 2014). Reviews of the literature reveal consistent negative themes expressed by breast cancer survivors with BCRL. See Figure 9-3 for an overview of the psychosocial impact of BCRL.

Patient and Family Education and Supportive Care

Patients and caregivers should be provided with emotional support and instructions regarding lymphedema prevention and risk reduction strategies. See Figure 9-4 for a list of non–evidence-based measures for minimizing lymph fluid accumulation and obstruction to lymph flow in the affected extremity (American Cancer Society, 2016; Mehrara, 2017; NCI, 2015; National Lymphedema Network, 2012). A systematic review of the literature to evaluate the evidence associating venipuncture in the affected arm to the development of BCRL concluded that "no good evidence" existed to link venipuncture to lymphedema (Jakes & Twelves, 2015, p. 455). The authors proposed that, where possible, venipuncture should be performed on the unaffected arm, but if necessary, the affected arm can be used as long as there is no preexisting lymphedema and venous access appears good (Jakes & Twelves, 2015).

Patient teaching topics include, as appropriate, recognizing the signs and symptoms of lymphedema onset or exacerbation, including subjective changes (arm heaviness, discomfort, numbness) and objective changes (arm redness, swelling, skin texture); self-

---

Figure 9-3. Psychosocial Impact of Breast Cancer–Related Lymphedema

- Negative emotional feelings: emotional distress, anxiety, depression, sadness, anger, hopelessness
- Negative social impact: marginalization, financial burden, perceived diminished sexual appeal
- Negative self-identity: body image disturbance, loss of pre-lymphedema identity, feelings of being old and unattractive, perceived diminished sexual appeal
- Social isolation and abandonment: lack of social, family, and professional support
- Nonsupportive work environment: insufficient health insurance

---

Note. Based on information from Fu & Kang, 2013; Fu et al., 2013; Ostby et al., 2014; Ridner et al., 2012.

Figure 9-4. Patient Education on Lymphedema Risk Reduction Measures

---

Recommendations for the Hand and Arm on the Affected Side
• Use your affected hand and arm in a normal way, but try to protect them from breaks in the skin due to cuts, scratches, or burns.
• Adhere to the following skin and nail care measures to prevent injury and infection:
 – Maintaining meticulous skin hygiene and nail care
 – Using skin moisturizer to keep skin moist
 – Pushing cuticles back after bathing while they are soft
 – Wearing loose rubber gloves when washing dishes or cleaning with harsh chemicals
 – Using oven mitts when holding hot pots and pans
 – Wearing protective gloves when gardening or playing golf or tennis
 – Applying sunscreen to your arm (at least SPF 30) prior to sun exposure
 – Using insect repellent on arm when necessary to avoid bites
 – Cleaning, applying antibacterial ointment, and covering small breaks in the skin
 – Observing for signs of infection (redness, swelling, tenderness)
 – Reporting skin changes or signs of infection promptly
• Other protective measures:
 – Maintaining optimal body weight
 – Elevating the arm above the level of the heart when possible
 – Initiating an exercise program as recommended

What to Avoid for the Hand and Arm on the Affected Side
• Actions that may obstruct circulation or cause blood to pool in the affected arm and hand, such as the following:
 – Puncturing the skin for medical procedures (e.g., blood draws, insertions of IV lines, vaccinations, injections)
 – Measuring blood pressure on the affected arm
 – Carrying heavy packages or hanging shoulder bags on the affected side
 – Wearing tight jewelry or constrictive clothing on the affected arm
 – Cutting nail cuticles on the affected hand
 – Soaking in hot tubs or applying local heat to the arm
 – Hanging the arm in a downward position for long periods

Note. Based on information from American Cancer Society, 2016; Mehrara, 2017; National Cancer Institute, 2015; National Lymphedema Network, 2012.

monitoring to recognize changes in arm volume or skin features and the importance of prompt reporting; meticulous skin care to decrease infection risk; exercise regimens and weight loss or weight maintenance strategies; lymphedema self-care management (CDT, intermittent pneumatic compression therapy, self-massage); and referrals to specialists and support organizations (see Figure 9-5). Nutritional guidance and strategies for reaching or maintaining optimal weight to prevent development or exacerbation of lymphedema should also be a focus of patient education (Armer et al., 2013).

Brachial Plexopathy

Overview

The brachial plexus consists of a network of nerves that originate from spinal nerve roots in the neck and upper thorax and terminate in multiple motor and sensory nerves that innervate muscles and skin of the shoulder and arm (Bromberg, 2017). Many factors can damage the nerves in the brachial plexus, including radiation therapy, surgery, and tumor, leading to brachial plexopathy, which is manifested by sen-

---

Figure 9-5. Organizations Providing Lymphedema Education and Resources

- American Cancer Society: www.cancer.org/treatment/treatments-and-side-effects/physical-side-effects/lymphedema.html
- American Lymphedema Framework Project: www.alfp.org
- Breastcancer.org: www.breastcancer.org/treatment/lymphedema
- Lymphatic Education and Research Network: www.lymphaticnetwork.org
- Lymphology Association of North America: www.clt-lana.org
- National Cancer Institute—Lymphedema (PDQ®): www.cancer.gov/about-cancer/treatment/side-effects/lymphedema/lymphedema-hp-pdq
- National Lymphedema Network: www.lymphnet.org
  - Lymphedema Risk Reduction Practices: www.lymphnet.org/pdfDocs/nlnriskreduction.pdf
  - Summary of Lymphedema Risk Reduction Practices: www.lymphnet.org/pdfDocs/nlnriskreduction_summary.pdf
- Oncology Nursing Society—Putting Evidence Into Practice (PEP) resource on lymphedema: www.ons.org/practice-resources/pep/lymphedema

---

sory and motor changes in the areas supplied by the affected nerves (Bromberg, 2017; McNeely et al., 2012). Brachial plexopathy, arm lymphedema, and impaired shoulder movement can occur independently but often are present together in an individual because of similar pathologies: nerve damage, tissue fibrosis, and vascular injury (McNeely et al., 2012).

Incidence

Brachial plexopathy is an uncommon condition. It occurs in approximately 0.4% of patients with cancer (Bromberg, 2017) and in 1%–2% of patients treated with radiation therapy that includes the brachial plexus (Stephenson, 2017). Breast cancer accounts for 40%–75% of cases (Stephenson, 2017). Incidence is highest in women treated with breast-conserving surgery and adjuvant radiation therapy for early-stage breast cancer (Bromberg, 2017). As long-term cancer survival increases, the incidence of brachial plexopathy may increase because of its lengthy latent period following radiation damage (Delanian, Lefaix, & Pradat, 2012).

Etiology

Adjuvant radiation therapy technique and dose, volume of tissue irradiated, and concomitant use of chemotherapy are associated with inducing radiation injury to the brachial plexus, especially when the treatment field includes the axillary and supraclavicular lymph nodes (Stephenson, 2017). Radiation-induced brachial plexopathy can develop acutely and be self-limited or can occur after a latent period of years to decades and be more serious and irreversible (Rutkove, 2016). In past decades, radiation-induced brachial plexopathy could be severe because of inadequate protection of the brachial plexus during treatment. However, with modern radiation therapy techniques, brachial plexopathy has become unusual, even with radiation to the supraclavicular and axillary regions (Hayes et al., 2012).

Axillary lymph node dissection can damage nerves in the brachial plexus, leading to plexopathy (Hayes et al., 2012). Injury to the intercostal brachial or thoracodorsal nerve causes axillary paresthesia, muscle dysfunction that impairs shoulder mobility, and pain (Hayes et al., 2012). Brachial plexopathy can also occur as a result of operative positioning (McNeely et al., 2012).

Breast or lung tumors or lymphoma can lead to brachial plexopathy as a result of direct local pressure on the brachial plexus or through invasion along nerves or tracking along connective tissue (Bromberg, 2017; Stephenson, 2017).

Pathophysiology

Radiation therapy can have toxic effects on the nerves in the brachial plexus from a variety of factors. Damage to nerve axons can occur subsequent to direct injury that results in demyelination, radiation-induced fibrosis that compresses nerves, and capillary network impairment that causes localized ischemia that damages axons and blood vessels in the area (Delanian et al., 2012; Stephenson, 2017). Failure of cellular proliferation in the irradiated area is also a contributing factor (Stephenson, 2017).

Manifestations

Limited movement in the arm or hand on the affected side, muscle weakness progressing to atrophy, and sensory changes (e.g., numbness, tingling) can occur, although not necessarily at the same time (Bromberg, 2017; McNeely et al., 2012). Muscle atrophy may not be recognized for several weeks. Tendon reflexes may be reduced in weak muscles. Sensory loss commonly involves the axillary nerve distribution but may be diffuse or reflect the distributions of other involved nerves (Bromberg, 2017).

Late-onset radiation-induced brachial plexopathy can appear long after treatment. The symptoms can be subtle and nonspecific and may not be recognized as significant by the patient or care provider (Stephenson, 2017). Late-onset brachial plexopathy can manifest as paresthesia, muscle weakness, and impaired reflexes in the affected arm and progress to chronic pain and paralysis of the arm (Rutkove, 2016).

The presence and intensity of pain can help distinguish brachial plexopathy that is a late side effect of radiation therapy from brachial plexopathy caused by cancer recurrence (Bromberg, 2017; Stephenson, 2017). Pain associated with radiation-induced brachial plexopathy usually is limited to the shoulder and proximal arm, is reported as mild to moderate in intensity, and occurs further along in the course of symptoms (Bromberg, 2017; Stephenson, 2017). Pain associated with recurrent cancer is more severe and occurs at symptom onset (Bromberg, 2017; Stephenson, 2017). Paresthesia and weakness in the arm are also more severe with radiation-induced brachial plexopathy than that caused by tumor (Bromberg, 2017).

Assessment

Clinical neurologic examination may be sufficient to diagnose brachial plexopathy (McNeely et al., 2012). The patient is questioned about the onset, presence, quality, and intensity of neurologic symptoms and cancer history and treatment (Stephenson, 2017). Musculoskeletal examination may reveal winged scapula or decreased shoulder external rotation and abduction that are indicative of damage to the upper trunk of the brachial plexus (Stephenson, 2017). Nerve conduction studies can be performed to assess distribution of abnormalities in the brachial plexus and exclude other diagnoses, such as carpal tunnel syndrome (Bromberg, 2017; Stephenson, 2017). Needle electromyography is the most sensitive test of motor nerve damage and can further localize the involved area. Abnormalities may not be apparent for up to three weeks after acute onset of brachial plexopathy (Bromberg, 2017). Imaging tests, including MRI, CT, or positron-emission tomography–CT, are performed to rule out recurrent or metastatic tumor (Bromberg, 2017; Stephenson, 2017).

Management

Early identification of brachial plexopathy is important so that the symptoms do not lead to permanent impairment. Rehabilitation (Stephenson, 2017) includes physical and occupational therapy. Physical therapy focuses on managing pain, strengthening muscles, and preserving range of motion. Occupational therapy consists of fine motor skill training and provision of adaptive equipment, as appropriate.

Symptoms and neurologic changes are monitored and electromyography or MRI is repeated, as necessary (Stephenson, 2017). Long-term follow-up of at least five years is recommended for patients treated with radiation therapy encompassing the brachial plexus (Hayes et al., 2012).

Premature Menopause

Overview

More than 25,000 women with breast cancer, or 11% of all women in this population, in the United States were expected to be younger than the age of 45 in 2014 (Howlader et al., 2017). Breast cancer in young women is typically treated aggressively with therapies (e.g., chemotherapy, hormonal therapy) that have toxic effects on the ovary and can lead to premature menopause (Pagani et al., 2015; Partridge et al., 2014). Premature menopause is associated with life-altering changes and diminished quality of life because of physiologic changes (risk of infertility, hot flashes, bone loss, vaginal dryness, weight gain) and psychosocial effects (altered body image, depression, sleep disturbances, sexual dysfunction) (Morgan, Anderson, Gourley, Wallace, & Spears, 2012; Partridge et al., 2014; Rosenberg & Partridge, 2013). Figure 9-6 provides a list of definitions pertinent to this topic.

Pathophysiology

The physiology of ovarian function begins at birth. A girl is born with her full complement of ovarian primordial follicles from which immature egg cells (oocytes) arise. No new follicles will be produced during her lifetime (Kort, Eisenberg, Millheiser, & Westphal, 2014). Between fetal life and menopause, the ovarian follicles progressively degenerate; hundreds of follicles are depleted with each menstrual cycle until so few are present that the woman becomes menopausal (Kort et al., 2014). Over time, the quality of the oocytes diminishes, and by age 37, the majority of oocytes originally present are no longer functional (de Pedro, Otero, & Martin, 2015).

Figure 9-6. Glossary

amenorrhea—Absence of menstrual cycles for more than three cycles or for six months in women who previously had menses. May be temporary, intermittent, or permanent.

menopause—Permanent cessation of menses due to a profound and permanent decrease in ovarian estrogen. This may result from aging, bilateral oophorectomy, or estrogen depletion therapies (e.g., chemotherapy, tamoxifen, ovarian suppression) that lead to hormone levels in the postmenopausal range.

ovarian reserve—Amount of primordial follicles within the ovaries from which mature eggs can develop. This reserve is not renewable and diminishes progressively with age.

premature ovarian failure—Amenorrhea of at least three months duration resulting from the premature depletion of functional ovarian follicles in women younger than 40 years. This may also be referred to as primary ovarian insufficiency, acute ovarian failure, or chemotherapy-related amenorrhea.

Note. Based on information from Morgan et al., 2012; National Comprehensive Cancer Network, 2017; Runowicz et al., 2016; Tomasi-Cont et al., 2014; Torino et al., 2012.

Chemotherapy agents can exert toxic effects on the ovary directly, by destroying ovarian follicles and decreasing the ovarian reserve, or indirectly, by damaging stromal connective tissue cells or the vascular supply to the ovary (Lambertini, Anserini, Levaggi, Poggio, & Del Mastro, 2013; Tomasi-Cont, Lambertini, Hulsbosch, Peccatori, & Amant, 2014). The toxic effects on ovarian function may occur immediately or after a long delay (Rosenberg & Partridge, 2013). An immediate effect is temporary amenorrhea due to loss of the growing follicle population. Menses may resume if ovarian reserve of resting primordial follicles is sufficient. With delayed effects, the loss of ovarian reserve may not become apparent for years. If menses do not resume for a year or longer after systemic therapy, ovarian function is unlikely to return, and the woman will be considered to have premature ovarian failure (Rosenberg & Partridge, 2013). Menstrual periods may return after chemotherapy, but ovarian reserve may still be inadequate to create a pregnancy. However, spontaneous pregnancies have been reported in women with chemotherapy-induced amenorrhea who have hormone levels associated with menopause (Vitek et al., 2014).

Risk Factors

Three factors are associated with the greatest risk for premature menopause: use of chemotherapy agents that are toxic to the ovaries and increased cumulative dose; age at initiation of chemotherapy; and use of tamoxifen as adjuvant antiestrogen therapy following chemotherapy (Lambertini et al., 2013; Morgan et al., 2012; Rosenberg & Partridge, 2013).

Chemotherapy agents associated with premature ovarian failure include the following:

- Cyclophosphamide, an alkylating agent (non–cell cycle specific) commonly used in breast cancer chemotherapy regimens, is highly toxic to the ovaries and confers the greatest risk for premature ovarian failure (Lambertini et al., 2013; Rosenberg & Partridge, 2013; Vitek et al., 2014).
- Cisplatin and carboplatin, platinum-containing compounds, damage DNA and can lead to apoptosis of ovarian cells (Lambertini et al., 2013).
- Doxorubicin, an anthracycline, has been reported to have stronger toxic effects on the ovaries than previously thought (Letourneau et al., 2012).

- Paclitaxel and docetaxel, taxane agents often used in breast chemotherapy regimens, increase the risk of premature ovarian failure when used in combination with doxorubicin (de Pedro et al., 2015; Lambertini et al., 2013).
- Irinotecan (topoisomerase I) and etoposide (topoisomerase II) bind to DNA, interfere with cell replication, and stimulate apoptosis in the ovary (Lambertini et al., 2013).
- Methotrexate and 5-fluorouracil, cell cycle–specific agents that may be used in breast cancer treatment regimens, are considered low risk for premature ovarian failure because they do not diminish ovarian reserve (Lambertini et al., 2013; Vitek et al., 2014).

Age at initiation of anticancer therapy correlates to greater risks. Women who are older when breast chemotherapy begins have lower ovarian reserve than younger women and therefore greater risk of infertility (Kort et al., 2014). For women treated with doxorubicin and docetaxel, amenorrhea lasting at least two years was experienced by approximately 61% of women younger than age 40 compared to almost 100% of women older than age 40 (Ganz et al., 2011). Resumption of menses following chemotherapy does not necessarily indicate fertility; 5% of those diagnosed at age 30, 32% diagnosed at age 35, and 80% diagnosed at age 40 remained infertile (Letourneau et al., 2012). Age-related declines in ovarian reserve also will occur in premenopausal women who take tamoxifen for the recommended period of five years, during which time they usually are advised not to become pregnant (Oktay, Turan, Bedoschi, Pacheco, & Moy, 2015).

Tamoxifen following chemotherapy is also associated with increased risk for infertility. Tamoxifen is the standard adjuvant endocrine therapy to suppress ovarian function in premenopausal women with early-stage estrogen receptor–positive breast cancer. Used alone, tamoxifen has been found to confer a low risk of premature menopause (de Pedro et al., 2015; Lambertini et al., 2013; Tomasi-Cont et al., 2014). However, results of a recent study revealed that young survivors of breast cancer who had ever used tamoxifen (median age was 32 years at therapy initiation) were much less likely to have a child in the years following treatment compared to similar women diagnosed with breast cancer who had never used tamoxifen. Reasons for this outcome were unclear (Shandley et al., 2017).

Tamoxifen taken after chemotherapy has been shown to increase the risk of infertility compared to chemotherapy alone (Lee et al., 2009). About 80% of premenopausal women who are treated with both chemotherapy and estrogen therapy will experience premature menopause in the year following diagnosis (Baber, Hickey, & Kwik, 2005). Fertility concerns have been reported to be an important reason that premenopausal women younger than age 45 refuse or discontinue tamoxifen therapy (Llarena, Estevez, Tucker, & Jeruss, 2015).

Evaluation of Ovarian Reserve

Transvaginal ultrasound can be used to count the number of antral (or resting) follicles to estimate ovarian reserve (de Pedro et al., 2015). Measurement of serum levels of anti-Müllerian hormone (AMH) has been shown to be a reliable biochemical marker of ovarian reserve, as AMH is proportional to the follicle count (Tomasi-Cont et al., 2014). AMH levels fall rapidly during chemotherapy, especially with the use of alkylating agents (e.g., cyclophosphamide) (Bozza et al., 2014).

Fertility Issues

Premenopausal women with breast cancer may be overwhelmed by the cancer diagnosis and not be thinking about or aware of future fertility issues at the outset of treatment (de Pedro et al., 2015). Women in developed countries have increasingly delayed initial childbirth until their 30s or 40s and may be diagnosed with breast cancer before they have started a family (de Pedro et al., 2015).

The First International Consensus Guidelines for Breast Cancer in Young Women (Partridge et al., 2014) include recommendations for healthcare providers to implement in the care of young women at risk for premature ovarian failure after a breast cancer diagnosis (Partridge et al., 2014). Interprofessional collaboration among healthcare providers (breast surgeons, medical oncologists, breast care nurses, social workers, psychologists, gynecologists, fertility specialists) is important to provide holistic care. Before beginning systemic treatment (chemotherapy or hormonal therapy), young women should be informed of the treatment-related risks of amenorrhea and premature menopause and referred to a fertility specialist, as appropriate. Young women should be told that even if they develop amenorrhea during therapy, they may still be able to become pregnant and should be counseled about appropriate nonhormonal contraception methods.

Options for Fertility Preservation

A variety of fertility preservation options are available to premenopausal women diagnosed with breast cancer (see Table 9-3).

Ovarian Suppression With Gonadotropin-Releasing Hormone Agonists

Gonadotropin-releasing hormone (GnRH) agonists (e.g., goserelin) are given during chemotherapy to protect the ovaries by suppressing ovarian function. Chemotherapy does not need to be delayed, unlike with cryopreservation procedures. This method of fertility preservation has been considered experimental in published practice guidelines (American College of Obstetricians and Gynecologists, 2014; Loren et al., 2013) but may become recognized as a standard therapy based on two large randomized clinical trials (Del Mastro & Lambertini, 2015; Lambertini, Ginsburg, & Partridge, 2015). Meta-analyses examining the benefits of GnRH agonists for preserving fertility in women being treated for breast cancer have produced conflicting results, and an additional patient-level meta-analysis is underway (Waks & Partridge, 2016). A panel of international experts has reported strong support for the use of ovarian suppression during chemotherapy to protect against premature ovarian failure and preserve fertility in young women being treated for hormone receptor–negative breast cancer (Coates et al., 2015).

Embryo Cryopreservation

Embryo cryopreservation is an established method of fertility preservation. A male sperm donor is required to fertilize the egg and create an embryo (Loren et al., 2013). The process involves ovarian hyperstimulation with hormones to stimulate follicle development and egg maturation, then egg retrieval and in vitro fertilization prior to freezing the embryos (Oktay et al., 2015). To protect women with estrogen receptor–positive breast cancer from the effects of excessive estrogen exposure on breast tissue during ovarian hyperstimulation, either tamoxifen, a selective estrogen receptor modulator with antagonist effect on the breast, or letrozole, an aromatase inhibitor, may be given

Table 9-3. Fertility Preservation Techniques for Premenopausal Women With Breast Cancer

Technique	Description	Status of Technique	Time Frame for Initiation of Chemotherapy	Surgery Involved
Cryopreservation				
• Embryo	Ovarian stimulation with hormone therapy, egg harvest, sperm used for in vitro fertilization, freezing of embryo	Established method	Delay of 2–6 weeks to allow for egg maturation and retrieval after hormonal stimulation	Yes
• Oocyte	Ovarian stimulation with hormone therapy, egg harvest, freezing of eggs without fertilization	Established method	Delay of 2–6 weeks to allow for egg maturation and retrieval after hormonal stimulation	Yes
• Ovarian tissue	Portion of ovary is removed and frozen for future use. Caution is necessary related to potential risk of reimplanting metastatic cancer cells.	Experimental[a]	No hormonal stimulation or delay in treatment	Yes
Ovarian suppression with gonadotropin-releasing hormone agonists	Use of hormones to temporarily suppress ovarian function during active treatment	Experimental[a,b]	No delay in treatment	No

[a] This method has been endorsed by an expert panel to preserve fertility in young women (Coates et al., 2015).

[b] This method has been recommended to be accepted as a standard therapy based on analysis of data from two large randomized clinical trials (Lambertini, Ginsburg, & Partridge, 2015).

Note. Based on information from Lambertini, Ceppi, et al., 2015; Lambertini, Ginsburg, & Partridge, 2015; Loren et al., 2013; Oktay et al., 2015; Tomasi-Cont et al., 2014; Waks & Partridge, 2016.

in combination with follicle-stimulating hormones (de Pedro et al., 2015; Lambertini, Ginsburg, & Partridge, 2015; Oktay et al., 2015). Chemotherapy initiation is generally delayed two to five weeks to allow for the ovarian stimulation and egg harvesting (Oktay et al., 2015).

Oocyte Cryopreservation

Oocyte cryopreservation is considered a standard fertility preservation option for women at risk of becoming infertile because of antitumor therapy or advancing age. No sperm source is required because the oocytes are stored unfertilized (American College of Obstetricians and Gynecologists, 2014; de Pedro et al., 2015). The techniques employed for egg maturation are the same as described for embryo cryopreservation, except that the harvested eggs are not fertilized in vitro prior to cryopreservation. Chemotherapy initiation is generally delayed two to five weeks to allow for the ovarian stimulation and egg harvesting.

Ovarian Tissue Cryopreservation

Cryopreservation of ovarian tissue is a surgical technique that involves removing a portion of the ovary and freezing it for future reimplantation or follicle aspiration (de Pedro et al., 2015). No hormonal stimulation is required, so there is no delay in initiation of systemic therapy. This technique should be avoided in women with a *BRCA* mutation because of the potential for transplanting ovarian tissue that may contain cancer cells (de Pedro et al., 2015). This method is considered experimental, and current guidelines recommend that it be carried out only in a clinical trial (Imbert et al., 2014; Loren et al., 2013). An expert panel has recently recommended that cryopreservation of ovarian tissue or oocytes be offered to women younger than 40 years of age who request fertility preservation (Coates et al., 2015).

Pregnancy After Breast Cancer

Retrospective evidence suggests that a spontaneous pregnancy after breast cancer does not increase the risk of disease recurrence regardless of tumor estrogen receptor status (Azim et al., 2013). Appropriate timing of a pregnancy is a concern for young women with early estrogen receptor–positive breast cancer for whom adjuvant endocrine therapy is recommended for 5–10 years. Ovarian reserve decreases with age; however, stopping endocrine therapy early to become pregnant may adversely affect prognosis (Pagani et al., 2015). Young women treated for breast cancer who are having difficulty conceiving after at least six months should be referred to a fertility specialist. Timely referral is crucial because ovarian reserve is rapidly lost in these women (Pagani et al., 2015). An international collaboration known as the POSITIVE trial (Pregnancy Outcome and Safety of Interrupting Therapy for women with endocrine responsIVE breast cancer) was recently initiated to investigate the risk of breast cancer recurrence when endocrine therapy is temporarily interrupted to attempt a pregnancy (National Institutes of Health, 2017). See Table 9-4 for a list of organizations that provide support and information about cancer-related infertility and sexuality issues.

Hot Flashes

Overview

Hot flashes are caused by the sudden onset of vasomotor changes that produce feelings of intense heat and profuse sweating and flushing in the face and chest and may be accompanied by heart palpitations and anxiety and followed by chills (Kaplan, 2015). In women treated for breast cancer, 65%–96% report experiencing vasomotor symptoms—a much higher incidence than in women going through natural menopause (Stan, Loprinzi, & Ruddy, 2013). Hot flashes can vary in frequency from several times a day to several times a month and in intensity from mild to very severe and can last for years (Kaplan, 2015). They are associated with psychological distress, interference with daily activities, and decreased quality of life related to lack of sleep, energy, and libido; these factors may lead to early discontinuation of endocrine therapy (Kadakia, Loprinzi, & Barton, 2012; Stan et al., 2013). Subjective assessments of hot flash frequency and intensity using self-report diaries are considered sufficient for clinical practice (Kaplan & Mahon, 2014).

Table 9-4. Selected Online Resources for Cancer-Related Infertility and Sexuality Issues

Organization	Topic	Website
American Association of Sexuality Educators, Counselors and Therapists	Finding a sexuality specialist	www.aasect.org
American Cancer Society	Sexual and fertility side effects of treatment	www.cancer.org/treatment/treatments-and-side-effects/physical-side-effects/fertility-and-sexual-side-effects/sexuality-for-women-with-cancer.html
American Society for Reproductive Medicine	Fact sheets and resource directory	www.asrm.org/resources/patient-resources
Breastcancer.org	Sex and intimacy	www.breastcancer.org/tips/intimacy
Cancer.Net	Dating, intimacy, sexuality, and fertility issues	www.cancer.net/navigating-cancer-care/dating-sex-and-reproduction
Livestrong	Fertility issues	www.livestrong.org/we-can-help/livestrong-fertility
	Female fertility preservation	www.livestrong.org/we-can-help/just-diagnosed/female-fertility-preservation
National Cancer Institute	Sexuality and reproductive issues	www.cancer.gov/about-cancer/treatment/side-effects/sexuality-fertility-women
National Comprehensive Cancer Network	Fertility issues, menopause, surveillance/follow-up	www.nccn.org/professionals/physician_gls/pdf/breast.pdf
North American Menopause Society	Menopause information and specialist directory	www.menopause.org/for-women
Oncofertility Consortium	Fertility resources for patients, educators, and healthcare providers	www.oncofertility.northwestern.edu (for healthcare providers) www.myoncofertility.org (for patients)
OncoLink	Sexuality and fertility issues	www.oncolink.org/support/sexuality-fertility
Oncology Nursing Society	On demand course on sexual dysfunction and infertility	www.ons.org/content/sexual-dysfunction-and-fertility-impairment
SaveMyFertility	Online handbooks and fact sheets for patients and healthcare providers	www.savemyfertility.org
Sexuality Information and Education Council of the United States	Sexuality information and education	www.siecus.org
Society for Sex Therapy and Research	Finding a sexuality specialist	https://sstarnet.org/find-a-therapist

Pathophysiology

The underlying physiology of hot flashes is not well understood and most likely is multifactorial (Kaplan, 2015). Normally, core body temperature is maintained within a narrow range controlled by the thermoregulatory center in the hypothalamus (Kaplan, 2015). Estrogen circulating in the blood interacts with the neurotransmitters serotonin and norepinephrine to regulate the actions of the thermoregulatory center (Shanafelt, Barton, Adjei, & Loprinzi, 2002). Increases in the core temperature above the set temperature range cause the hypothalamus to stimulate compensatory vascular responses to dissipate body heat (vasodilation and profuse sweating), which are characteristics of hot flashes (Kaplan & Mahon, 2014). Core temperatures below the set range lead to heat conservation responses (vasoconstriction and chills) (Dalal & Zhukovsky, 2006; Krause & Nakajima, 2015). Abrupt withdrawal of estrogen is thought to result in dysfunction of the hypothalamic thermoregulatory center so that even small, transient increases in the core body temperature cause an outsized heat loss response felt as hot flashes (Freedman, 2005; Krause & Nakajima, 2015).

Risk Factors

Younger women treated for breast cancer may experience premature menopause because of factors discussed previously. Higher cumulative doses and longer duration of chemotherapy agents toxic to the ovaries increase the risk of early menopause and are associated with higher incidence of vasomotor symptoms (Morrow, Mattair, & Hortobagyi, 2011). Adjuvant endocrine therapies given to suppress ovarian function in women with estrogen receptor–positive breast cancer (tamoxifen for premenopausal women and aromatase inhibitors for postmenopausal women) are associated with hot flashes, especially tamoxifen. Of women treated with tamoxifen, 50%–70% report hot flashes (Stan et al., 2013). Discontinuing hormone replacement therapy abruptly following breast cancer diagnosis can result in hot flashes (Stan et al., 2013).

Management

Pharmacologic Interventions

Hormone replacement therapy is very effective in alleviating hot flashes in postmenopausal women but is contraindicated in women with a history of breast cancer because of increased risk of recurrence (Stan et al., 2013). Systematic reviews of the evidence have categorized only two interventions as "likely to be effective" in reducing the frequency and severity of hot flashes in women with breast cancer. Both are nonhormonal pharmacologic agents: venlafaxine, a selective serotonin reuptake inhibitor antidepressant, and gabapentin, an anticonvulsant (Kaplan & Mahon, 2014; Kaplan et al., 2011; Ramaswami et al., 2015).

Venlafaxine (75 mg per day) does not interfere with the efficacy of tamoxifen therapy and is reported to be the recommended drug for first-line treatment of hot flashes in women with breast cancer (Ramaswami et al., 2015). Patients preferred venlafaxine over gabapentin (900 mg per day) because gabapentin caused adverse side effects (e.g., somnolence, disorientation, headache, peripheral edema).

Paroxetine, a selective serotonin reuptake inhibitor antidepressant, was approved in 2013 as the first nonhormonal treatment for the treatment of moderate to severe hot flashes associated with menopause (U.S. Food and Drug Administration [FDA], 2013). Caution is advised in using paroxetine for women with tamoxifen-induced hot flashes (National Comprehensive Cancer Network®, 2017). Paroxetine is a strong inhibitor of the CYP2D6 enzyme system that mediates the conversion of tamoxifen to its active form, endoxifen, and thus can compromise the effectiveness of tamoxifen (Kaplan & Mahon, 2013). Mortality from breast cancer was elevated in women taking both tamoxifen and paroxetine because of reduced efficacy of tamoxifen (Kelly et al., 2010).

Clonidine, a centrally acting alpha-adrenergic agonist, has been reported to moderately reduce hot flashes in women with breast cancer. However, the authors of a systematic review rated clonidine as "effectiveness not established" because of conflicting study results (Kaplan & Mahon, 2014). In addition, clonidine has significant side effects, including dry mouth, constipation, and insomnia, that limit its usefulness (Krause & Nakajima, 2015).

Nonpharmacologic Interventions

Lifestyle modifications for hot flash relief may be helpful but are not evidence-based (Kaplan & Mahon, 2014). Examples include keeping the room cool; avoiding spices, caffeine, and hot fluids; using a fan and cooling pillows; and dressing in layers. Systematic reviews of several nonpharmacologic interventions to manage hot flashes, including acupuncture, hypnosis, cognitive-behavioral approaches, yoga, and relaxation therapy, ranked the evidence as "effectiveness not established." Use of homeopathic remedies and soy supplements were ranked as "effectiveness unlikely" (Kaplan & Mahon, 2014; Kaplan et al., 2011). The placebo effect has been found to be strongly associated with positive outcomes in studies of hot flash interventions. Participants who received the placebo intervention in several randomized clinical trials reported significant reductions in hot flash activity. Thus, the placebo effect is important to consider when reviewing data about hot flash interventions (Kaplan & Mahon, 2014; Kaplan et al., 2011).

Bone Loss

Overview

Bone loss (osteoporosis) occurs in up to 80% of women treated for breast cancer (Runowicz et al., 2016), with a prevalence five times greater than what occurs with normal aging (Partridge et al., 2014). Conditions that lead to increased bone loss in women treated for breast cancer include chemotherapy-induced premature menopause, use of antiestrogen therapies and ovarian suppression drugs, aging and natural menopause, and cancer metastasis to bone (Hadji et al., 2011).

Pathophysiology

Bone is a dynamic tissue that is continually being remodeled by specialized bone cells: osteoblasts that build bone, and osteoclasts that break down (resorb) bone. Normally these two processes are maintained in balance so that bone loss and bone formation are in equilibrium (Coleman, Body, Aapro, Hadji, & Herrstedt, 2014). Imbalances in normal bone remodeling promote osteoporosis, a chronic condition characterized by low bone mineral density and increased fracture risk (Coleman et al., 2014; Partridge et al., 2014). The presence of circulating estrogen reduces bone breakdown by inhibiting osteoclastic activity and stimulating osteoblasts to form bone. Conditions that decrease estrogen levels lead to greater bone loss and osteoporosis (Partridge et al., 2014).

Risk Factors

Modifiable risk factors include smoking; excess alcohol, cola, and coffee intake; sedentary lifestyle; muscle weakness; low body weight; low calcium levels; and vitamin D deficiency (Runowicz et al., 2016; Stan et al., 2013).

Nonmodifiable risk factors include age older than 50 years, personal or family history of fractures, Caucasian or Asian background, female gender, small build, and late menarche (Stan et al., 2013).

Decreased estrogen levels can occur as a result of treatment-related factors such as bilateral oophorectomy, chronic glucocorticoid use, and cancer therapies, including chemotherapy-induced premature menopause, use of drugs to inhibit ovarian function (GnRH agonists, such as goserelin), and antiestrogen therapies (Coleman et al., 2014; Stan et al., 2013). Antiestrogen therapies are the treatment of choice for women with early-stage estrogen receptor–positive breast cancer: tamoxifen if they are premenopausal, or aromatase inhibitors if they are postmenopausal, used alone or in sequence for up to 10 years (de Pedro et al., 2015). Tamoxifen has weak bone-protecting properties, but aromatase inhibitors, which rapidly deplete estrogen, are associated with increased risk for osteoporosis and bone fractures (Coleman et al., 2014; de Pedro et al., 2015; Hadji et al., 2011).

Assessment

American Cancer Society/American Society of Clinical Oncology guidelines for osteoporosis screening for breast cancer survivors include recommendations for both postmenopausal and premenopausal women. In postmenopausal women, they recommend dual-energy x-ray absorptiometry (DEXA) scan to measure bone mineral density at baseline and every two years for those taking aromatase inhibitors, or yearly if major risk factors change. In premenopausal women, they recommend DEXA scans at baseline and every two years for those taking tamoxifen or a GnRH agonist and in women who have chemotherapy-induced premature menopause (Runowicz et al., 2016).

Management

Pharmacologic interventions with bone antiresorptive agents include bisphosphonates and denosumab. Bisphosphonates are a group of drugs that inhibit the bone-resorbing actions of osteoclasts. They are used in oral or IV form to reduce bone loss and fracture risk in women receiving hormonal therapies (Hadji et al., 2011). Bisphosphonate therapy is indicated for postmenopausal women with estrogen receptor–positive breast cancer taking aromatase inhibitors and for premenopausal women receiving endocrine therapy that includes ovarian suppression (Gralow et al., 2013; Stan et al., 2013). In addition, recent clinical practice guidelines recommend that a bisphosphonate (either zoledronic acid 4 mg IV every six months or clodronate 1,600 mg PO per day) be considered as adjuvant therapy for appropriate postmenopausal patients with nonmetastatic breast cancer, as this treatment has been found to increase survival in these patients (Dhesy-Thind et al., 2017).

Adverse side effects associated with bisphosphonate therapy include the following:

- Oral administration: Esophagitis is the most frequent toxicity of oral bisphosphonates. Treatment adherence is generally low because the patient has to fast before and after taking the drug and sit upright for 30 minutes afterward to avoid esophageal irritation (Hadji et al., 2011).
- IV administration: Nephrotoxicity is the most common toxicity. Increased hydration and serial measures of serum creatinine are mandatory during treatment (Coleman et al., 2014).
- Oral and IV administration: Uncommon but serious adverse events include osteonecrosis of the jaw, which is exposed necrotic bone in the jaw persisting for more than eight weeks, and atypical femoral fractures, which are stress fractures that occur with little or no trauma (Coleman et al., 2014; Early Breast Cancer Trialists' Collaborative Group, 2015).

Denosumab is a monoclonal antibody targeted against osteoclastic bone resorption. It has FDA approval for the treatment of postmenopausal osteoporosis, aromatase inhibitor–induced bone loss, and breast cancer metastatic to bone (Partridge et al., 2014). Denosumab is also approved to treat hypercalcemia in patients who have not had an adequate response to bisphosphonate therapy (Amgen Inc., 2017). Pathologic destruction of bone leading to hypercalcemia is often associated with advanced breast cancer (Kaplan, 2018). Adverse events associated with denosumab include symptomatic hypocalcemia, osteonecrosis of the jaw, and atypical femoral fractures (Amgen Inc., 2017).

Patient Education

Healthcare professionals should provide their patients with information regarding prevention of further bone loss. This includes making lifestyle modifications such as increasing weight-bearing exercise and physical activity, avoiding smoking, and limiting alcohol consumption. Another prevention strategy is supplementing with calcium and vitamin D. Individuals older than age 50 and younger patients who are at risk for cancer treatment–associated bone loss should get 1,200 mg of calcium and 800–1,000 IU vitamin D3 per day (Gralow et al., 2013; Runowicz et al., 2016). Healthcare providers should emphasize the importance of complying with antiresorptive drug therapy and reporting adverse effects (Hadji et al., 2011). Finally, bone mineral density monitoring should be scheduled, as appropriate (Hadji et al., 2011).

Weight Gain

Overview

Weight gain is common among women during and after chemotherapy for breast cancer. The average gain is 2.5–6.2 kg (5.5–13.7 lbs) (Stan et al., 2013). Premenopausal women and women treated with multiagent chemotherapy regimens are reported to gain more than the average amount of weight. Women receiving estrogen therapy alone (without chemotherapy) had lesser weight gains (Stan et al., 2013). Weight gain after breast cancer diagnosis is associated with decreased quality of life and increased risk of comorbid conditions, including lymphedema, cardiovascular disease, diabetes, degenerative joint disease, gallstones, and functional decline (Demark-Wahnefried et al., 2015; Stan et al., 2013). Obesity has been reported to be associated with an approximately 30% increase in the risk of breast of breast cancer recurrence and shorter overall breast cancer survival compared to normal-weight women with breast cancer (Coates et al., 2015; Goodwin, 2016; Playdon et al., 2015). Maintaining body weight in a healthy range after menopause may help prevent the development of hormone-positive breast cancers (Vrieling, Buck, Kaaks, & Chang-Claude, 2010).

Pathophysiology

BMI is the most commonly used measure to define where an adult falls on a scale of body weight. A BMI of 18.5–24.9 kg/m^2 represents a healthy weight; 25–29.9 kg/m^2 is considered overweight; and obesity starts at 30 kg/m^2 (Centers for Disease Control and Prevention, 2017). However, BMI has limitations because it is a measure of both lean muscle mass and fat, and adult weight gain is mostly made up of increased body fat (Vrieling et al., 2010).

Weight gain following chemotherapy is characterized by sarcopenic obesity, in which fat mass increases and lean muscle mass decreases (Stan et al., 2013). After menopause, estrogen is synthesized mainly in the adipose tissue; thus, fatter women have higher levels of circulating estrogen than lean postmenopausal women (Vrieling et al., 2010). Estrogen synthesis in premenopausal women occurs mainly in the ovaries. However, premenopausal women who are overweight or obese may have low circulating estrogen and progesterone levels because their menstrual cycles are more likely to be anovulatory (ovulation does not occur) and they have increased liver clearance of estrogen (Vrieling et al., 2010). Obesity in postmenopausal women may be associated with hyperinsulinemia and insulin resistance, both factors that are thought to promote hormone receptor–positive breast cancer (Vrieling et al., 2010).

Risk Factors

Chemotherapy is a risk factor for weight gain after breast cancer diagnosis. The hormonal changes associated with treatment-induced ovarian failure and abrupt onset of premature menopause may lead to reduced metabolism (Demark-Wahnefried et al., 2015). Emotional distress and increased fatigue due to chemotherapy may lead to overeating, reduced physical activity and exercise, and decreased resting energy expenditure—all of which can contribute to obesity (Demark-Wahnefried et al., 2015; Stan et al., 2013).

Weight gain throughout adult life is associated with higher risk for developing breast cancer (Playdon et al., 2015). Weight gain in postmenopausal women is associated with a higher risk for developing hormone receptor–positive breast cancer (Vrieling et al., 2010). Weight gain after diagnosis of breast cancer is associated with higher all-cause mortality rates compared with weight maintenance, especially if the amount of weight gained was 10% of body weight or more (Playdon et al., 2015).

Management

Experts recommend prevention of weight gain after breast cancer diagnosis to help improve treatment outcomes and overall health (Coates et al., 2015; Demark-Wahnefried et al., 2015; Playdon et al., 2015; Runowicz et al., 2016). Weight management, exercise, and healthy diet are key features of health promotion and are associated with reduced risk of cancer recurrence (Demark-Wahnefried et al., 2015; Runowicz et al., 2016).

Recommendations for cancer survivors based on American Cancer Society guidelines include the following (Rock et al., 2012; Runowicz et al., 2016):

- Weight management: Maintain healthy weight or lose weight if overweight or obese.
- Physical activity: Avoid sedentary lifestyle. Exercise should include moderate-intensity aerobic exercise at least 150 minutes per week and strength training at least twice per week.
- Healthy diet: Consume mostly vegetables, fruits, and whole grains. Eat at least two and a half cups of vegetables and fruits daily. Avoid refined grain products and limit red meat and processed meats.
- Limited alcohol intake: Although recommendations include a maximum of one drink per day for women, authors of a recent study analyzing 30 years of data from more than 88,000 women concluded that "for women who have never smoked, risk of alcohol related cancers (mainly breast cancer) increases even within the range of up to one alcoholic drink a day" (Cao, Willett, Rimm, Stampfer, & Giovannucci, 2015, p. 1).

Vaginal Atrophy

Overview

Vaginal atrophy typically occurs in women following menopause or oophorectomy related to the dramatic reduction in estrogen production. However, younger women who experience early menopause or estrogen suppression as a result of antineoplastic or antiestrogenic therapies are also at risk for vaginal atrophy. The condition also may be termed *vulvovaginal atrophy* or *atrophic vaginitis* because of the dryness, thinning, and inflammation of the vaginal epithelium that occurs secondary to estrogen loss (Bachmann & Santen, 2016).

Pathophysiology

Vaginal atrophy is common in women who are treated for breast cancer with estrogen-depleting therapies. Without the stimulation of estrogen, the normally thick vaginal mucosa becomes thin and pale and more prone to inflammation (Tan, Bradshaw, & Carr, 2012). The vaginal tissue loses elasticity and vaginal secretions and lubrication decrease, factors that contribute to dyspareunia (Stan et al., 2013; Tan et al., 2012). Vaginal pH increases, leading to greater risk of vaginal infections (Stan et al., 2013).

Risk Factors

Risk factors for vaginal atrophy include use of chemotherapy agents toxic to the ovaries, drugs to suppress ovarian function, and aromatase inhibitors (Krause & Nakajima, 2015; Krychman & Millheiser, 2013; Tan et al., 2012). Aromatase inhibitors are reported to cause a much higher incidence of vaginal dryness, dyspareunia (pain with sexual intercourse), and loss of libido compared to tamoxifen therapy (Rosenberg et al., 2014).

Clinical Manifestations

Signs of vaginal atrophy include vaginal walls that are smooth, shiny, and red and may be friable and bleed easily (Tan et al., 2012). Symptoms of vaginal atrophy include dry vaginal and vulvar tissues, pruritus, dyspareunia with intercourse, and increased risk of vaginal infections (Bachmann & Santen, 2016; Krause & Nakajima, 2015). Symptoms usually progress and worsen with continuing estrogen depletion (Bachmann & Santen, 2016).

Management

Early intervention is important to prevent progression to chronic vaginal atrophy and discomfort and to help restore vaginal lubrication, natural pH, and tissue elasticity (Rosenberg et al., 2014). Water-based lubricants (e.g., Astroglide®, K-Y Jelly®) and moisturizers (e.g., Replens®, K-Y Liquibeads®) are effective in alleviating vaginal dryness and dyspareunia (Stan et al., 2013; Tan et al., 2012). Water-based lubricants do not damage latex products such as condoms, diaphragms, or cervical caps; petroleum-based lubricants should not be used with these products (Krychman & Millheiser, 2013). Moisturizers, which are used to replace vaginal secretions, are effective if used several times a week. Lubricants generally are used when needed to facilitate sexual intercourse (Stan et al., 2013; Tan et al., 2012).

Ospemifene (60 mg per day), an oral selective estrogen receptor modulator with estrogenic effects, received FDA approval in 2013 to treat moderate to severe dyspareunia due to vulvar and vaginal atrophy in postmenopausal women (Shionogi Inc., 2015). However, the drug is not recommended for women with known or suspected breast cancer or with a history of breast cancer due to lack of adequate studies in this population. A boxed warning indicates that the drug increases the risk of endometrial cancer in a woman with a uterus who uses unopposed estrogens.

Vaginal estrogen preparations are more effective than nonhormonal therapies, but generally they are not recommended for women with a breast cancer history because of concerns about systemic absorption and cancer recurrence (Stan et al., 2013). However, low-dose vaginal estrogens are minimally absorbed and may be considered for women with breast cancer who have not achieved relief from nonhormonal therapies for severe dyspareunia due to vaginal atrophy. These products include the estradiol vaginal ring (Estring®), estradiol vaginal tablet (Vagifem®), and vaginal conjugated estrogens (Premarin® vaginal cream) (Krychman & Millheiser, 2013; Stan et al., 2013; Tan et al., 2012). Data regarding the safety and efficacy of these agents in this population are lacking. However, women receiving aromatase inhibitors to treat estrogen receptor–positive breast cancer should be cautioned to avoid vaginal estrogens or to use them for the briefest period after being counseled about the potential risks for cancer recurrence (Stan et al., 2013).

Intravaginal dehydroepiandrosterone (DHEA) has shown some efficacy in treating sexual dysfunction due to vaginal atrophy in postmenopausal women without causing changes in systemic hormone levels. DHEA is an androgen released by the adrenal glands that is converted to estrogen in target tissues and is the major source of estrogen in postmenopausal women (Tan et al., 2012). An intravaginal product called Intrarosa™, whose active ingredient is DHEA (known as prasterone), is FDA-approved to treat postmenopausal women experiencing moderate to severe pain (dyspareunia) during sexual intercourse due to vulvar and vaginal atrophy (U.S. FDA, 2016). More data are needed to determine the safety and efficacy of DHEA in women with a breast cancer history (Krychman & Millheiser, 2013; Stan et al., 2013; Tan et al., 2012).

Patient Education

When discussing issues surrounding vaginal atrophy, healthcare providers should provide patients with education and advice on treatments to alleviate the problem.

- Explain that over-the-counter vaginal moisturizers and lubricants are effective for vaginal dryness and should be used for initial therapy; instruct how to apply (Schover, 2014).
- Explain that hormone replacement therapy is not recommended to relieve vaginal atrophy in women with a breast cancer history (Stan et al., 2013).
- Suggest that women who have not experienced relief from over-the-counter products ask their healthcare provider about low-dose vaginal estrogen preparations (Stan et al., 2013).
- Explain that remaining sexually active or using a vaginal dilator may help prevent severe vaginal atrophy (Schover, 2014).

Sexual Dysfunction

Overview

Sexuality is an integral part of life and is influenced by physical, psychological, emotional, and sociocultural factors (Bober & Varela, 2012; Krychman & Millheiser, 2013). Treatments for breast cancer may negatively affect sexuality by causing changes in body image and sensation (surgery and radiation), inducing hormonal changes and premature menopause (chemotherapy, estrogen therapy, ovarian suppression), and causing hair loss and fatigue (chemotherapy) (Bober & Varela, 2012; Krychman & Millheiser, 2013; Stan et al., 2013). Sexual dysfunction is a common and distressing effect of breast cancer therapies and encompasses lack of sexual energy, reduced sexual desire, decreased arousal and orgasm, vaginal dryness, and painful intercourse (dyspareunia) (Bober & Varela, 2012; Krychman & Millheiser, 2013; Stan et al., 2013).

Risk Factors

Adjuvant chemotherapy is a major factor affecting sexuality, as it can lead to estrogen deficiency with associated menopausal symptoms (e.g., hot flashes, vaginal atrophy), hair loss from the head and body, fatigue, nausea, and peripheral neuropathy (Krychman & Millheiser, 2013). Breast surgery can lead to loss of a breast, scarring, and diminished sensation in the breast and nipple (Bober & Varela, 2012).

Younger age (50 years or younger) at the time of breast cancer diagnosis appears to increase the risk for sexual dysfunction related to the presence of vaginal pain, body image changes, and fatigue. These factors have been found to be independently associated with sexual dysfunction (Rosenberg et al., 2014). Body image changes are associated with breast surgery, including mastectomy and reconstruction procedures, weight gain, and hair loss. In addition, breast surgery or loss of childbearing potential secondary to treatment-induced infertility may have a negative impact on the patient's self-esteem, dating, and romantic partnerships (Krychman & Millheiser, 2013).

Assessment

A careful patient history and physical examination are important to assess for comorbid conditions (e.g., diabetes) and use of drugs, such as antidepressants and antihypertensives, that can negatively affect sexual response (Krychman & Millheiser, 2013). The responsibility for initiating a discussion about sexual dysfunction, taking into account cultural mores, lies with the healthcare provider. This is important because the patient may be embarrassed or reluctant to reveal her situation or distress (Stan et al., 2013). The presence of sexual dysfunction should be assessed regularly using objective findings or patient self-report (Stan et al., 2013). Unfortunately, oncology nurses and other healthcare providers may not feel comfortable discussing sexual issues with patients because they may lack the appropriate preparation and knowledge about support resources or have concerns about embarrassing the patient or invading her privacy (Kaplan & Pacelli, 2011; Stan et al., 2013). Two communication models can provide nurses with guidance and confidence in addressing sexuality issues with patients: the PLISSIT model (Annon, 1976) and the BETTER model (Mick, Hughes, & Cohen, 2003) (see Figures 9-7 and 9-8).

Management

Interventions for sexual dysfunction due to cancer treatment should incorporate the expertise of a team of specialists, including oncologists, oncology nurses, psychologists, social workers, sexual counselors, and gynecologists, as appropriate (Krychman & Millheiser, 2013; Runowicz et al., 2016). An intravaginal insert containing DHEA (Intrarosa) recently gained FDA approval for treating dyspareunia due to menopausal vaginal atrophy (U.S. FDA, 2016). Culturally appropriate sexual counseling should be available for individuals or couples and should focus on open communication, problem solving, coping strategies, and alternative methods of sexual expression and intimacy (Bober & Varela, 2012; Rosenberg et al., 2014). Interventions to alleviate treatment-related fatigue and improve appearance and body image through use of

---

Figure 9-7. The PLISSIT Model

P = Permission
The nurse gives the patient permission to express concerns and feelings related to her personal sexual issues and reassurance that her issues are shared by others in the same situation.

LI = Limited Information
The nurse provides the patient with limited information specific to her situation and sexual concerns, such as how her breast cancer treatments can negatively affect her sexual functioning, libido, and body image.

SS = Specific Suggestions
The nurse provides specific suggestions to help the patient manage or compensate for sexual dysfunction, such as interventions to provide vaginal lubrication or diminish fatigue, and explains alternate methods of expressing closeness and intimacy, such as cuddling or massage.

IT = Intensive Therapy
The nurse refers the patient to a sexuality specialist after the prior three steps have not resolved the patient's problems and a higher level of intervention is indicated.

Note. Based on information from Annon, 1976; Katz, 2005; Mick, 2007.

From "The Sexuality Discussion: Tools for the Oncology Nurse," by M. Kaplan and R. Pacelli, 2011, *Clinical Journal of Oncology Nursing, 15,* p. 16. Copyright 2011 by Oncology Nursing Society. Adapted with permission.

Figure 9-8. The BETTER Model

B = Bring up the topic of sexuality with the patient. Nurses initiate this conversation and assure the patient that her sexual function is an acceptable area for discussion.

E = Explain that sexuality is a quality-of-life issue and thus is important for the nurse to address.

T = Tell the patient about outside resources that can provide information and guidance and provide a list.

T = Time the discussion of sexuality according to the patient's readiness to share and receive information.

E = Educate the patient about how cancer therapy side effects can have a profound effect on her interest and ability to perform sexually.

R = Record the sexuality discussion in the patient's healthcare record.

Note. Based on information from Mick et al., 2003, 2004.

From "The Sexuality Discussion: Tools for the Oncology Nurse," by M. Kaplan and R. Pacelli, 2011, *Clinical Journal of Oncology Nursing, 15,* p. 16. Copyright 2011 by Oncology Nursing Society. Adapted with permission.

---

breast prostheses or wigs, as well as increased physical activity and weight loss, may be helpful (Rosenberg et al., 2014; Runowicz et al., 2016). Use of testosterone has not shown benefit in the treatment of sexual dysfunction (Stan et al., 2013).

Patient Education

Nurses can use structured communication models to help guide the sexuality discussion with patients and their sexual partners. Two models that lend themselves to this discussion are the PLISSIT and BETTER models, as mentioned previously (Kaplan & Pacelli, 2011). Explain to patients and their partners that alternative forms of sexual expression and physical intimacy are acceptable, while being sensitive to their cultural and personal values (Bober & Varela, 2012; Krychman & Millheiser, 2013). Refer patients to appropriate support organizations and resources (see Table 9-4).

Summary

Symptom distress can adversely alter the experience of women diagnosed with breast cancer. Close review of the most commonly experienced side effects from treatment shows clear but complex interrelationships. Even minor symptoms can serve as a constant reminder of the cancer diagnosis. Nurses should be familiar with evidence-based resources for current information on symptom management, including the Oncology Nursing Society Putting Evidence Into Practice resources (www .ons.org/practice-resources/pep) and the National Comprehensive Cancer Network resources (www.nccn.org) for symptom management. Careful assessment at follow-up visits can result in the early detection of symptoms so that management can be implemented promptly with the goal of improved quality of life. Education regarding cancer treatment side effects should be provided to all healthcare professionals involved in the care of these patients, including those in the primary care setting. Doing so will help to lessen patients' anxiety, avoid misconceptions, and reduce patients' fear of recurrence.

References

American Cancer Society. (2016, July 7). For people at risk of lymphedema. Retrieved from http://www .cancer.org/treatment/treatments-and-side-effects/physical-side-effects/lymphedema/for-people-at -risk-of-lymphedema.html

American College of Obstetricians and Gynecologists. (2014). Committee Opinion No. 584: Oocyte cryo-preservation. *Obstetrics and Gynecology, 123,* 221–222. doi:10.1097/01.AOG.0000441355.66434.6d

Amgen Inc. (2017, May). *Xgeva® (denosumab) injection, for subcutaneous use* [Package insert]. Thousand Oaks, CA: Author.

Annon, J.S. (1976). The PLISSIT model: A proposed conceptual scheme for the behavioral treatment of sexual problems. *Journal of Sex Education and Therapy, 2*(1), 1–15.

Armer, J.M., Hulett, J.M., Bernas, M., Ostby, P., Stewart, B.R., & Cormier, J.N. (2013). Best-practice guide-lines in assessment, risk reduction, management, and surveillance for post-breast cancer lymphedema. *Current Breast Cancer Reports, 5,* 134–144. doi:10.1007/s12609-013-0105-0

Azim, H.A., Jr., Kroman, N., Paesmans, M., Gelber, S., Rotmensz, N., Ameye, L., … Peccatori, F.A. (2013). Prognostic impact of pregnancy after breast cancer according to estrogen receptor status: A multi-center retrospective study. *Journal of Clinical Oncology, 31,* 73–79. doi:10.1200/JCO.2012.44.2285

Baber, R., Hickey, M., & Kwik, M. (2005). Therapy for menopausal symptoms during and after treatment for breast cancer: Safety considerations. *Drug Safety, 28,* 1085–1100. doi:10.2165/00002018-200528120 -00004

Bachmann, G., & Santen, R.J. (2016, June 28). Clinical manifestations and diagnosis of genitourinary syndrome of menopause (vulvovaginal atrophy) [Literature review current through September 2017]. Retrieved from http://www.uptodate.com/contents/clinical-manifestations-and-diagnosis-of -genitourinary-syndrome-of-menopause-vulvovaginal-atrophy

Bar Ad, V., Dutta, P.R., Solin, L.J., Hwang, W.-T., Tan, K.S., Both, S., … Harris, E.E.R. (2012). Time-course of arm lymphedema and potential risk factors for progression of lymphedema after breast conserva-tion treatment for early stage breast cancer. *Breast Journal, 18,* 219–225. doi:10.1111/j.1524-4741.2012 .01229.x

Basta, M.N., Fox, J.P., Kanchwala, S.K., Wu, L.C., Serletti, J.M., Kovach, S.J., … Fischer, J.P. (2016). Com-plicated breast cancer–related lymphedema: Evaluating health care resource utilization and associ-ated costs of management. *American Journal of Surgery, 211,* 133–141. doi:10.1016/j.amjsurg.2015.06.015

Basta, M.N., Gao, L.L., & Wu, L.C. (2014). Operative treatment of peripheral lymphedema: A systematic meta-analysis of the efficacy and safety of lymphovenous microsurgery and tissue transplantation. *Plas-tic and Reconstructive Surgery, 133,* 905–913. doi:10.1097/PRS.0000000000000010

Bernas, M. (2013). Assessment and risk reduction in lymphedema. *Seminars in Oncology Nursing, 29,* 12–19. doi:10.1016/j.soncn.2012.11.003

Bober, S.L., & Varela, V.S. (2012). Sexuality in adult cancer survivors: Challenges and intervention. *Jour-nal of Clinical Oncology, 30,* 3712–3719. doi:10.1200/JCO.2012.41.7915

Boughey, J.C., Hoskin, T.L., Cheville, A.L., Miller, J., Loprinzi, M.D., Thomsen, K.M., … Degnim, A.C. (2014). Risk factors associated with breast lymphedema. *Annals of Surgical Oncology, 21,* 1202–1208. doi:10.1245/s10434-013-3408-5

Bozza, C., Puglisi, F., Lambertini, M., Osa, E.-O., Manno, M., & Del Mastro, L. (2014). Anti-Müllerian hor-mone: Determination of ovarian reserve in early breast cancer patients. *Endocrine-Related Cancer, 21,* R51–R65. doi:10.1530/ERC-13-0335

Bromberg, M.B. (2017, May 31). Brachial plexus syndromes [Literature review current through Septem-ber 2017]. Retrieved from http://www.uptodate.com/contents/brachial-plexus-syndromes

Brown, L.C., Mutter, R.W., & Halyard, M.Y. (2015). Benefits, risks, and safety of external beam radiation therapy for breast cancer. *International Journal of Women's Health, 7,* 449–458. doi:10.2147/IJWH.S55552

Cao, Y., Willett, W.C., Rimm, E.B., Stampfer, M.J., & Giovannucci, E.L. (2015). Light to moderate intake of alcohol, drinking patterns, and risk of cancer: Results from two prospective US cohort studies. *BMJ, 351,* h4238. doi:10.1136/bmj.h4238

Centers for Disease Control and Prevention. (2017, August 29). About adult BMI. Retrieved from https:// www.cdc.gov/healthyweight/assessing/bmi/adult_bmi

Chang, C.J., & Cormier, J.N. (2013). Lymphedema interventions: Exercise, surgery, and compression devices. *Seminars in Oncology Nursing, 29,* 28–40. doi:10.1016/j.soncn.2012.11.005

Coates, A.S., Winer, E.P., Goldhirsch, A., Gelber, R.D., Gnant, M., Piccart-Gebhart, M., … Senn, H.-J. (2015). Tailoring therapies—Improving the management of early breast cancer: St. Gallen International Expert Consensus on the Primary Therapy of Early Breast Cancer 2015. *Annals of Oncology, 26,* 1533–1546. doi:10.1093/annonc/mdv221

Coleman, R., Body, J.J., Aapro, M., Hadji, P., & Herrstedt, J. (2014). Bone health in cancer patients: ESMO clinical practice guidelines. *Annals of Oncology, 25*(Suppl. 3), iii124–iii137. doi:10.1093/annonc/mdu103

Cormier, J.N., Rourke, L., Crosby, M., Chang, D., & Armer, J. (2012). The surgical treatment of lymphedema: A systematic review of the contemporary literature (2004–2010). *Annals of Surgical Oncology, 19,* 642–651. doi:10.1245/s10434-011-2017-4

Dalal, S., & Zhukovsky, D.S. (2006). Pathophysiology and management of hot flashes. *Journal of Supportive Oncology, 4,* 315–320, 325.

Dayan, J.H., Dayan, E., & Smith, M.L. (2015). Reverse lymphatic mapping: A new technique for maximizing safety in vascularized lymph node transfer. *Plastic and Reconstructive Surgery, 135,* 277–285. doi:10 .1097/PRS.0000000000000822

Delanian, S., Lefaix, J.-L., & Pradat, P.-F. (2012). Radiation-induced neuropathy in cancer survivors. *Radiotherapy and Oncology, 105,* 273–282. doi:10.1016/j.radonc.2012.10.012

Del Mastro, L., & Lambertini, M. (2015). Temporary ovarian suppression with gonadotropin-releasing hormone agonist during chemotherapy for fertility preservation: Toward the end of the debate? *Oncologist, 20,* 1233–1235. doi:10.1634/theoncologist.2015-0373

Demark-Wahnefried, W., Rogers, L.Q., Alfano, C.M., Thomson, C.A., Courneya, K.S., Meyerhardt, J.A., … Ligibel, J.A. (2015). Practical clinical interventions for diet, physical activity, and weight control in cancer survivors. *CA: A Cancer Journal for Clinicians, 65,* 167–189. doi:10.3322/caac.21265

de Pedro, M., Otero, B., & Martin, B. (2015). Fertility preservation and breast cancer: A review. *Ecancermedicalscience, 9,* 503. doi:10.3332/ecancer.2015.503

Dhesy-Thind, S., Fletcher, G.G., Blanchette, P.S., Clemons, M.J., Dillmon, M.S., Frank, E.S., … Van Poznak, C.H. (2017). Use of adjuvant bisphosphonates and other bone-modifying agents in breast cancer: A Cancer Care Ontario and American Society of Clinical Oncology clinical practice guideline. *Journal of Clinical Oncology, 35,* 2062–2081. doi:10.1200/JCO.2016.70.7257

DiSipio, T., Rye, S., Newman, B., & Hayes, S. (2013). Incidence of unilateral arm lymphoedema after breast cancer: A systematic review and meta-analysis. *Lancet Oncology, 14,* 500–515. doi:10.1016/S1470 -2045(13)70076-7

Dominick, S.A., Madlensky, L., Natarajan, L., & Pierce, J.P. (2013). Risk factors associated with breast-cancer related lymphedema in the WHEL Study. *Journal of Cancer Survivorship, 7,* 115–123. doi:10.1007 /s11764-012-0251-9

Early Breast Cancer Trialists' Collaborative Group. (2015). Adjuvant bisphosphonate treatment in early breast cancer: Meta-analyses of individual patient data from randomised trials. *Lancet, 386,* 1353–1361. doi:10.1016/S0140-6736(15)60908-4

Feldman, J.L., Stout, N.L., Wanchai, A., Stewart, B.R., Cormier, J.N., & Armer, J.M. (2012). Intermittent pneumatic compression therapy: A systematic review. *Lymphology, 45,* 13–25.

Freedman, R.R. (2005). Pathophysiology and treatment of menopausal hot flashes. *Seminars in Reproductive Medicine, 23,* 117–125. doi:10.1055/s-2005-869479

Fu, M.R., Deng, J., & Armer, J.M. (2014). Putting evidence into practice: Cancer-related lymphedema: Evolving evidence for treatment and management from 2009–2014. *Clinical Journal of Oncology Nursing, 18*(6, Suppl. 3), 68–79. doi:10.1188/14.CJON.S3.68-79

Fu, M.R., & Kang, Y. (2013). Psychosocial impact of living with cancer-related lymphedema. *Seminars in Oncology Nursing, 29,* 50–60. doi:10.1016/j.soncn.2012.11.007

Fu, M.R., Ridner, S.H., Hu, S.H., Stewart, B.R., Cormier, J.N., & Armer, J.M. (2013). Psychosocial impact of lymphedema: A systematic review of literature from 2004 to 2011. *Psycho-Oncology, 22,* 1466–1484. doi:10.1002/pon.3201

Ganz, P.A., Land, S.R., Geyer, C.E., Cecchini, R.S., Costantino, J.P., Pajon, E.R., … Swain, S.M. (2011). Menstrual history and quality-of-life outcomes in women with node-positive breast cancer treated with adjuvant therapy on the NSABP B-30 trial. *Journal of Clinical Oncology, 29,* 1110–1116. doi:10.1200/JCO.2010.29.7689

Goodwin, P.J. (2016). Obesity and breast cancer outcomes: How much evidence is needed to change practice? *Journal of Clinical Oncology, 34,* 646–648. doi:10.1200/JCO.2015.64.7503

Gralow, J.R., Biermann, J.S., Farooki, A., Fornier, M.N., Gagel, R.F., Kumar, R., … Van Poznack, C.H. (2013). NCCN task force report: Bone health in cancer care. *Journal of the National Comprehensive Cancer Network, 11*(Suppl. 3), S1–S50.

Hadji, P., Aapro, M.S., Body, J.J., Bundred, N.J., Brufsky, A., Coleman, R.E., … Lipton, A. (2011). Management of aromatase inhibitor-associated bone loss in postmenopausal women with breast cancer: Practical guidance for prevention and treatment. *Annals of Oncology, 22,* 2546–2555. doi:10.1093/annonc/mdr017

Hayes, S.C., Johansson, K., Stout, N.L., Prosnitz, R., Armer, J.M., Gabram, S., & Schmitz, K.H. (2012). Upper-body morbidity after breast cancer: Incidence and evidence for evaluation, prevention, and management with a prospective surveillance model of care. *Cancer, 118*(Suppl. 8), 2237–2249. doi:10.1002/cncr.27467

Helyer, L.K., Varnic, M., Le, L.W., Leong, W., & McCready, D. (2010). Obesity is a risk factor for developing postoperative lymphedema in breast cancer patients. *Breast Journal, 16,* 48–54. doi:10.1111/j.1524 -4741.2009.00855.x

Howlader, N., Noone, A.M., Krapcho, M., Miller, D., Bishop, K., Kosary, C.L., ... Cronin, K.A. (Eds.). (2017, June). *SEER cancer statistics review, 1975–2014.* Retrieved from http://seer.cancer.gov/csr/1975_2014

Imbert, R., Moffa, F., Tsepelidis, S., Simon, P., Delbaere, A., Devreker, F., ... Demeestere, I. (2014). Safety and usefulness of cryopreservation of ovarian tissue to preserve fertility: A 12-year retrospective analysis. *Human Reproduction, 29,* 1931–1940. doi:10.1093/humrep/deu158

International Society of Lymphology. (2013). The diagnosis and treatment of peripheral lymphedema: 2013 Consensus Document of the International Society of Lymphology. *Lymphology, 46,* 1–11.

Jakes, A.D., & Twelves, C. (2015). Breast cancer-related lymphoedema and venepuncture: A review and evidence-based recommendations. *Breast Cancer Research and Treatment, 154,* 455–461. doi:10.1007/s10549 -015-3639-1

Kadakia, K.C., Loprinzi, C.L., & Barton, D.L. (2012). Hot flashes: The ongoing search for effective interventions. *Menopause, 19,* 719–721. doi:10.1097/gme.0b013e3182578d31

Kaplan, M. (2015). Hot flashes. In C.G. Brown (Ed.), *A guide to oncology symptom management* (2nd ed., pp. 421–447). Pittsburgh, PA: Oncology Nursing Society.

Kaplan, M. (2018). Hypercalcemia of malignancy. In C.H. Yarbro, D. Wujcik, & B.H. Gobel (Eds.), *Cancer nursing: Principles and practice* (8th ed., pp. 1107–1134). Burlington, MA: Jones & Bartlett Learning.

Kaplan, M., & Mahon, S.M. (2013). Tamoxifen benefits and CYP2D6 testing in women with hormone-receptor-positive breast cancer. *Clinical Journal of Oncology Nursing, 17,* 174–179. doi:10.1188/13.CJON .174-179

Kaplan, M., & Mahon, S.M. (2014). Hot flash management: Update on the evidence for patients with cancer. *Clinical Journal of Oncology Nursing, 18*(6, Suppl. 3), 59–67. doi:10.1188/14.CJON.S3.59-67

Kaplan, M., Mahon, S.M., Cope, D., Keating, E., Hill, S., & Jacobson, M. (2011). Putting evidence into practice: Evidence-based interventions for hot flashes resulting from cancer therapies. *Clinical Journal of Oncology Nursing, 15,* 149–157. doi:10.1188/11.CJON.149-157

Kaplan, M., & Pacelli, R. (2011). The sexuality discussion: Tools for the oncology nurse. *Clinical Journal of Oncology Nursing, 15,* 15–17. doi:10.1188/11.CJON.15-17

Karaca-Mandic, P., Hirsch, A.T., Rockson, S.G., & Ridner, S.H. (2015). The cutaneous, net clinical, and health economic benefits of advanced pneumatic compression devices in patients with lymphedema. *JAMA Dermatology, 151,* 1187–1193. doi:10.1001/jamadermatol.2015.1895

Katz, A. (2005). The sounds of silence: Sexuality information for cancer patients. *Journal of Clinical Oncology, 23,* 238–241. doi:10.1200/JCO.2005.05.101

Kelly, C.M., Juurlink, D.N., Gomes, T., Duong-Hua, M., Pritchard, K.I., Austin, P.C., & Paszat, L.F. (2010). Selective serotonin reuptake inhibitors and breast cancer mortality in women receiving tamoxifen: A population based cohort study. *BMJ, 340,* c693. doi:10.1136/bmj.c693

Kort, J.D., Eisenberg, M.L., Millheiser, L.S., & Westphal, L.M. (2014). Fertility issues in cancer survivorship. *CA: A Cancer Journal for Clinicians, 64,* 118–134. doi:10.3322/caac.21205

Krause, M.S., & Nakajima, S.T. (2015). Hormonal and nonhormonal treatment of vasomotor symptoms. *Obstetrics and Gynecology Clinics of North America, 42,* 163–179. doi:10.1016/j.ogc.2014.09.008

Krychman, M., & Millheiser, L.S. (2013). Sexual health issues in women with cancer. *Journal of Sexual Medicine, 10*(Suppl. 1), 5–15. doi:10.1111/jsm.12034

Kwan, M.L., Cohn, J.C., Armer, J.M., Stewart, B.R., & Cormier, J.N. (2011). Exercise in patients with lymphedema: A systematic review of the contemporary literature. *Journal of Cancer Survivorship, 5,* 320– 336. doi:10.1007/s11764-011-0203-9

Kwan, M.L., Darbinian, J., Schmitz, K.H., Citron, R., Partee, P., Kutner, S.E., & Kushi, L.H. (2010). Risk factors for lymphedema in a prospective breast cancer survivorship study: The Pathways Study. *Archives of Surgery, 145,* 1055–1063. doi:10.1001/archsurg.2010.231

Lambertini, M., Anserini, P., Levaggi, A., Poggio, F., & Del Mastro, L. (2013). Fertility counseling of young breast cancer patients. *Journal of Thoracic Disease, 5*(Suppl. 1), S68–S80. doi:10.3978/j.issn.2072-1439 .2013.05.22

Lambertini, M., Ceppi, M., Poggio, F., Peccatori, F.A., Azim, H.A., Jr., Ugolini, D., ... Del Mastro, L. (2015). Ovarian suppression using luteinizing hormone-releasing hormone agonists during chemotherapy to preserve ovarian function and fertility of breast cancer patients: A meta-analysis of randomized studies. *Annals of Oncology, 26,* 2408–2419. doi:10.1093/annonc/mdv374

Lambertini, M., Ginsburg, E.S., & Partridge, A.H. (2015). Update on fertility preservation in young women undergoing breast cancer and ovarian cancer therapy. *Current Opinion in Obstetrics and Gynecology, 27,* 98–107. doi:10.1097/GCO.0000000000000138

Lasinski, B.B. (2013). Complete decongestive therapy for treatment of lymphedema. *Seminars in Oncology Nursing, 29,* 20–27. doi:10.1016/j.soncn.2012.11.004

Lawenda, B.D., Mondry, T.E., & Johnstone, P.A. (2009). Lymphedema: A primer on the identification and management of a chronic condition in oncologic treatment. *CA: A Cancer Journal for Clinicians, 59,* 8–24. doi:10.3322/caac.20001

Lee, S., Kil, W.J., Chun, M., Jung, Y.-S., Kang, S.Y., Kang, S.-H., & Oh, Y.-T. (2009). Chemotherapy-related amenorrhea in premenopausal women with breast cancer. *Menopause, 16,* 98–103. doi:10.1097/gme.0b013e3181844877

Letourneau, J.M., Ebbel, E.E., Katz, P.P., Oktay, K.H., McCulloch, C.E., Ai, W.Z., ... Rosen, M.P. (2012). Acute ovarian failure underestimates age-specific reproductive impairment for young women undergoing chemotherapy for cancer. *Cancer, 118,* 1933–1939. doi:10.1002/cncr.26403

Llarena, N.C., Estevez, S.L., Tucker, S.L., & Jeruss, J.S. (2015). Impact of fertility concerns on tamoxifen initiation and persistence. *Journal of the National Cancer Institute, 107,* djv202. doi:10.1093/jnci/djv202

Loren, A.W., Mangu, P.B., Beck, L.N., Brennan, L., Magdalinski, A.J., Partridge, A.H., ... Oktay, K. (2013). Fertility preservation for patients with cancer: American Society of Clinical Oncology clinical practice guideline update. *Journal of Clinical Oncology, 31,* 2500–2510. doi:10.1200/JCO.2013.49.2678

McNeely, M.L., Binkley, J.M., Pusic, A.L., Campbell, K.L., Gabram, S., & Soballe, P.W. (2012). A prospective model of care for breast cancer rehabilitation: Postoperative and postreconstructive issues. *Cancer, 118*(Suppl. 8), 2226–2236. doi:10.1002/cncr.27468

Mehrara, B. (2017, September 22). Breast cancer-associated lymphedema [Literature review current through September 2017]. Retrieved from http://www.uptodate.com/contents/breast-cancer-associated-lymphedema

Mick, J.M. (2007). Sexuality assessment: 10 strategies for improvement. *Clinical Journal of Oncology Nursing, 11,* 671–675. doi:10.1188/07.CJON.671-675

Mick, J.M., Hughes, M., & Cohen, M.Z. (2003). Sexuality and cancer: How oncology nurses can address it BETTER [Abstract 180]. *Oncology Nursing Forum, 30*(Suppl. 2), 152–153.

Mick, J.M., Hughes, M., & Cohen, M.Z. (2004). Using the BETTER model to assess sexuality. *Clinical Journal of Oncology Nursing, 8,* 84–86. doi:10.1188/04.CJON.84-86

Morgan, S., Anderson, R.A., Gourley, C., Wallace, W.H., & Spears, N. (2012). How do chemotherapeutic agents damage the ovary? *Human Reproduction Update, 18,* 525–535. doi:10.1093/humupd/dms022

Morrow, P.K.H., Mattair, D.N., & Hortobagyi, G.N. (2011). Hot flashes: A review of pathophysiology and treatment modalities. *Oncologist, 16,* 1658–1664. doi:10.1634/theoncologist.2011-0174

National Cancer Institute. (2015, April 29). *Lymphedema (PDQ®)* [Patient version]. Retrieved from http://www.cancer.gov/about-cancer/treatment/side-effects/lymphedema/lymphedema-pdq

National Comprehensive Cancer Network. (2017). *NCCN Clinical Practice Guidelines in Oncology (NCCN Guidelines®): Breast cancer* [v.2.2017]. Retrieved from http://www.nccn.org/professionals/physician_gls/pdf/breast.pdf

National Institutes of Health. (2017, September 11). Pregnancy Outcome and Safety of Interrupting Therapy for Women With Endocrine Responsive Breast Cancer (POSITIVE) [ClinicalTrials.gov identifier: NCT02308085]. Retrieved from https://clinicaltrials.gov/ct2/show/NCT02308085?term=NCT02308085&rank=1

National Lymphedema Network. (2012, May). Position statement of the National Lymphedema Network: Summary of lymphedema risk reduction practices. Retrieved from http://www.lymphnet.org/pdfDocs/nlnriskreduction_summary.pdf

National Lymphedema Network. (2013, November). Position statement of the National Lymphedema Network: Exercise. Retrieved from http://www.lymphnet.org/pdfDocs/nlnexercise.pdf

Oktay, K., Turan, V., Bedoschi, G., Pacheco, F.S., & Moy, F. (2015). Fertility preservation success subsequent to concurrent aromatase inhibitor treatment and ovarian stimulation in women with breast cancer. *Journal of Clinical Oncology, 33,* 2424–2429. doi:10.1200/JCO.2014.59.3723

Ostby, P.L., Armer, J.M., Dale, P.S., Van Loo, M.J., Wilbanks, C.L., & Stewart, B.R. (2014). Surveillance recommendations in reducing risk of and optimally managing breast cancer-related lymphedema. *Journal of Personalized Medicine, 4,* 424–447. doi:10.3390/jpm4030424

O'Toole, J., Jammallo, L.S., Miller, C.L., Skolny, M.N., Specht, M.C., & Taghian, A.G. (2013). Screening for breast cancer-related lymphedema: The need for standardization. *Oncologist, 18,* 350–352. doi:10 .1634/theoncologist.2012-0387

Pagani, O., Ruggeri, M., Manunta, S., Saunders, C., Peccatori, F., Cardoso, F., … Partridge, A.H. (2015). Pregnancy after breast cancer: Are young patients willing to participate in clinical studies? *Breast, 24,* 201–207. doi:10.1016/j.breast.2015.01.005

Partridge, A.H., Pagani, O., Abulkhair, O., Aebi, S., Amant, F., Azim, H.A., Jr., … Cardoso, F. (2014). First international consensus guidelines for breast cancer in young women (BCY1). *Breast, 23,* 209–220. doi:10.1016/j.breast.2014.03.011

Paskett, E.D., Dean, J.A., Oliveri, J.M., & Harrop, J.P. (2012). Cancer-related lymphedema risk factors, diagnosis, treatment, and impact: A review. *Journal of Clinical Oncology, 30,* 3726–3733. doi:10.1200/JCO.2012.41.8574

Patricolo, G.E., Armstrong, K., Riutta, J., & Lanni, T. (2015). Lymphedema care for the breast cancer patient: An integrative approach. *Breast, 24,* 82–85. doi:10.1016/j.breast.2014.10.004

Penha, T.R.L., Ijsbrandy, C., Hendrix, N.A.M., Heuts, E.M., Voogd, A.C., von Meyenfeldt, M.F., & van der Hulst, R.R.W.J. (2013). Microsurgical techniques for the treatment of breast cancer–related lymphedema: A systematic review. *Journal of Reconstructive Microsurgery, 29,* 99–106. doi:10.1055/s-0032-1329919

Phillips, J. (2014, October). Breast cancer lymphedema hand/arm measurements. *Lymphedema Management Special Interest Group Newsletter, 25*(2). Retrieved from http://onsopcontent.ons.org/Publications /SIGNewsletters/lym/lym25.2.html#story2

Playdon, M.C., Bracken, M.B., Sanft, T.B., Ligibel, J.A., Harrigan, M., & Irwin, M.L. (2015). Weight gain after breast cancer diagnosis and all-cause mortality: Systematic review and meta-analysis. *Journal of the National Cancer Institute, 107,* djv275. doi:10.1093/jnci/djv275

Ramaswami, R., Villarreal, M.D., Pitta, D.M., Carpenter, J.S., Stebbing, J., & Kalesan, B. (2015). Venlafaxine in management of hot flashes in women with breast cancer: A systematic review and meta-analysis. *Breast Cancer Research and Treatment, 152,* 231–237. doi:10.1007/s10549-015-3465-5

Ridner, S.H. (2013). Pathophysiology of lymphedema. *Seminars in Oncology Nursing, 29,* 4–11. doi:10.1016 /j.soncn.2012.11.002

Ridner, S.H., Fu, M.R., Wanchai, A., Stewart, B.R., Armer, J.M., & Cormier, J.N. (2012). Self-management of lymphedema: A systematic review of the literature from 2004 to 2011. *Nursing Research, 61,* 291–299. doi:10.1097/NNR.0b013e31824f82b2

Rock, C.L., Doyle, C., Demark-Wahnefried, W., Meyerhardt, J., Courneya, K.S., Schwartz, A.L., … Gansler, T. (2012). Nutrition and physical activity guidelines for cancer survivors. *CA: A Cancer Journal for Clinicians, 62,* 242–274. doi:10.3322/caac.21142

Rodrick, J.R., Poage, E., Wanchai, A., Stewart, B.R., Cormier, J.N., & Armer, J.M. (2014). Complementary, alternative, and other noncomplete decongestive therapy treatment methods in the management of lymphedema: A systematic search and review. *PM&R, 6,* 250–274. doi:10.1016/j.pmrj.2013.09.008

Rosenberg, S.M., & Partridge, A.H. (2013). Premature menopause in young breast cancer: Effects on quality of life and treatment interventions. *Journal of Thoracic Disease, 5*(Suppl. 1), S55–S61. doi:10.3978 /j.issn.2072-1439.2013.06.20

Rosenberg, S.M., Tamimi, R.M., Gelber, S., Ruddy, K.J., Bober, S.L., Kereakoglow, S., … Partridge, A.H. (2014). Treatment-related amenorrhea and sexual functioning in young breast cancer survivors. *Cancer, 120,* 2264–2271. doi:10.1002/cncr.28738

Runowicz, C.D., Leach, C.R., Henry, N.L., Henry, K.S., Mackey, H.T., Cowens-Alvarado, R.L., … Ganz, P.A. (2016). American Cancer Society/American Society of Clinical Oncology breast cancer survivorship care guideline. *CA: A Cancer Journal for Clinicians, 66,* 43–73. doi:10.3322/caac.21319

Rutkove, S.B. (2016, December 9). Overview of upper extremity peripheral nerve syndromes [Literature review current through September 2017]. Retrieved from http://www.uptodate.com/contents/overview -of-upper-extremity-peripheral-nerve-syndromes

Schover, L.R. (2014). Premature ovarian failure is a major risk factor for cancer-related sexual dysfunction. *Cancer, 120,* 2230–2232. doi:10.1002/cncr.28735

Shah, C., Arthur, D., Riutta, J., Whitworth, P., & Vicini, F.A. (2012). Breast-cancer related lymphedema: A review of procedure-specific incidence rates, clinical assessment aids, treatment paradigms, and risk reduction. *Breast Journal, 18,* 357–361. doi:10.1111/j.1524-4741.2012.01252.x

Shanafelt, T.D., Barton, D.L., Adjei, A.A., & Loprinzi, C.L. (2002). Pathology and treatment of hot flashes. *Mayo Clinic Proceedings, 77,* 1207–1218. doi:10.4065/77.11.1207

Shandley, L.M., Spencer, J.B., Fothergill, A.C., Mertens, A., Manatunga, A., Paplomata, E., & Howards, P.P. (2017). Impact of tamoxifen therapy on fertility in breast cancer survivors. *Fertility and Sterility, 107,* 243–252.e5. doi:10.1016/j.fertnstert.2016.10.020

Shih, Y.-C.T., Xu, Y., Cormier, J.N., Giordano, S., Ridner, S.H., Buchholz, T.A., … Elting, L.S. (2009). Incidence, treatment costs, and complications of lymphedema after breast cancer among women of working age: A 2-year follow-up study. *Journal of Clinical Oncology, 27,* 2007–2014. doi:10.1200/JCO.2008.18.3517

Shionogi Inc. (2015). *Osphena® (ospemifene)* [Package insert]. Florham Park, NJ: Author.

Stan, D., Loprinzi, C.L., & Ruddy, K.J. (2013). Breast cancer survivorship issues. *Hematology/Oncology Clinics of North America, 27,* 805–827. doi:10.1016/j.hoc.2013.05.005

Stephenson, R.O. (2017, May 18). Radiation-induced brachial plexopathy. Retrieved from http://emedicine.medscape.com/article/316497-overview

Stuiver, M.M., ten Tusscher, M.R., Agasi-Idenburg, C.S., Lucas, C., Aaronson, N.K., & Bossuyt, P.M.M. (2015). Conservative interventions for preventing clinically detectable upper-limb lymphoedema in patients who are at risk of developing lymphoedema after breast cancer therapy. *Cochrane Database of Systematic Reviews, 2015*(2). doi:10.1002/14651858.CD009765.pub2

Tan, O., Bradshaw, K., & Carr, B.R. (2012). Management of vulvovaginal atrophy-related sexual dysfunction in postmenopausal women: An up-to-date review. *Menopause, 19,* 109–117. doi:10.1097/gme.0b013e31821f92df

Tomasi-Cont, N., Lambertini, M., Hulsbosch, S., Peccatori, A.F., & Amant, F. (2014). Strategies for fertility preservation in young early breast cancer patients. *Breast, 23,* 503–510. doi:10.1016/j.breast.2014.05.024

Torino, F., Barnabei, A., De Vecchis, L., Appetecchia, M., Strigari, L., & Corsello, S.M. (2012). Recognizing menopause in women with amenorrhea induced by cytotoxic chemotherapy for endocrine-responsive early breast cancer. *Endocrine-Related Cancer, 19,* R21–R33. doi:10.1530/ERC-11-0199

U.S. Food and Drug Administration. (2013, June 28). *FDA approves the first non-hormonal treatment for hot flashes associated with menopause* [News release]. Retrieved from https://wayback.archive-it.org/7993/20161023125652/http://www.fda.gov/NewsEvents/Newsroom/PressAnnouncements/ucm359030.htm

U.S. Food and Drug Administration. (2016, November 17). *FDA approves Intrarosa for postmenopausal women experiencing pain during sex* [News release]. Retrieved from http://www.fda.gov/NewsEvents/Newsroom/PressAnnouncements/ucm529641.htm

Vitek, W.S., Shayne, M., Hoeger, K., Han, Y., Messing, S., & Fung, C. (2014). Gonadotropin-releasing hormone agonists for the preservation of ovarian function among women with breast cancer who did not use tamoxifen after chemotherapy: A systematic review and meta-analysis. *Fertility and Sterility, 102,* 808–815.e1. doi:10.1016/j.fertnstert.2014.06.003

Vrieling, A., Buck, K., Kaaks, R., & Chang-Claude, J. (2010). Adult weight gain in relation to breast cancer risk by estrogen and progesterone receptor status: A meta-analysis. *Breast Cancer Research and Treatment, 123,* 641–649. doi:10.1007/s10549-010-1116-4

Waks, A.G., & Partridge, A.H. (2016). Fertility preservation in patients with breast cancer: Necessity, methods, and safety. *Journal of the National Comprehensive Cancer Network, 14,* 355–363. Retrieved from http://www.jnccn.org/content/14/3/355.long

Warren, L.E.G., Miller, C.L., Horick, N., Skolny, M.N., Jammallo, L.S., Sadek, B.T., … Taghian, A.G. (2014). The impact of radiation therapy on the risk of lymphedema after treatment for breast cancer: A prospective cohort study. *International Journal of Radiation Oncology, Biology, Physics, 88,* 565–571. doi:10.1016/j.ijrobp.2013.11.232

CHAPTER 10

Breast Navigation

Sharon Gentry, RN, MSN, AOCN®, CBCN®, CBEC, ONN-CG

Introduction

Patient navigation is used to guide patients through the cancer care continuum. Patients become active participants in their care as they journey alongside a navigator during care transitions to recognize and overcome logistical barriers, assimilate medical information for informed treatment decisions, and receive emotional support during critical times.

History of Breast Navigation

Origins

The origin of breast navigation can be traced to Dr. Harold P. Freeman. In response to the results of a 1989 American Cancer Society (ACS) report titled *Report to the Nation: Cancer in the Poor*, which found that poor people face significant barriers to accessing cancer care services, Freeman partnered with ACS in 1990 to create the first patient navigation program in the Harlem neighborhood of New York City (Freeman, Muth, & Kerner, 1995). Breast cancer was the original focus of Freeman's patient navigation program in response to the high rate of late-stage diagnosis among African American women at Harlem Hospital (Freeman, 2006). More than half of his clients presented with stage III and IV breast cancer, which contributed to the high death rate in this population (Freeman, 2013). The fundamental goal of his navigation concept was to assist patients with abnormal findings on screening examinations or a diagnosis of cancer by eliminating barriers to timely cancer screening, diagnosis, and treatment by circumnavigating the hospital and human services bureaucracies (Freeman, 2006). Navigators were to be an active part of the community they served and to be familiar with the healthcare system so they could relate to their patients. A retrospective study of Freeman's combination of patient navigation with free or low-cost screening mammograms resulted in an increase in early-stage diagnosis as well as an increase in five-year survival from 39% to 70% (Oluwole et al., 2003).

Subsequently, navigation has expanded across the care continuum from outreach and prevention to survivorship and end of life (Freeman & Rodriguez, 2011). With the interconnection of psychosocial issues to breast care, navigation has evolved to include outcomes on screening, diagnosis, treatment, adherence, and quality of life that involve psychological, social, and physical support systems (Robinson-White, Conroy, Slavish, & Rosenzweig, 2010).

Freeman and Rodriguez (2011) defined principles of patient navigation to support this healthcare delivery system. This patient-centered approach across the continuum can integrate a fragmented system with breast care coordination supported by distinct boundaries on navigator scope of practice, time frame of involvement, and cost-effectiveness of the service. These principles should be taken into consideration when implementing a breast navigation program.

Evolution

In the 1990s, Johns Hopkins Hospital in Baltimore, Maryland, was initiating institutionwide efforts to address the 40% no-show rate for screening mammograms from their community population that comprised mainly low-income African American women (Shockney, Haylock, & Cantril, 2013). Cancer registry data showed many newly diagnosed patients presenting with stage III and IV disease, and 15% arrived initially in the emergency department with pain. Delays related to providers and systems were barriers to patients' ability to receive follow-up care or planned treatment. Lillie Shockney, as the administrative director, used survivor volunteers as well as faith-based community leaders to gather personal perspectives of patients' experiences and expectations. At first, lay navigators were used to help patients access resources for care, but upon recognizing the deficit in patient education, psychosocial support, and barrier assessment, a nurse navigator role was implemented at the point of diagnosis (Shockney et al., 2013). Today, certified volunteer lay navigators and survivor navigators continue to work alongside nurse navigators to optimize breast care services. A key to a successful, efficient breast care delivery system is the operations management process map tool. It is crucial for any administrator or navigator to identify the specific delays, inefficiencies, and communication barriers to breast care across a system (Kapp & Pratt-Chapman, 2015). Program leaders, interprofessional team members, and patients can be a part of the analysis. Once the initial care is mapped in relation to time between care transitions and who performs the care, the program leadership can address inefficiencies, delays, duplications, and gaps in care by redefining roles, altering the care process, and improving care coordination (Shockney et al., 2013). Shockney's (2010a) institution significantly increased timeliness to care throughout the continuum and most notably reduced the start time to chemotherapy by two weeks by using this process. Navigators also are encouraged to use this tool to evaluate the entire care process (Shockney, 2011).

Breast Navigation Training

Nursing navigation evolved from utilization review (UR) nurses in the 1970s, who performed retrospective reviews to identify hospitalized days that lacked medical necessity, to utilization management (UM) nurses in the 1980s, who completed concurrent reviews to alert physicians when more documentation was needed to justify additional hospital days (Shockney, 2010a). The change from retrospective to concurrent review allowed communication between nurses and physicians, but barriers to treatment and inefficiencies in care were not addressed by systemic changes.

In the 1990s, case management nurses took the place of UR and UM nurses and became part of an interprofessional team to proactively address barriers to efficient care, facilitate communication, and provide disease-specific education with links to community resources for effective care (Shockney, 2010a).

At the end of the 1990s, most breast cancer care shifted to ambulatory care, creating the opportunity for nurses to coordinate and prepare patients to receive care in multiple outpatient facilities. Judy Kneece, RN, saw this as an opening to implement a program of education and support for patients with breast cancer at Baptist Medical Center in South Carolina. The program revolved around a breast health specialist that supported patients during their entire breast cancer experience (Perry, 1992). In 1994, Kneece began EduCare, Inc., a breast health publishing and training company to prepare nurses to successfully navigate patients in an interprofessional manner (EduCare Inc., n.d.; Kneece, 1994). In 1999, Lexington Medical Center in South Carolina redesigned their breast care delivery around the concept of a breast health educator to provide education, support, and anticipatory guidance from diagnosis through treatment (Kneece, 2008). The wait time for a diagnostic mammogram went from two weeks to 24 hours, and 95% of patients received their breast biopsy pathology results within 24 hours (Kneece, 2008).

Since EduCare's conception, Kneece has trained more than 2,300 nurses across the United States and holds national strategic planning workshops for breast center administrators (J. Kneece, personal communication, November 12, 2015). COPE Library is an online resource of more than 400 educational breast health–related topics and EduCare training, as well as printable resources, and can be accessed for an annual fee (www.educareinc.com/index.php).

Initial Funding for Breast Navigation

Funding for the first breast navigation positions was supported by grants from ACS, the Avon Foundation for Women, Susan G. Komen, and the National Breast Cancer Foundation (Shockney, 2010a). Grants and healthcare system foundation support continue to be the primary funding sources for many programs. President George W. Bush signed into law the Patient Navigator Outreach and Chronic Disease Prevention Act of 2005. The legislation authorized $25 million in grants through the Health Resources and Services Administration, the Office of Rural Health Policy, the National Cancer Institute (NCI), and the Indian Health Service to establish patient navigator programs to empower, educate, and assist patients in disparate communities to move through complicated healthcare systems (Hopkins & Mumber, 2009). The NCI Center to Reduce Cancer Health Disparities, along with ACS and the Avon Foundation for Women, used funding from the 2005 act to sponsor a nine-site Patient Navigation Research Program (PNRP) to evaluate and test the efficacy and cost-effectiveness of patient navigation in breast, colorectal, cervical, and prostate cancers in randomized groups of racial, ethnic minority and low socioeconomic populations (Freund et al., 2008; NCI, 2015). In 2006, the Centers for Medicare and Medicaid Services (CMS) funded six navigation service projects for breast, cervical, colorectal, lung, and prostate cancers to study the impact of navigation on satisfaction, cancer care utilization, and clinical outcomes using randomized clinical trials (Mitchell, Bir, Hoover, & Subramanian, 2012). The demonstration of the project's effectiveness at reducing cancer screening disparities and cost, as well as improving participants' satisfaction with the services, can be accessed at https://innovation.cms.gov/Files/reports/CPTD-Final.pdf.

Accreditation Agencies

National Accreditation Program for Breast Centers

In 2008, the National Accreditation Program for Breast Centers (NAPBC) was conceived to establish evidence-based standards for the management of patients with breast cancer or benign breast disease and to provide a process for elected cancer programs to monitor compliance. It was the first organization to include a standard for breast navigation (Bensenhaver & Winchester, 2014). Standard 2.2 states that a "patient navigation process is in place to guide the patient with a breast abnormality through provided and referred services" (NAPBC, 2014, p. 35). The standard recognizes that breast navigation will be different based on community needs but that the process must include "consistent care coordination throughout the continuum of care and an assessment of the physical, psychological and social needs of the patient. The anticipated results are enhanced patient outcomes, increased satisfaction, and reduced costs of care" (NAPBC, 2014, p. 35).

Commission on Cancer

The American College of Surgeons Commission on Cancer (2015) addresses the patient navigation process in Standard 3.1, which is as follows:

> A patient navigation process, driven by a triennial Community Needs Assessment, is established to address health care disparities and barriers to cancer care. Resources to address identified barriers may be provided either on-site or by referral. (p. 54)

This standard is different from NAPBC's criterion in that it is inclusive of all cancers and that the navigation process is driven by the cancer committee with possible modifications annually.

Navigator Roles in Breast Navigation

The American College of Surgeons Commission on Cancer (2015) states that navigation services will be dependent on the identified barriers to care. NAPBC (2014) gives more direction for breast care, specifying that navigation should be provided by a professional (nurse or social worker) or a trained nonprofessional who is overseen by a professional for patient assessment, program management, and patient education.

The Oncology Nursing Society, the Association of Oncology Social Work, and the National Association of Social Workers issued a joint position statement on patient navigation that reflects the NAPBC position calling for trained nonprofessionals to have supervision by nurses or social workers (Oncology Nursing Society, 2010). In 2008, the Advisory Board Company Oncology Roundtable, a private membership group that studies issues relevant to oncology, defined the roles as being dictated by the goals of the program, the scope of service, and individual navigator qualifications (Advisory Board Company Oncology Roundtable, 2008). Freeman (2012) called for proficiency in the role with providers who are navigating to administer care that requires their level of education and experience and to not perform services that do not require their skill set.

The National Consortium of Breast Centers (2016) distinguishes six types of breast navigators:

- Diagnostic imaging/treatment technicians
- Management/social workers
- Advocates
- Clinical navigators, such as certified medical assistants and licensed practical or vocational nurses
- Providers, such as physicians or advanced-degree nurses
- RNs

The George Washington University Cancer Institute, along with national patient navigation stakeholders and experts, developed a framework for delineating navigation roles (Willis et al., 2013), with three distinct roles: community (community health workers), community/healthcare institution (patient navigators), and healthcare institution (nurses and social workers).

Willis et al. (2013) clarified that patient navigators are lay navigators who have received professional training as dictated by their healthcare institution. The framework includes 12 agreed-upon functional domains for navigation and describes the role differences and similarities for each domain (see Table 10-1). The framework is a tool for administrators to use when looking at the level of navigation required to meet the program needs in their specific healthcare system. Using the various skilled roles, studies have shown positive breast healthcare outcomes, such as a decrease in patients lost to follow-up after an abnormal screening, a decrease in time to cancer diagnostics and treatment, identification of and reduction in barriers to care, facilitation of care to decrease missed appointments, and higher patient satisfaction with care (Browne, Darnell, Savage, & Brown, 2015; Kiely, 2014; Lorhan et al., 2013; Marchand, 2010; McVay, Toney, & Kautz, 2014; Meade et al., 2014).

Models of Navigation

Breast navigation programs are created to meet the needs of the patients in the healthcare institution that develops the program. Depending on the goals of the program, the model may reflect breast disease–specific care throughout the continuum or it may stand alone for outreach, diagnostic, and treatment services or survivorship.

Outreach

Outreach navigators must be knowledgeable about breast screening, signs and symptoms, screening guidelines, and resources for screening and diagnostic follow-up, as well as how to collaborate with community partners (Thomas & Peters, 2014).

The George Washington University Cancer Institute was one of the nine site demonstration projects selected by PNRP funding for outreach navigation. The project focused on breast cancer and navigated 1,047 women between 2006 and 2010 at nine hospitals or clinics in the District of Columbia. Navigated women reached diagnostic resolution 17 days quicker than non-navigated women. For those who required a breast biopsy, the diagnostic time was 31 days shorter in navigated women (Hoffman et al., 2012). The program included a citywide effort for outreach where unaffiliated clinical and community sites worked together to conduct training, shared informa-

Table 10-1. Patient Navigation Framework: Navigator Function Across Domains

Domain	Community (Community Health Worker)	Community/ Healthcare Institution (Patient Navigator)	Healthcare Institution (Nurse Navigator/ Social Work Navigator)
Professional Roles and Responsibilities: *The knowledge base and skills needed to perform job-related duties and tasks, including understanding scope of practice, supporting evaluation efforts, and identifying and exercising self-care strategies.* *The following general skills are required:* • *Organizational skills* • *Office skills* • *Interpersonal skills* • *Time management* • *Problem solving* • *Multitasking* • *Critical thinking*	General knowledge base on health issues such as cancer, diabetes, obesity, heart disease, stroke, HIV/AIDS, and other chronic diseases. Active documentation in client record. Conduct evaluation focused on community needs assessment and health behaviors.	Knowledge of cancer screening, diagnosis, treatment, and survivorship and related physical, psychological, and social issues. Active documentation of encounter with patient, barriers to care, and resources or referrals to resolve barriers, which may be noted in the client record and/or the medical record. Conduct evaluation focused on barriers to care, health disparities, and quality indicators.	Knowledge and maintenance of knowledge (e.g., license, certification, continuing education) of cancer clinical impacts on patient, caregivers, and families and ability to intervene (e.g., symptom management, assessment of functional status and psychosocial health). Active documentation in medical record. Conduct evaluation focused on clinical outcomes and quality indicators.
Community Resources: *Ongoing identification, coordination, and referral to resources such as individuals, organizations, and services in the community.*	Provide referral to evidence-based health promotion programs. Provide assistance accessing health insurance.	Provide assistance with scheduling appointments and facilitate request and follow-up with specialist or supportive care based on clinical referral. Provide assistance accessing health insurance, copay programs, patient assistance programs, and financial assistance.	Focus on clinically oriented resources, such as referrals for second opinions, treatment or testing that may not be offered at the patient's institution, as well as supportive or specialty referrals within or external to the institution (specific to nurse navigators). Provide assistance in identifying community resources to access psychosocial support throughout treatment (specific to social work navigators).

(Continued on next page)

Table 10-1. Patient Navigation Framework: Navigator Function Across Domains *(Continued)*

Domain	Community (Community Health Worker)	Community/ Healthcare Institution (Patient Navigator)	Healthcare Institution (Nurse Navigator/ Social Work Navigator)
Patient Empowerment: *Identifying problems and resources to help patients solve problems and be part of the decision-making process.* *An important facilitator of patient empowerment is development of good patient rapport.*	Motivate individual and community to make positive changes in health behaviors. Activate and empower individuals and communities to self-advocate and make healthy decisions.	Assist patient with identifying administrative, structural, social, and practical issues to participate in decision-making and solutions. Empower patients by ensuring they know all their options; identify their preferences and priorities, and assist them to access healthcare services and self-manage their health. Educate patients on their rights and preferences and ensure they are able to participate in the decision-making process throughout their care and into survivorship or end-of-life care.	Assist patients in decision-making regarding diagnostic testing and treatment options (specific to nurse navigators). Provide patients with strategies to cope with disease, treatment, and stress (specific to social work navigators).
Communication: *Ensuring appropriate communication with patient, healthcare and service providers, and community.*	Facilitate communication with community about access and utilization of the healthcare system.	Assist patient and provider with communicating expectations, needs, and perspectives.	Provide translation and communication of clinical information. Provide counseling through one-on-one communication and serve as conduit between patient and providers to address emotional and psychosocial needs of patients (specific to social work navigators).

(Continued on next page)

Table 10-1. Patient Navigation Framework: Navigator Function Across Domains *(Continued)*

Domain	Community (Community Health Worker)	Community/ Healthcare Institution (Patient Navigator)	Healthcare Institution (Nurse Navigator/ Social Work Navigator)
Barriers to Care/Health Disparities: *Identifying and addressing barriers to care and reducing health disparities as defined by age, disability, education, ethnicity, gender, sexual identification, geographic location, income, or race in populations that often bear a greater burden of disease than the general population.*	Address barriers to accessing the healthcare system. Focus on reduction of general health disparities.	Address structural, cultural, social, emotional, and administrative barriers to care. Focus on reduction of cancer health disparities in medically underserved patients and timely access to care across the continuum.	Address clinical and service delivery barriers to care. Provision of services to at-risk populations, which may be defined by individual need, high acuity, or high volume at institutional level.
Education, Prevention, and Health Promotion: *Promoting healthy behaviors and lifestyle, including integrative and wellness approaches.*	Provide general health promotion at the individual and community level, including physical activity, healthy eating habits, stress reduction, sunscreen use, tobacco cessation, and reduction of other risky behaviors to reduce risk of cancer and chronic disease.	Educate patients on practical concerns and next steps in treatment with regard to what to expect. Identify the educational needs of patients to advocate on their behalf with the care team. Inform patients of the importance and benefits of clinical trials and connect them to additional resources.	Assess educational needs of patient. Identify the educational needs of patients to advocate on their behalf with the care team. Inform patients of the importance and benefit of clinical trials and connect them with additional resources. Provide clinical education about diagnosis, treatment, side effects, and posttreatment care (specific to nurse navigators). Educate patients and caregivers on their biopsychosocial concerns regarding their diagnosis and treatment (specific to social work navigators).

(Continued on next page)

Table 10-1. Patient Navigation Framework: Navigator Function Across Domains
(Continued)

Domain	Community (Community Health Worker)	Community/ Healthcare Institution (Patient Navigator)	Healthcare Institution (Nurse Navigator/ Social Work Navigator)
Ethics and Professional Conduct: *Understanding scope of practice and professional boundaries, assuring confidentiality, and following legal requirements. Maintaining and adhering to the professional standards. Bringing accountability, responsibility, and trust to the individuals the profession services.*	Abide by state-defined scope of practice.	Understand difference in scope of practice between licensed professionals and non-licensed professionals.	Abide by the ethical principles in the profession's scope of practice and code of conduct according to licensure.
Cultural Competency: *Healthcare services that recognize, respect, and respond to cultural and social differences within the context of beliefs, practices, behaviors, and needs of diverse community and/or population served.*	Act as a community/cultural liaison and mediator between community and healthcare system using culturally appropriate education materials.	Provide navigation services in a culturally competent manner (e.g., National Culturally and Linguistically Appropriate Services [CLAS] Standards in Health and Health Care). Educate providers to increase their understanding of community's history, culture, and needs, as well as the cultural appropriateness of their approaches and educational materials.	Provide clinical care and education materials in culturally competent manner.
Outreach: *Providing healthcare education to individuals and communities that address health disparities.*	Work with the community to identify education needs and opportunities.	Educate on cancer-related topics to reduce fears and barriers related to cancer screening. Effectively link patients referred from the community to resources that can improve coordination and timeliness to treatment.	Consult and counsel patients on their unique risks.

(Continued on next page)

Table 10-1. Patient Navigation Framework: Navigator Function Across Domains
(Continued)

Domain	Community (Community Health Worker)	Community/Healthcare Institution (Patient Navigator)	Healthcare Institution (Nurse Navigator/Social Work Navigator)
Care Coordination: *A method of organizing patient care activities to facilitate the appropriate delivery of healthcare services.*	Provide case management, service coordination, and system navigation.	Identify the pathway in the continuum and document the next steps to ensure the patient's optimal outcomes. Identify unmet needs and facilitate cancer care resources to eliminate barriers along the cancer continuum.	Assess and facilitate coordination of psychosocial and medical/clinical care along the care continuum.
Psychosocial Support Services/Assessment: *Providing and/or connecting patients to resources for psychosocial support services.*	Identify resources in the community for emotional and social support.	Administer distress screening and provide assistance with administrative, practical, or social issues identified.	Screen and assess for psychosocial distress. Provide psychosocial support services such as counseling (specific to social work navigators).
Advocacy: *Advocating on behalf of patient within the community and healthcare system.*	Speak up for individual and community needs.	Educate providers on individual preferences of care and needs.	Assure patients' needs and preferences are integrated into treatment and care delivery.

Note. From "Development of a Framework for Patient Navigation: Delineating Roles Across Navigator Types," by A. Willis, E. Reed, M. Pratt-Chapman, H. Kapp, E. Hatcher, V. Vaitones, … C. Washington, 2013, *Journal of Oncology Navigation and Survivorship, 4*(6), pp. 22–24. Copyright 2013 by Academy of Oncology Nurse and Patient Navigators. Reprinted with permission.

---

tion about community resources, and increased communication among navigators (Patierno et al., 2010). The outreach process at George Washington University Cancer Institute involves a patient and a nurse navigator working together to ensure fast-track services for at-risk women in the community, reduced times for additional testing, and improved tracking to decrease the number of women lost to follow-up (see Figure 10-1).

Arias (2012) described how she conducted a systematic evaluation in three separate Midwest hospitals that are part of a privately owned healthcare system to optimize their outreach regional imaging and oncology patient navigation services. After two years of implementing nurse, radiologic technologist, and volunteer navigation, their regional imaging volume increased 10%, with one hospital experiencing a 30% volume uptake. The turnaround time from screening mammogram to diagnostic mammogram dropped by six days, and the retention rates of women in the system for breast biopsies increased from 25% to 77%.

Cascella and Keren (2012) used nurse and lay navigation in Connecticut's highest identified breast mortality community to encourage breast cancer screening. The nurse trained the bilingual lay survivor navigators who interacted with the women in the community as the women came to a local church's food pantry. The monthly outreach with navigators who spoke their language allowed women to schedule and complete their mammograms. This culturally appropriate outreach promoted community awareness as well as increased screening.

Treatment

Treatment navigation encompasses the trajectory from an abnormal result through diagnosis and treatment (Freeman & Rodriguez, 2011). Treatment navigation consists of interprofessional care with specialists for diagnostic workup and treatment planning. Francks, Iverson, and Miller (2014) described the role of a nurse navigator in this stage of care as requiring experience in breast cancer care; knowledge of breast cancer treatment guidelines, including the National

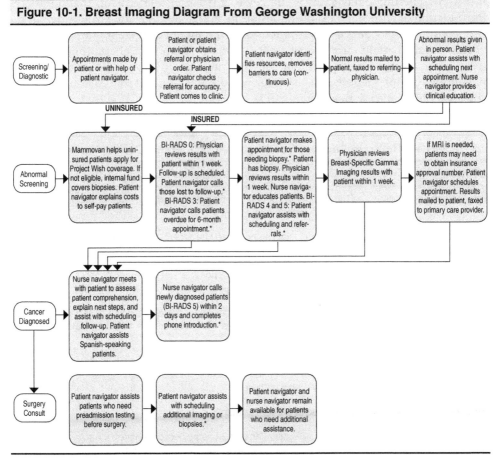

Figure 10-1. Breast Imaging Diagram From George Washington University

* Indicates QI priority

BI-RADS—Breast Imaging Reporting and Data System; MRI—magnetic resonance imaging; QI—quality improvement

Note. Figure courtesy of Mandi Pratt-Chapman. Used with permission.

Comprehensive Cancer Network® (NCCN®) guidelines; familiarity with clinical trials and research; understanding of appropriate genetic testing; awareness of breast care resources and ancillary services synchronization; and a thorough understanding of interprofessional team roles to facilitate referrals and coordination of care. Table 10-2 shows common ancillary services around breast cancer treatment navigation and suggested times to refer. Blaseg (2009) described a treatment continuum model with an oncology RN for every cancer type and all patients receiving automatic referrals to the dietitian, social worker, financial counselor, and interprofessional tumor conference, with referral to other supportive services such as genetics, lymphedema, and research as appropriate. Figure 10-2 is an overview of the Novant Health Greater Winston Breast Nurse Navigator (NHGWBNN) treatment model, which has been recognized as decreasing outpatient migration (Advisory Board Company Oncology Roundtable, 2011). To strategically align breast nurse navigation upstream in the patient experience, the critical element of diagnosis disclosure is completed by the radiologist at the breast imaging center with the breast nurse navigator present. The breast nurse navigator in the imaging center is responsible for following up with all biopsied diagnostic breast patients (see Figure 10-3). The nurse navigator is the key to a trusting relationship that allows the introduction of clinical trials, prehabilitation, and genetics at an earlier stage in the care continuum. Evidence-based practices in the model are telephone calls to each chemotherapy patient after their first treatment or change in chemotherapy agents to decrease emergency department use (Sprandio, 2010) and a diet consult for all patients with triple-negative breast cancer to discuss a low-fat diet to enhance survivorship (Chlebowski & Blackburn, 2014).

Table 10-2. Timing of Ancillary Services Used With Breast Cancer Management

Service	When to Refer
Lymphedema specialist	Prior to (ideally) or after lymph node sampling or with development of any signs of lymphedema
Dietitian	Before the initial chemotherapy treatment or with any concerns regarding weight or healthy eating
Social worker	With identification of any psychosocial needs, financial concerns, coping concerns, or assistance needed related to travel or lodging
Financial counselor	Before chemotherapy or radiation for preauthorization of services and for any concerns about finances, lack of insurance, or insurance coverage
American Cancer Society programs	Individualized according to the patient needs
Wig boutique	Before alopecia develops
Survivorship programs	At the end of active treatment
Fertility specialist	With the determination of the chemotherapy regimen for any woman younger than age 40 or man younger than age 50

Note. From "Breast Cancer Navigation" (p. 127), by B. Francks, M.L. Iverson, and J. Miller in K.D. Blaseg, P. Daugherty, and K.A. Gamblin (Eds.), *Oncology Nurse Navigation: Delivering Patient-Centered Care Across the Continuum,* 2014, Pittsburgh, PA: Oncology Nursing Society. Copyright 2014 by Oncology Nursing Society. Reprinted with permission.

Figure 10-2. Novant Health Greater Winston Breast Nurse Navigator Treatment Model

Novant Health Greater Winston Breast Nurse Navigator (NHGWBNN) Program

▼

NHGWBNN Community Outreach				
NC Northwest Komen Education Committee	Pink Ribbon Talk Committee	Pink Broomstick speaker	Race for the Cure	Speak at schools, civic organizations, churches, groups, etc.

▼

All Novant Health Greater Winston Breast Clinic Pathology	
Benign pathology—Nurse navigator calls with results and discusses recommendations of the radiologist – 6 month or 1 yr follow-up	**Benign high-risk pathology** (atypical ductal hyperplasia, radial scars, papillomas)—Nurse navigator sees patient and arranges surgical follow-up as advised by radiologist

▼

Genetic Clinic offered to all high-risk patients.

▼

Positive breast cancer pathology

▼

Radiologist shares diagnosis with NHGWBNN present.
All patients referred from outside sources (surgeon, RT, Med Onc) will be offered NHGWBNN services at initial consult

▼

Patient receives appointment with 1) surgeon, 2) radiation oncologist, and/or 3) medical oncologist							
Breast cancer education packet	Genetic Clinic for all high-risk patients	Prehabilitation assessment	Resource specialist	Psychologist	Transportation	Family assessment	Neoadjuvant clinical trials

▼

NHGWBNN calls patient one week after diagnosis if patient has not been contacted at clinic visit. NHGWBNN calls patient the day after the initial surgical visit. Postsurgery garments are discussed with all mastectomy patients.

▼

Surgery (Patient could receive neoadjuvant therapy at this point and loop back into surgery.)

▼

See day of surgery (at all SLN injections) and/or day after surgery
Pink Broomstick Program referral completed.

▼

Call 3 business days after surgery.
Are follow-up care appointments scheduled? Continue to assess needs.

▼

Weekly Breast Cancer Multidisciplinary Board Review new cases. Clinical trial eligibility discussed for all patients.
Navigator selects cases based on pathology, or other team members request cases for presentation. Information is shared with patient's team after meeting.

▼

Call 10 days and 3 weeks after surgery. Continue to assess needs.
Lymphedema class or 1:1 PT evaluation if needed; prosthesis information reinforced if mastectomy; further surgery for reconstructive needs; clinical trials; Muscles In Motion

▼

Diet Consult—All triple-negatives offered diet consult.

▼

Follow-Up Care—Call or meet depending on treatment track.

Note. Figure courtesy of Novant Health Derrick L. Davis Cancer Center Oncology Breast Advisory Committee. Used with permission.

Figure 10-3. Novant Health Derrick L. Davis Cancer Center Oncology Breast Advisory Committee Standards of Care

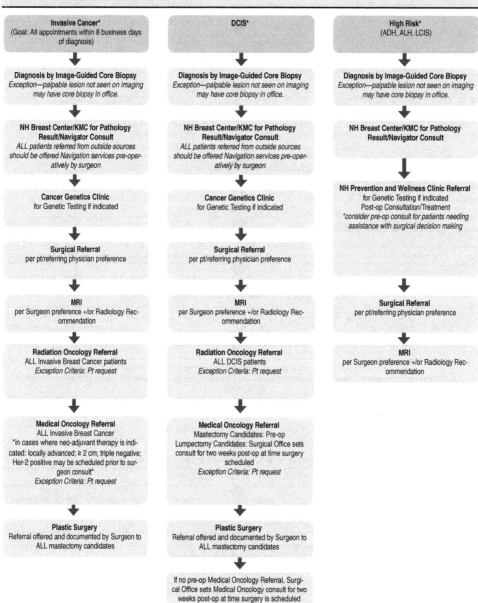

* All recommendations based upon National Comprehensive Cancer Network Guidelines (www.nccn.org) and National Accreditation Program for Breast Centers Standards for Accreditation (www.napbc-breast.org).

ADH—atypical ductal hyperplasia; ALH—atypical lobular hyperplasia; DCIS—ductal carcinoma in situ; KMC—Kernersville Medical Center; LCIS—lobular carcinoma in situ; MRI—magnetic resonance imaging; NH—Novant Health; pt—patient

Note. Figure courtesy of Novant Health Derrick L. Davis Cancer Center Oncology Breast Advisory Committee. Used with permission.

Survivorship

Survivorship navigation is a new field, as institutions have different resources to create these programs. Nurse navigators can assume a role in survivorship care because they understand the specific risks related to the different treatment modalities and can connect patients to critical resources and specialty care, as well as facilitate patient-centered communication and care among healthcare providers (Pratt-Chapman, 2015). Blaseg, Kile, and Salner (2011) described the following benefits a survivorship navigator may offer

- Supporting and "navigating" patients during their transition from active treatment through recovery and beyond
- Improving patient satisfaction and health outcomes
- Establishing relationships with primary care physicians and facilitating communication between the oncologists and the primary care physicians
- Educating patients about the treatment summary and survivorship plan
- Ensuring that the psychosocial, financial, physical, and spiritual needs of patients continue to be met. (p. 32)

Sibley Memorial Hospital of Johns Hopkins Medicine uses a nurse practitioner and navigator model to discuss a survivorship care plan that includes current side effects, as well as a plan for future care, during a wellness transition visit (Goetz, 2014). Prior to the transition visit, the breast nurse navigators ask newly diagnosed patients what their life goals were and then share these goals with the treatment team so they can possibly be recovered post-treatment (Shockney, 2015). The transition visit is an opportunity to review the patient's life goals and makes the survivorship care plan "more of a life plan rather than solely being medically oriented" (Shockney, 2015, p. 109). See Figure 10-4 for an illustrative depiction of the work flow process.

Blaseg et al. (2011) described an NCI Community Cancer Centers Program nurse practitioner–led navigation model pilot where patients with breast cancer are seen four to six weeks after their primary treatment. Patients receive a treatment summary created by CNExT registry software and individual counseling on their plan and resources for support services, as well as information on wellness and lifestyle modifications. The nurse practitioner becomes a point of contact for the survivors, and the nurse practitioner services are billable to help generate revenue for a sustainable model.

Another survivorship navigation model uses a bachelor of science nurse/oncology-certified nurse to create the American Society of Clinical Oncology Cancer Treatment Summary and care plans (Blaseg et al., 2011). The creation takes 10 minutes to one hour, and the navigator monitors the schedule to identify patients who need a treatment summary developed or may get a referral for a disease-specific navigator. The navigator performs a survivorship consultation and will make any needed referrals. The navigator also follows up as necessary by telephone call or is available for any post-treatment needs at follow-up clinical appointments.

Klein and Hawkins (2015) described a community-based oncology practice that used a single advanced practice nurse visit to provide survivorship care with a treatment summary and a survivorship care plan to women who had completed adjuvant treatment for breast cancer. Using the Confidence in Survivorship Information Questionnaire and the Patient Satisfaction With Cancer Care tools (NCI, n.d.), the researchers found that patients showed improved knowledge in all domains.

Figure 10-4. Breast Cancer Survivorship Workflow—Survivorship Care Plan

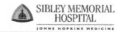
SIBLEY MEMORIAL
HOSPITAL
JOHNS HOPKINS MEDICINE

Breast cancer patient completes active treatment (surgery/radiation and/or chemo).

Rad/onc or surgeon refers patient to NP for survivorship transition visit (consult) preferably 6 or more weeks after treatment completion.

NP and patient meet and review: Staging and Path; treatment received (surgery, chemo, rad, hormonal); potential long-term side effects; Follow-up schedule; Health maintenance goals/schedule; any existing side effects (comprehensive); current lifestyle behaviors assessment including exercise, diet, alcohol consumption, vit d, sleep, support system, work stress.

Together NP and Patient create a Health Promotion Plan by looking at what current behaviors could be tweaked and what short and long term goals would be reasonable, and what strategies could be used to help the patient meet those goals.

Occasionally we set up a close follow-up (2–4 weeks) especially if there are significant adverse symptoms or we need more time to complete the Survivorship Care Plan (SCP).

NP documents the SCP and Health Promotion Plan in an EPIC SCP template, where certain data auto-populates, e.g. demographic information, provider names and BMI. The final product is visible under EPIC note, but in addition the completed template is copied into a specially formatted Word document in order to print an attractive copy.

Administrative staff mails a cover letter, the SCP, a list of resources including integrative health services, local upcoming survivorship events, as well as an evaluation form and a business reply envelope to the patient. Copies of the SCP are sent to the referring physician, the PCP, as well as any other physician the patient specifies.

Survivorship navigator receives evaluations and follows up with patient with any concerns, as does NP where relevant. The form and process are continually improved based on feedback.

BMI—body mass index; NP—nurse practitioner; PCP—primary care provider

Note. Figure copyright 2016 by Maureen Ross, NP, and Pamela Goetz, BA. Used with permission.

Outcomes of Breast Navigation

Navigation in breast cancer care has produced many positives outcomes since its inception in the 1990s (Paskett, Harrop, & Wells, 2011; Wells et al., 2008). The outcomes cover the entire continuum of breast care and use diverse roles in care delivery across many different populations (Robinson-White et al., 2010).

Increased Participation in Breast Cancer Screening

From Freeman's initial study in 1990, breast navigation has improved participation in cancer screening (Freeman, 2013). Han, Lee, Kim, and Kim (2009)

used indigenous lay navigators to improve breast cancer screening rates, as well as rates of clinical breast examination (23%) and breast self-examination (36%), in Korean American women who had not completed a mammogram in the past two years. Another study using a culturally modified navigator model in which navigators recruited patients from their respective settings and during culturally specific community events consisted of face-to-face and telephone contact to promote mammography use for women who had not been screened in 18 months or more. This resulted in a 55% annual rescreening rate (Burhansstipanov et al., 2010).

Clark et al. (2009) used case management to increase mammography screening by 25% in an African American population at high risk for inadequate cancer screening by addressing barriers of transportation, housing, and language and encouraging screening and follow-up of abnormal tests. Three internal medical practice groups at an academic safety net hospital in Boston, Massachusetts, used trained patient navigators to interact directly with patients as part of the primary care team to assist in overcoming barriers to screening and to coordinate care for mammography scheduling (Phillips et al., 2011). After nine months, mammogram adherence was greater in the navigated population, which was largely racial and ethnic minorities who either had public or no health insurance.

Braun et al. (2015) reported on a randomized controlled trial using lay navigators to increase cancer screening for a group of Asian and Pacific Islander Medicare beneficiaries who lived on a medically underserved island. With the use of community navigators to provide outreach education and scheduling, mammography screening increased by 20%.

Improved Timeliness and Completion of the Workup of Abnormal Breast Findings

Women perceive a breast diagnostic evaluation as threatening and have a higher level of satisfaction with the healthcare experience when providers give information and create a supportive environment (Harding, 2014). Young, single women with a lower education level and a perception of having little social support experience higher stress during this phase (Harding, 2014).

Harding and McCrone (2013) reported on a qualitative study among non-navigated women undergoing breast diagnostic evaluation that showed women experienced difficulties with lack of information, not knowing how to move through the healthcare system, and unhappiness with the communication received. Harding (2014) suggested that a "critical component of a support program is to have a nurse available to women throughout the diagnostic phase to fulfill pivotal roles of providing information, facilitating communication with health care providers, and offering psychosocial support" (p. 489).

Paskett et al. (2012) used female, college-educated lay navigators in Ohio to call breast or cervical screening participants within five days to identify individual barriers to care and then provided social actions such as listening, providing education and referrals, and scheduling. The resolution of an abnormal screening finding was 36% higher in the navigated group than in the comparison group.

The Denver PNRP (Raich, Whitley, Thorland, Valverde, & Fairclough, 2012) had a 92% breast diagnostic resolution rate in the navigated population versus 77% in the control patients with patient navigators using telephone, email, or in-person communication. The patient navigator assessed practical barriers, social support, and the patient's intention to complete the care recommended, as well as provided education, scheduling, and personal one-on-one support at appointments if language, fear, or lack of social support was identified.

The San Antonio PNRP (Dudley et al., 2012) teamed up a *promotora*, a lay Hispanic/ Latino community member with specialized training to provide basic health education in the community, with a patient navigator (public health RN, dental hygienist, social worker, or business administrator) in a study of poor Hispanic women. The mean time to diagnosis was 36 days for the navigated group versus 53 days for the control group. This case management navigation model used the promotora's skills in overcoming cultural and socioeconomic barriers that were identified in the assessment and allowed the patient navigator to develop a care plan and focus on interventions for medical-related barriers.

Markossian, Darnell, and Calhoun (2012) assisted low-income minority women with two master's-prepared social workers and two lay navigators as a patient navigation model in a federally qualified health center network to reach breast diagnostic resolution within 60 days. They found that 83% of the navigated group experienced a shorter time to results versus 52% in the non-navigated group.

A common tool in decreasing resolution time with navigation is the identification of barriers to care. PNRP researchers (Katz et al., 2014) described the PNRP tool as a predefined list divided into patient-, system-, or other-focused difficulties, and navigators recorded actions that were taken to address the identified difficulties. Tejeda et al. (2013) took the PNRP tool and divided the eight PNRP factors into three levels of influence—intrapersonal, interpersonal, and institutional—with a fourth factor of "unknown" to capture additional barriers.

Krok-Schoen, Brewer, et al. (2015) suggested that this barrier identification can be used by programs seeking American College of Surgeons Commission on Cancer compliance with navigation to identify patient populations that are most likely to have care barriers and need patient navigation. Krok-Schoen, Kurta, et al. (2015), from the Ohio PNRP, demonstrated that time to resolution for breast, cervical, or colorectal abnormalities was influenced by patient socioeconomic factors rather than clinic type (academic medical center or federally qualified health center).

Ramachandran et al. (2015) looked at the impact of barriers to care for timely outcomes in resolution of abnormal breast and cervical screening results. They found that the number of barriers identified by the navigator for each patient was reflective of the time to resolve the screening abnormality. Women with two barriers experienced a delay of two weeks, and those with three or more saw a seven-month delay. This suggested that intensive navigation could focus on patients with the greatest need.

Tejeda et al. (2013) looked at barriers between African American and Latina women and found that no single patient characteristic predicted what type of barrier a woman would have in obtaining a workup of a breast abnormality. Their study pointed out that patient navigators can best address intrapersonal level barriers, such as finances, transportation, comorbidities, and beliefs, but may be less able to remove institutional level barriers, such as system problems in scheduling care.

Koh, Nelson, and Cook (2011) used a nurse navigation model with the PNRP tool to study what patient barriers were addressed by the program and how much time was spent on them. The largest time-consuming barriers were related to employment issues, attitudes toward providers, and perceptions or beliefs about tests or treatment. By spending the majority of nursing time on education needs, 71% of the barriers were completely resolved by the time treatment was started. This information was helpful when analyzed for program development for more staff and expected caseload. In defining the roles for a patient navigation framework, Willis et al. (2013) pointed out that community navigators focused on barriers related to accessing the healthcare system and addressing general health disparities, while healthcare institution navigators such as nurses and social workers addressed clinical and service delivery barriers at the institutional or systemic level (see Table 10-3).

Table 10-3. Patient Barriers

Level of Influence	Category	Barrier	Questions to Ask
Intrapersonal	Finance	Insurance	Does the patient have insurance? Is paying for health care a concern? Is the patient able to pay for all needed medications at one time? Are there other financial needs (e.g., food, housing) that delay health care?
		Housing	Is housing a concern at this time?
	Transportation	Lack of transportation	Can the patient get from home to the site of health care? Is the patient aware of any transportation assistance? Family? Friends? Is the patient traveling out of the area during the healthcare treatment time? Is the distance to the healthcare facility a concern?
	Comorbidities	Disability	Does the patient have a mental or medical disability? If so, what is the current care and provider?
		Comorbidity	Does the patient have one or more medical comorbidities? If so, what is the current care and provider?
	Attitudes, beliefs, perceptions	Fear	Does the patient have a fear of tests or treatment? Has the patient had an unpleasant experience with health care or a provider? Are there cultural beliefs the healthcare team needs to be aware of? What is the patient's perception about receiving health care? Are there other issues that take precedence over receiving health care?

(Continued on next page)

Table 10-3. Patient Barriers *(Continued)*

Level of Influence	Category	Barrier	Questions to Ask
Interpersonal	Family, employment, communication	Family	Does the patient have a social support system through family or friends? Who is the primary caregiver? Is the caregiver local? Is there child care available? Are family or friends available to provide assistance during health care? Is there a need for other family care during treatment?
		Employment	Are there work issues that will make health care difficult?
	Communication	Literacy	Can the patient understand oral and written information from the healthcare team? Is there a lack of understanding after healthcare information is given to the patient?
		Language	Is an interpreter needed for the patient?
Institutional	Healthcare system	Logistics	Are healthcare facilities too far for the patient to travel? Are the hours of operation inconvenient?
		Delays	Are there problems with scheduling care? Are there too long phone delays, either waiting on the phone or waiting for a call? Is there a concern with office wait time? Is there confusion over rescheduled appointments?
	Unknown	–	Do any other cited barriers to care exist?

Note. Based on information from Katz et al., 2014; Tejeda et al., 2013.

Improved Timeliness in Breast Cancer Treatment

Once a breast cancer diagnosis is confirmed, the patient begins a complex process of staging and treatment decision making. Byers (2012) stated that a navigator requires advanced clinical skills to support patients undergoing cancer treatment. The nurse navigator knows the healthcare system and the community and has communication skills to educate, advocate, and counsel according to the patient's education level, as well as insight to facilitate timely, comprehensive care as a member of the interprofessional team. Patient navigators continue to assess and address logistical barriers to care such as transportation, child care, financial difficulties, and scheduling of appointments (Haideri & Moormeier, 2011; Madore, Kilbourn, Valverde, Borrayo, & Raich, 2014; Ramirez et al., 2014).

Among a navigated group of patients with breast cancer at a safety net hospital, Haideri and Moormeier (2011) noted a large shift from women having no insurance to becoming enrolled in Medicaid as navigators advocated financial resources and provided assistance in the application process. Communication advocacy, such as translation, and promotion and assessment of understanding of treatment adherence recommendations were common tasks. As far as timeliness, the underserved Latina navigated group had a higher percentage to start treatment within 30 days (Ramirez et al., 2014), and the urban safety net population had a nine-day decrease in time to definitive therapy (Haideri & Moormeier, 2011).

One study originating from PNRP data and another from the Massachusetts General Hospital Avon Breast Care Program supported the use of lay navigation to improve care following a breast cancer diagnosis (Ko et al., 2014; Raj, Ko, Battaglia, Chabner, & Moy, 2012). Ko et al. (2014) compiled PNRP data to show that patient-navigated participants who were eligible for hormone therapy were more likely to start treatment than non-navigated eligible patients.

A decrease in time to treatment has been supported when a nurse navigator evaluates internal processes of wait time and targets specific interventions. A decrease of two days from biopsy to specialist consultation and a decrease of four days from diagnostic biopsy to initiation of treatment have been observed (Koh et al., 2011). Basu et al. (2013) looked at time from diagnosis to consultation after implementing a breast nurse navigation program and noted a two-day decrease in time. Clinical decision making in nurse navigation was instrumental in scheduling other necessary appointments such as genetics, plastic surgeons, and additional testing where appropriate for comprehensive evaluation and care.

Studies have supported using a nurse navigator to improve breast care as measured by the Breast Cancer Care Quality Indicators by assessing the measures before and after navigation implementation (Donelan et al., 2011; Weber, Mascarenhas, Bellin, Raab, & Wong, 2012). The indicators a navigator would influence, such as education, removal of barriers, improved patient decision making and timely appropriate treatment after surgery, generated an improvement in patient compliance percentage (Weber et al., 2012). Donelan et al. (2011) showed an increase in the number of young women starting chemotherapy within eight weeks of surgery, as well as a survivorship difference, when women followed up with their annual mammogram. Raj et al. (2012) showed that patient navigation that is culturally representative of the community promotes quality care in concordance with the American Society of Clinical Oncology/NCCN quality measures.

Nurse navigators observe care patterns on a daily basis and have the skills to perform a gap analysis in the healthcare continuum. Campbell, Craig, Eggert, and Bailey-Dorton (2010) observed a nurse navigator's influence on timeliness to care from diagnosis through treatment for all patients with breast cancer by better preparing patients for treatment, utilizing resources to decrease barriers to care, and mobilizing financial assistance.

Christensen and Bellomo (2014) worked with the Intermountain Southwest Cancer Center in 2011 and through a gap analysis identified a decrease from 14 days to 7 days in the appointment time for a medical oncology appointment. The navigation team developed a navigation pathway (see Table 10-4) for newly diagnosed patients with breast cancer and was able to reduce the time interval between medical oncologist referral and treatment initiation by 10 days. Part of the process was a patient and family appointment with the nurse navigator three days prior to the medical oncologist visit that would address barriers to care and provide education and psychosocial support, as well as proactively prepare them for the medical oncology visit. Molecular testing, such as estrogen, progesterone, and HER2 status can be initiated if appropriate so that results will be ready for the medical oncologist. The nurse navigator refer-

Table 10-4. Oncology Nurse Navigation Pathway

Referral to Medical Oncology	Care Coordination	New Patient Education	Medical Oncology Consult	Active Treatment Begins	Active Treatment Complete	Survivorship and Surveillance	Transition Care
Oncology scheduler makes appointments for new patient education and medical oncology consult.	Navigator and medical oncologists meet weekly and one-on-one as needed to discuss patient cases and order staging studies, molecular profiling, and other tests as needed.	Navigator meets with patient and family to discuss oncology basics, staging studies, and resources. Barriers to care are identified and addressed.	Oncology scheduler makes appointment for chemotherapy education with the patient, family, and navigator prior to first day of treatment.	Navigator meets with patient and family members as needed during treatment and provides brief visits through rounds in the chemotherapy room.	Oncology scheduler makes appointment for end-of-treatment visits with the navigator. Treatment summary and care plan are reviewed. Referrals to cancer rehab and other services as needed.	Navigator encourages and facilitates support group. Also contacts patient at 3- and 6-month intervals and yearly thereafter.	Navigator assists with palliative care, hospice, and end-of-life education, resources, and support.

Note. From "Using a Nurse Navigation Pathway in the Timely Care of Oncology Patients," by D. Christensen and C. Bellomo, 2014, *Journal of Oncology Navigation and Survivorship, 5*(3), p. 15. Copyright 2014 by Academy of Oncology Nurse and Patient Navigators. Reprinted with permission.

ences the NCCN guidelines and facilitates appropriate staging studies via the medical oncologist. Additional time savings were seen in the medical oncology visits, which were reduced by 24 minutes when patients met with the nurse navigator.

Because genetic risk assessment and genomic testing can influence surgical and treatment decisions for a patient with breast cancer, this assessment and testing, as well as the results, need to be completed in a timely manner to avoid care delays. Navigators can identify women early in the process who might benefit from seeing a credentialed genetics professional for further evaluation (Bellcross, Leadbetter, Alford, & Peipins, 2013; Malone, Bruno, Hayden, & Carlson, 2014; Mays et al., 2012; Rahm, Sukhanova, Ellis, & Mouchawar, 2007). It is within the scope of oncology nurses to recognize and refer to genetic services so that informed treatment decisions of care are made based on the patient's risk of recurrence. Omission of this step can lead to legal action against a provider (Shockney, 2010b).

Knowles and Nelson (2015) described a new concept to improve population health in which they used part of the employment of a diagnostic nurse navigator in a community medical center to create a program for patients not diagnosed with breast cancer but who are at high risk according to evidence-based models to calculate lifetime risk. The program referred women with increased risk to a genetics professional. Barke and Freivogel (2017) described the complexity of this process, which is enhanced with the involvement of a genetic counselor, and discussed different risk models and recommendations. Hughes (2017) shared the community screening model, which was implemented in a pilot project that combined nurse navigation with genetic counselors. The program then implemented a Women's Risk Assessment Survey process that feeds into a Cancer Prevention and Wellness Clinic.

Genomic testing is increasing as individual tumor genetic makeup is being analyzed. McAllister and Schmitt (2015) observed barriers for timely test ordering in patients with breast cancer and developed a quality improvement project to address the gap for eligible patients. The nurse navigator initiated a tracking tool to identify all patients eligible for Oncotype DX® testing and worked with an advanced practice nurse who ordered the test as soon as surgical pathology was available. The results were improved compliance with NCCN genomic testing recommendations (from 26% to 88%), reduced ordering time by more than two weeks, and decreased reporting time from five weeks to three weeks. This, in turn, allowed for earlier chemotherapy initiation. The nurse navigator was able to educate patients on the test and result implications and schedule the medical oncology visit when results were available.

Improved Access to Palliative and Supportive Care

NCCN (2017) defined palliative care as

> health care that focuses on effective management of pain and other distressing symptoms . . . . The goal of palliative care is to anticipate, prevent, and reduce suffering and to support the best possible quality of life for patients and their families, regardless of the stage of the disease or need for other therapies. Palliative care begins at diagnosis and should be delivered concurrently with disease-directed, life-prolonging therapies. (p. PAL-1)

Hauser et al. (2011) proposed the role of navigation in palliative care as assessing for symptoms that lead to patient distress and acting as a conduit for action with the interprofessional team to alleviate uncontrolled symptoms. Navigators can empower patients and families to discuss patient goals with proactive conversations and refer them to palliative care clinics if available.

Fischer, Cervantes, Fink, and Kutner (2015) showed how a culturally tailored patient navigation program for Latinos with advanced medical illness increased advance care planning and promoted discussions on pain management. Navigated patients who used hospice services had longer lengths of stay in hospice than the non-navigated group.

Greater Patient Adherence

Nurse navigators have a role to help patients adhere to and complete their care, including completing years of endocrine therapy. Navigators provide valuable education as well as repeat, clarify, reinforce, and validate the material given to the patient from multiple sources (Korber, Padula, Gray, & Powell, 2011). During treatment, the navigator is seen as the primary source to help assess symptoms and provide management suggestions. Throughout the care, the nurse is pivotal in obtaining appointments and medical and social support services, but, most importantly, coordination in a timely manner is valued. Navigators may be very helpful in assisting older women with accessing care across the breast cancer trajectory, especially in the areas of knowledge deficits, comorbidities that add complications to care, and multiple appointments with healthcare professionals (Pieters, Heilemann, Grant, & Maly, 2011).

Increase in Clinical Trial Participation

Navigators can increase minority accrual to clinical trials as recommended by the NCI Community Cancer Centers Program by educating about trials, advocating for trials in treatment decisions, and being a liaison between the research team and patients (Gonzalez et al., 2011). Also, navigators remove barriers to clinical trial enrollment for underserved populations (St. Germain et al., 2014).

The Radiation Research Program piloted a unique model titled the Cancer Disparities Research Partnership program to increase access to NCI clinical trials for six communities with large health disparities (Wong et al., 2014). A community outreach/education and patient navigation program was structured where navigators informed patients about clinical trials, reduced the number of missed appointments, and addressed other barriers to clinical trial participation.

Rapid City Regional Hospital in South Dakota used the documentation of this critical role of navigation to receive additional funding from Susan G. Komen to assist patients with breast cancer in accessing clinical trials. American Indian/Native American, Hispanic/Latino, African American, and the urban/rural poor were the targeted populations that experienced navigation, with 46% participating in a prevention or treatment clinical trial. McClung et al. (2013) showed an increase in clinical trial participation with the use of bilingual Chinese cancer survivors as patient navigators to positively change patients' attitudes toward clinical trials and empower them to actively participate in treatment decisions.

Nurse navigators can promote the introduction of a clinical trial at an earlier stage in the care continuum. When NHGWBNN strategically aligned the greater Winston-Salem breast nurse navigator upstream in the patient experience at the time of diagnosis, a primary objective was to promote clinical trial participation as each patient was evaluated for neoadjuvant chemotherapy. Within one year, clinical trial participation increased by 20.4% (Calcutt-Flaherty, Gentry, & Mathis, 2014). Holmes, Major, Lyonga, Alleyne, and Clayton (2012) specifically designed a community nurse navigation program that increased African American participation in breast clinical trials from 3% to 7%.

Enhanced Psychosocial Support

Navigation can decrease anxiety, provide emotional support, and facilitate patient-centered understanding for positive psychosocial outcomes. Psychosocial support with community or patient navigators revolves around the navigator's ability to provide logistical support, such as completing paperwork for insurance, billing, and housing; providing emotional support with frequent contact; and being physically there in a consistent relational sense (Carroll et al., 2010; Gabitova & Burke, 2014; Madore et al., 2014; Rousseau et al., 2014).

Gabitova and Burke (2014) used hospital-experienced bilingual lay navigators with strong communication skills to decrease emotional distress in a breast clinic by being the constant person through all visits. Navigation provided patients with the physical presence of social support that linked them to community resources and knew the patients on a personal level, which made the patients feel like they had an "insider" on their team (Carroll et al., 2010). Rousseau et al. (2014) reported that lay navigation assisted patients to be more involved in their care because the navigator was a neutral party in the care process. Even in those who had supportive family, patients could share their feelings without having to worry about upsetting family members.

Nurses bring in another level of navigation care by screening for distress, assessing psychosocial needs, and providing counseling as part of their role. Patients with a nurse navigator may have a lower level of distress reflected in a lower anxiety score and higher satisfaction score (Ferrante, Chen, & Kim, 2008; Harding, 2015). The use of anticipatory guidance with information made patients feel better prepared and cultivated a sense of caring and safety as patients encountered difficulties throughout the treatment phase (Pedersen, Hack, McClement, & Taylor-Brown, 2014).

The majority of studies that look at navigation and psychosocial care for patients with breast cancer discuss common themes of the navigators' physical presence as well as a source of knowledge for education and problem solving (Korber et al., 2011; Wagner et al., 2014).

Higher Patient Satisfaction

Patient satisfaction can measure the value of the breast navigation role and has been described as "soft revenue" because patients who are pleased with their care will be prone to stay in the healthcare system for other aspects of care, whereas disgruntled patients will leave the system (Sein, 2011). The patient's perception of care carries weight in the community, as this word-of-mouth testimonial regarding the care given by the navigator and the institution can influence care choices for others in the local area. No consensus exists in the literature on the best assessment for patient satisfaction because each system's focus on navigation and outcomes are unique to the individual program. In recognition of this fact, ACS hosted a National Patient Navigation Leadership Summit in 2010, and a Patient-Reported Outcomes Measures Working Group devised measures to evaluate outcomes that are valued by patients. The measures can be found at www.ncbi.nlm.nih.gov/pmc/articles/PMC4407470 (Fiscella et al., 2011).

Koh et al. (2011) adapted the validated Satisfaction With Hospital Care Questionnaire (Likert scale) to measure patient satisfaction at a breast tertiary care facility and found that patient satisfaction was very high in navigated care. The analysis of this study is an example of how the patient voice can direct change in the system of care, as this program has an opportunity to reprocess the nurse navigator time to education and reallocate the non-nursing duties of appointment scheduling, record keeping, and direction giving.

Another Likert scale was developed and used to study breast cancer navigation and patient satisfaction in a community setting (Hook, Ware, Siler, & Packard, 2012). A panel of expert cancer specialists developed the Nurse Navigation Patient Satisfaction Survey, which explored educational needs, emotional management, user-friendliness of the navigation services, and satisfaction with the service navigator (non-nurse) program, as well as overall satisfaction with the navigation model of care. Overall, participants reported they were highly satisfied.

Breast cancer care navigators were evaluated in British Columbia with a system-developed Likert scale with open-ended questions for qualitative comments to assess how patients perceived care (Trevillion, Singh-Carlson, Wong, & Sherriff, 2015); 95% of the patients responded positively to education, proactive preparation, emotional support, and ease of navigation access.

A qualitative format without the restraint of a restricted questionnaire in evaluating breast cancer care can highlight the role of nurse navigation even months after diagnosis (Pieters et al., 2011). Korber et al. (2011) used a semistructured, open-ended questionnaire to identify barriers and enhancers of breast cancer care completion. The nurse navigator was acknowledged as a valuable role in the specific points of education and emotional and physical support, as well as being a constant presence in the care.

Improved Sustainability and Cost-Effectiveness

The sustainability of patient navigation programs depends on the ability to demonstrate their economic value and the establishment of cost-effectiveness by systemic goals, such as reducing no-show rates, avoiding test duplication, enhancing retention rates, or increasing referrals to other programs in the system.

Whitley et al. (2011) described five categories of core and optional cost measures in a patient navigation program: program costs, human capital costs, direct medical costs, direct nonmedical costs, and indirect costs. They provided a thorough list of cost metrics for each category. They used an example of a year's charges versus actual costs for a patient with breast cancer and showed more than $43,000 in revenue that might offset the cost of a navigation program. Cost-effectiveness analysis compares alternative interventions to evaluate the added costs of a new program, such as navigation versus the status quo for the given target populations (Pratt-Chapman & Willis, 2013).

Markossian and Calhoun (2011) looked at how costs of breast cancer navigation can be justified by survival benefits and lifetime breast cancer–attributable cost savings. They concluded that if a navigated patient received a breast cancer diagnosis six months earlier than compared to usual care, then this program is cost-effective for $95,625 per life year saved.

Donaldson et al. (2012) showed that a breast cancer patient navigation program versus standard care based in a community setting with a low-income population can have a cost-effectiveness ratio of $511 to $2,080 per breast cancer resolution completed.

Henrico Doctors' Hospital used a gap analysis to recognize the need for a nurse navigator to be placed earlier in the breast continuum. This change decreased the breast patient outmigration rate from 240 to 28, and the financial impact to the system was $350,000 in billable services or procedures in one year (Desimini et al., 2011).

In 2011, Novant Health Derrick L. Davis Cancer Center published a report showing that the annual revenue captured from breast nurse navigation in decreasing outmigration was $436,000 (Advisory Board Company Oncology Roundtable, 2011). A systemic change in 2013 of placing a nurse navigator with the patient at the time of diagnosis dropped the rate further and brought in $272,500 of revenue to the healthcare system (Calcutt-Flaherty et al., 2014).

Intermountain Southwest Cancer Center in Utah showed a cost–benefit analysis (see Table 10-5) by medical oncologists experiencing a 24-minute reduction in clinical visit time with a newly diagnosed patient with breast cancer when the patient had received an educational visit with a nurse navigator (Christensen & Bellomo, 2014). This was a cost savings of $277,953 annually to the system. This allowed the medical oncologist to see an additional clinic patient each day. The additional revenue of $207,360 plus the decrease in time had the potential to bring in $485,312 to the system annually.

In the future, breast navigation programs will need to continue to use quality benchmark measures for sustainability and identify outcomes that provide a proven foundation for the program and demonstrate a return on investment. A business perspective will need to be embraced from outreach to survivorship while not losing the voice of the patient. Goals may include removing barriers from access through treatment, promoting treatment adherence via NCCN guidelines, and decreasing emergency department visits as well as hospital readmissions. With the growth in cancer survivorship, the focus will shift to wellness and prevention and navigation of successful follow-up plans for a healthier population. Figure 10-5 has examples of resources on breast navigation sustainability measures.

Table 10-5. Cost–Benefit Analysis

New Patient Consult (NPC) Metrics	Prenavigation Pathway	Postnavigation Pathway
Time in minutes	80	60
Per clinic day	12	12
Cost per consult	$408	$270
Total cost per day	$4896	$3240
Number of clinic days per year	192	192
Total NPC cost per year	**$940,032**	**$662,080**
Total cost-savings per year		**$277,952**
Additional revenue potential[a]		**$207,360**
Total cost-savings + revenue potential		**$485,312**

[a] Additional revenue by seeing 1 new patient per day per 4 oncologists.

Note. From "Using a Nurse Navigation Pathway in the Timely Care of Oncology Patients," by D. Christensen and C. Bellomo, 2014, *Journal of Oncology Navigation and Survivorship, 5*(3), p. 17. Copyright 2014 by Academy of Oncology Nurse and Patient Navigators. Reprinted with permission.

Figure 10-5. Resources for Breast Navigation Sustainability

- Academy of Oncology Nurse and Patient Navigators (www.aonnonline.org/metrics-source-document): 35 standardized navigation metrics in the areas of business performance/return on investment, clinical outcomes, and patient experience
- Advisory Board Company (www.advisory.com): Topics such as navigation, patient experience, care transformation, performance improvement, and population health
- Agency for Healthcare Research and Quality (www.ahrq.gov): Reports on healthcare quality and disparities, priority populations, and healthcare cost and utilization
- American Society of Clinical Oncology Institute for Quality (www.instituteforquality.org): Guidelines that can address specific clinical situations in breast cancer care or patient-centered oncology practice
- Health Resources and Services Administration (https://datawarehouse.hrsa.gov/tools/tools.aspx): Toolkit of objective tools and resources to assist organizations in quality improvement efforts with proven strategies and techniques to effectively support new or existing programs
- Institute for Healthcare Improvement (www.ihi.org/Pages/default.aspx): Topics such as improvement capability, person- and family-centered care, patient safety, and quality, cost, and value
- National Quality Measures for Breast Centers (http://www2.nqmbc.org): Quality initiative of the National Consortium of Breast Centers for programs to become a Certified Quality Breast Center™ or a Certified Quality Breast Center of Excellence™

To promote navigation sustainability and program effectiveness, the Academy of Oncology Nurse and Patient Navigators (AONN, n.d.) executed a comprehensive literature search on the topic of navigation value. The project team recognized three main categories of measure as standardized national metrics: business performance or return on investment (ROI), clinical outcomes, and patient experience (Strusowski et al., 2017). The team developed 35 baseline metrics that any navigation program could evaluate and monitor, despite the individuality of the patient navigation program, to demonstrate sustainability.

Certification

NAPBC accreditation does not require certification in navigation or nursing but recommends it in nursing and stresses that care should be given by nurses with breast disease knowledge and experience (NAPBC, 2014). The American College of Surgeons Commission on Cancer (2015) also encourages oncology nursing certification and, to achieve a commendation rating, 25% of oncology nurses employed must hold oncology nursing certification. Certification is a way to measure competency against a set of standards in a specialized field. Different certification processes exist for navigators in breast care, with some generalized for navigation and others specific to breast care.

General Oncology Navigation Certification

In 2016, AONN launched a general oncology navigator certification examination for nurses, as well as a general patient navigator beta examination (AONN, n.d.). These certification examinations are for anyone involved in navigation as outlined in the framework for navigation role delineation and core competencies for oncology patient navigators (Pratt-Chapman, Willis, & Masselink, 2015; Willis et al., 2013). The individual designations are oncology nurse navigator–certified generalist (ONN-CG) and oncology patient navigator–certified generalist (OPN-CG). This certification may be most appropriate for a navigator that has to cover breast navigation as well as other oncology tumor sites.

The criteria for taking the nurse navigator test include having an active AONN membership, an RN licensure in good standing, and a job description and reference letter signed and dated by the employer to AONN, as well as a curriculum vitae reflecting at least three years of direct navigation experience. The patient navigator criteria include having an active AONN membership and demonstrating one year of practice in patient navigation documented by submission of a résumé and letter from the patient navigator's supervisor or employer.

AONN has core competency domain learning modules with references on its website for nurses and patient navigators and encourages them to complete the free George Washington University Cancer Institute Oncology Patient Navigator Training. Recertification is achieved with annual AONN-designated navigation continuing education units and AONN membership.

Breast Cancer–Specific Navigator Certification

The National Consortium of Breast Centers offers a breast cancer–specific certification for six different levels of caregivers in breast care (National Consortium of Breast Centers, 2016):
- Certified navigator–breast imaging (CN-BI): Intended for all technologists from diagnostics to treatments
- Certified navigator–breast management (CN-BM): Targets social workers and managers of navigators
- Certified navigator–breast advocate (CN-BA): Captures all volunteers and lay navigators
- Certified navigator–breast clinical (CN-BC): Focuses on certified medical assistants, technicians, and licensed practical nurses

- Certified navigator–breast provider (CN-BP): Includes breast care diagnosticians, nurse practitioners, physicians, physician assistants, and breast care PhDs
- Certified navigator–breast nurse (CN-BN): Includes all RNs in the breast care continuum

Certification eligibility requirements can be found at http://www2.bpnc.org/certification.

Certified Breast Care Nurse

In 2009, the Oncology Nursing Certification Corporation started offering a certified breast care nurse (CBCN®) certification that is only for RNs and incorporates the entire spectrum of the breast care continuum (Oncology Nursing Certification Corporation, n.d.). Eligibility requirements include the following:
- Current RN license in the United States, its territories, or Canada
- One year of experience as an RN within the three years prior to test application
- At least 1,000 hours of breast care nursing within 30 months of application
- Completion of 10 hours of breast care continuing nursing education within the three years prior to application, of which five hours can be continuing medical education

The examination is computer-based testing at Prometric test centers throughout the year. The certification is valid for four years, and renewal can be completed by a combination of practice hours, testing, and completion of an individualized learning needs assessment.

Summary

Breast cancer navigation has evolved from the original intent of decreasing barriers to care to the present aim of promoting quality outcomes from outreach through survivorship and end-of-life services. The breast navigator lives in two worlds—the organization of care and the patients' sphere. Fillion et al. (2012) described this as a bidimensional component that the navigator serves by fostering continuity that is systems oriented and facilitates patient-centered care and empowerment for patient and caregivers. The navigator has knowledge of the complexities of the care system in order to engage the breast cancer care team proactively to create seamless care for optimal outcomes. A common task held in high regard by patients is education about the breast care process, as navigators clarify, reinforce, and validate information on a personal level in the context of the patients' life. The supportive role of identifying potential or real barriers to care, mobilizing resources to overcome barriers, and consistently being present and accessible develops a close relationship of trust and promotes patient satisfaction.

The reliable point of contact through the breast care continuum allows promotion of timely access to care and transition to the next phase of care. The administrative support in performing gap analysis and qualitative initiatives can lead to the establishment of best practices that reduce diagnostic and care delays, as well as promote the value and efficiency of breast navigation. This patient-centered value embedded in evidence-based navigation outcomes supports quality in service and a remarkable patient experience that in turn creates a stronger system of care.

References

Academy of Oncology Nurse and Patient Navigators. (n.d.). Certification. Retrieved from https://www
.aonnonline.org/certification

Advisory Board Company Oncology Roundtable. (2008). *Elevating the patient experience: Building successful patient navigation, multidisciplinary care, and survivorship programs.* Retrieved from https://www.advisory
.com/Research/Oncology-Roundtable/Studies/2008/Elevating-the-Patient-Experience

Advisory Board Company Oncology Roundtable. (2011). *Maximizing the value of patient navigation: Lessons for optimizing program performance.* Retrieved from https://www.advisory.com/research/oncology
-roundtable/studies/2011/maximizing-the-value-of-patient-navigation

American Cancer Society. (1989). *Report to the nation: Cancer in the poor.* Atlanta, GA: Author.

American College of Surgeons Commission on Cancer. (2015). *Cancer program standards: Ensuring patient-centered care* (2016 ed.). Retrieved from https://www.facs.org/quality-programs/cancer/coc/standards

Arias, J. (2012). Patient navigation: Blending imaging and oncology in breast cancer. *Journal of Oncology Navigation and Survivorship, 3*(1), 16–21. Retrieved from https://issuu.com/aonn/docs/jons-feb2012

Barke, L.D., & Freivogel, M.E. (2017). Breast cancer risk assessment models and high-risk screening. *Radiologic Clinics, 55,* 457–474. doi:10.1016/j.rcl.2016.12.013

Basu, M., Linebarger, J., Gabram, S.G.A., Patterson, S.G., Amin, M., & Ward, K.C. (2013). The effect of nurse navigation on timeliness of breast cancer care at an academic comprehensive cancer center. *Cancer, 119,* 2524–2531. doi:10.1002/cncr.28024

Bellcross, C.A., Leadbetter, S., Alford, S.A., & Peipins, L.A. (2013). Prevalence and healthcare actions of women in a large health system with a family history meeting the 2005 USPSTF recommendation for *BRCA* genetic counseling referral. *Cancer Epidemiology, Biomarkers and Prevention, 22,* 728–735. doi:10
.1158/1055-9965.EPI-12-1280

Bensenhaver, J., & Winchester, D.P. (2014). Surgical leadership and standardization of multidisciplinary breast center care: The evolution of the National Accreditation Program for Breast Centers. *Surgical Oncology Clinics of North America, 23,* 609–616. doi:10.1016/j.soc.2014.03.005

Blaseg, K. (2009). Patient navigation at Billings Clinic: An NCI Community Cancer Centers Program (NCCCP) pilot site. *ACCC's cancer care patient navigation: A call to action* (pp. 15–24). Rockville, MD: Association of Community Cancer Centers.

Blaseg, K., Kile, M., & Salner, A. (2011, May/June). Survivorship and palliative care: A comprehensive approach to a survivorship care plan. *Oncology Issues,* pp. 26–37.

Braun, K.L., Thomas, W.L., Jr., Domingo, J.-L.B., Allison, A.L., Ponce, A., Kamakana, P.H., … Tsark, J.U. (2015). Reducing cancer screening disparities in Medicare beneficiaries through cancer patient navigation. *Journal of the American Geriatrics Society, 63,* 365–370. doi:10.1111/jgs.13192

Browne, T., Darnell, J., Savage, T.E., & Brown, A. (2015). Social workers as patient navigators: A review of the literature. *Social Work Research, 39,* 158–166. doi:10.1093/swr/svv017

Burhansstipanov, L., Dignan, M.B., Schumacher, A., Krebs, L.U., Alfonsi, G., & Apodaca, C.C. (2010). Breast screening navigator programs within three settings that assist underserved women. *Journal of Cancer Education, 25,* 247–252. doi:10.1007/s13187-010-0071-4

Byers, T. (2012). Assessing the value of patient navigation for completing cancer screening. *Cancer Epidemiology, Biomarkers and Prevention, 21,* 1618–1619. doi:10.1158/1055-9965.EPI-12-0964

Calcutt-Flaherty, J., Gentry, S., & Mathis, L. (2014). Supporting evidence-based practice in nurse navigation [Abstract presented at the Fifth Annual Navigators and Survivorship Conference in Orlando, Florida]. *Journal of Oncology Navigation and Survivorship, 5*(4), 37.

Campbell, C., Craig, J., Eggert, J., & Bailey-Dorton, C. (2010). Implementing and measuring the impact of patient navigation at a comprehensive community cancer center. *Oncology Nursing Forum, 37,* 61–68. doi:10.1188/10.ONF.61-68

Carroll, J.K., Humiston, S.G., Meldrum, S.C., Salamone, C.M., Jean-Pierre, P., Epstein, R.M., & Fiscella, K. (2010). Patients' experiences with navigation for cancer care. *Patient Education and Counseling, 80,* 241–247. doi:10.1016/j.pec.2009.10.024

Cascella, S., & Keren, J. (2012). Mujer a mujer/woman to woman: Using a unique venue for culturally appropriate outreach and navigation in an underserved area to increase screening. *Journal of Oncology Navigation and Survivorship, 3*(2), 20–26.

Chlebowski, R.T., & Blackburn, G.L. (2014). Final survival analysis from the randomized Women's Intervention Nutrition Study (WINS) evaluating dietary intervention as adjuvant breast cancer therapy [Abstract]. *Cancer Research, 75*(Suppl. 9), Abstract No. S5-08. doi:10.1158/1538-7445.SABCS14-S5-08

Christensen, D., & Bellomo, C. (2014). Using a nurse navigation pathway in the timely care of oncology patients. *Journal of Oncology Navigation and Survivorship, 5*(3), 13–18.

Clark, C.R., Baril, N., Kunicki, M., Johnson, N., Soukup, J., Ferguson, K., … Bigby, J. (2009). Addressing social determinants of health to improve access to early breast cancer detection: Results of the Boston REACH 2010 Breast and Cervical Cancer Coalition Women's Health Demonstration Project. *Journal of Women's Health, 18,* 677–690. doi:10.1089/jwh.2008.0972

Desimini, E.M., Kennedy, J.A., Helsley, M.F., Shiner, K., Denton, C., Rice, T.T., … Lewis, M.G. (2011, September/October). Making the case for nurse navigators. *Oncology Issues,* pp. 26–33. Retrieved from https://www.accc-cancer.org/oncology_issues/articles/SO11/SO11-Making-the-Case-for-Nurse-Navigators.pdf

Donaldson, E.A., Holtgrave, D.R., Duffin, R.A., Feltner, F., Funderburk, W., & Freeman, H.P. (2012). Patient navigation for breast and colorectal cancer in 3 community hospital settings: An economic evaluation. *Cancer, 118,* 4851–4859. doi:10.1002/cncr.27487

Donelan, K., Mailhot, J.R., Dutwin, D., Barnicle, K., Oo, S.A., Hobrecker, K., … Chabner, B.A. (2011). Patient perspectives of clinical care and patient navigation in follow-up of abnormal mammography. *Journal of General Internal Medicine, 26,* 116–122. doi:10.1007/s11606-010-1436-4

Dudley, D.J., Drake, J., Quinlan, J., Holden, A., Saegert, P., Karnad, A., & Ramirez, A. (2012). Beneficial effects of a combined navigator/promotora approach for Hispanic women diagnosed with breast abnormalities. *Cancer Epidemiology, Biomarkers and Prevention, 21,* 1639–1644. doi:10.1158/1055-9965.EPI-12-0538

EduCare, Inc. (n.d.). About our company. Retrieved from http://www.educareinc.com/about.php

Ferrante, J.M., Chen, P.-H., & Kim, S. (2008). The effect of patient navigation on time to diagnosis, anxiety, and satisfaction in urban minority women with abnormal mammograms: A randomized controlled trial. *Journal of Urban Health, 85,* 114–124. doi:10.1007/s11524-007-9228-9

Fillion, L., Cook, S., Veillette, A.-M., Aubin, M., de Serres, M., Rainville, F., … Doll, R. (2012). Professional navigation framework: Elaboration and validation in a Canadian context [Online exclusive]. *Oncology Nursing Forum, 39,* E58–E69. doi:10.1188/12.ONF.E58-E69

Fiscella, K., Ransom, S., Jean-Pierre, P., Cella, D., Stein, K., Bauer, J.E., … Walsh, K. (2011). Patient-reported outcome measures suitable to assessment of patient navigation. *Cancer, 117*(Suppl. S17), 3601–3615. doi:10.1002/cncr.26260

Fischer, S.M., Cervantes, L., Fink, R.M., & Kutner, J.S. (2015). Apoyo con Cariño: A pilot randomized controlled trial of a patient navigator intervention to improve palliative care outcomes for Latinos with serious illness. *Journal of Pain and Symptom Management, 49,* 657–665. doi:10.1016/j.jpainsymman.2014.08.011

Francks, B., Iverson, M.L., & Miller, J. (2014). Breast cancer navigation. In K.D. Blaseg, P. Daugherty, & K.A. Gamblin (Eds.), *Oncology nurse navigation: Delivering patient-centered care across the continuum* (pp. 121–136). Pittsburgh, PA: Oncology Nursing Society.

Freeman, H.P. (2006). Patient navigation: A community centered approach to reducing cancer mortality. *Journal of Cancer Education, 21*(Suppl. 1), S11–S14. doi:10.1207/s15430154jce2101s_4

Freeman, H.P. (2012). The origin, evolution, and principles of patient navigation. *Cancer Epidemiology, Biomarkers and Prevention, 21,* 1614–1617. doi:10.1158/1055-9965.EPI-12-0982

Freeman, H.P. (2013). The history, principles, and future of patient navigation: Commentary. *Seminars in Oncology Nursing, 29,* 72–75. doi:10.1016/j.soncn.2013.02.002

Freeman, H.P., Muth, B.J., & Kerner, J.F. (1995). Expanding access to cancer screening and clinical follow-up among the medically underserved. *Cancer Practice, 3,* 19–30.

Freeman, H.P., & Rodriguez, R.L. (2011). History and principles of patient navigation. *Cancer, 117*(Suppl. S17), 3537–3540. doi:10.1002/cncr.26262

Freund, K.M., Battaglia, T.A., Calhoun, E., Dudley, D.J., Fiscella, K., Paskett, E., … Roetzheim, R.G. (2008). National Cancer Institute Patient Navigation Research Program: Methods, protocol, and measures. *Cancer, 113,* 3391–3399. doi:10.1002/cncr.23960

Gabitova, G., & Burke, N.J. (2014). Improving healthcare empowerment through breast cancer patient navigation: A mixed methods evaluation in a safety-net setting. *BMC Health Services Research, 14,* 407. doi:10.1186/1472-6963-14-407

Goetz, P. (2014). Quality outcomes and performance improvement committee. *Journal of Oncology Navigation and Survivorship, 5*(2), 6–7.

Gonzalez, M., Berger, M., Bryant, D., Ellison, C., Harness, J., Krasna, M., … Wilkinson, K. (2011, March/April). Using a minority matrix and patient navigation to improve accrual to clinical trials. *Oncology Issues,* pp. 59–60.

Haideri, N.A., & Moormeier, J.A. (2011). Impact of patient navigation from diagnosis to treatment in an urban safety net breast cancer population. *Journal of Cancer, 2*, 467–473. doi:10.7150/jca.2.467

Han, H.-R., Lee, H., Kim, M.T., & Kim, K.B. (2009). Tailored lay health worker intervention improves breast cancer screening outcomes in non-adherent Korean-American women. *Health Education Research, 24*, 318–329. doi:10.1093/her/cyn021

Harding, M.M. (2014). Incidence of distress and associated factors in women undergoing breast diagnostic evaluation. *Western Journal of Nursing Research, 36*, 475–494. doi:10.1177/0193945913506795

Harding, M.M. (2015). Effect of nurse navigation on patient care satisfaction and distress associated with breast biopsy [Online exclusive]. *Clinical Journal of Oncology Nursing, 19*, E15–E20. doi:10.1188/15.CJON.E15-E20

Harding, M.M., & McCrone, S. (2013). Experiences of non-navigated women undergoing breast diagnostic evaluation [Online exclusive]. *Clinical Journal of Oncology Nursing, 17*, E8–E12. doi:10.1188/13.CJON.E8-E12

Hauser, J., Sileo, M., Araneta, N., Kirk, R., Martinez, J., Finn, K., … Rodrigue, M.K. (2011). Navigation and palliative care. *Cancer, 117*(Suppl. S17), 3583–3589. doi:10.1002/cncr.26266

Hoffman, H.J., LaVerda, N.L., Young, H.A., Levine, P.H., Alexander, L.M., Brem, R., … Patierno, S.R. (2012). Patient navigation significantly reduces delays in breast cancer diagnosis in the District of Columbia. *Cancer Epidemiology, Biomarkers and Prevention, 21*, 1655–1663. doi:10.1158/1055-9965.EPI-12-0479

Holmes, D.R., Major, J., Lyonga, D.E., Alleyne, R.S., & Clayton, S.M. (2012). Increasing minority patient participation in cancer clinical trials using oncology nurse navigation. *American Journal of Surgery, 203*, 415–422. doi:10.1016/j.amjsurg.2011.02.005

Hook, A., Ware, L., Siler, B., & Packard, A. (2012). Breast cancer navigation and patient satisfaction: Exploring a community-based patient navigation model in a rural setting. *Oncology Nursing Forum, 39*, 379–385. doi:10.1188/12.ONF.379-385

Hopkins, J., & Mumber, M.P. (2009). Patient navigation through the cancer care continuum: An overview. *Journal of Oncology Practice, 5*, 150–152, doi:10.1200/JOP.0943501

Hughes, S.K. (2017). A pathway for identifying women at increased risk for breast cancer and providing personalized management and risk reduction. *Oncology Issues, 32*(2), 38–45. Retrieved from http://www.nxtbook.com/nxtbooks/accc/oncologyissues_20170304/index.php?startid=38#/40

Kapp, H., & Pratt-Chapman, M. (2015). Patient experience mapping: A quality improvement tool for patient navigators. *Journal of Oncology Navigation and Survivorship, 6*(1), 20–24.

Katz, M.L., Young, G.S., Reiter, P.L., Battaglia, T.A., Wells, K.J., Sanders, M., … Paskett, E.D. (2014). Barriers reported among patients with breast and cervical abnormalities in the Patient Navigation Research Program: Impact on timely care. *Women's Health Issues, 24*, e155–e162. doi:10.1016/j.whi.2013.10.010

Kiely, D. (2014). Timeliness in breast cancer care as an indicator of quality. *Clinical Journal of Oncology Nursing, 18*, 82–88. doi:10.1188/14.CJON.82-88

Klein, S.H., & Hawkins, S.Y. (2015). Transitioning patients after breast cancer treatment: Implementing survivorship care plans. *Journal of Oncology Navigation and Survivorship, 6*(5), 20–27.

Kneece, J.C. (1994, March/April). Fulfilling a mission. *Cope*, pp. 6–7.

Kneece, J.C. (2008). Breast health navigator: A paradigm shift in breast health care. *Seminars in Breast Disease, 11*, 13–19. doi:10.1053/j.sembd.2008.04.004

Knowles, M., & Nelsen, R. (2015). Recognizing the importance of a diagnostic breast health navigator. Abstract presentation at the Sixth Annual Navigation and Survivorship Conference. *Journal of Oncology Navigation and Survivorship, 6*(4), 59–60.

Ko, N.Y., Darnell, J.S., Calhoun, E., Freund, K.M., Wells, K.J., Shapiro, C.L., … Battaglia, T.A. (2014). Can patient navigation improve receipt of recommended breast cancer care? Evidence from the National Patient Navigation Research Program. *Journal of Clinical Oncology, 32*, 2758–2764. doi:10.1200/JCO.2013.53.6037

Koh, C., Nelson, J.M., & Cook, P.F. (2011). Evaluation of a patient navigation program. *Clinical Journal of Oncology Nursing, 15*, 41–48. doi:10.1188/11.CJON.41-48

Korber, S.F., Padula, C., Gray, J., & Powell, M. (2011). A breast navigator program: Barriers, enhancers, and nursing interventions. *Oncology Nursing Forum, 38*, 44–50. doi:10.1188/11.ONF.44-50

Krok-Schoen, J.L., Brewer, B.M., Young, G.S., Weier, R.C., Tatum, C.M., DeGraffinreid, C.R., & Paskett, E.D. (2015). Participants' barriers to diagnostic resolution and factors associated with needing patient navigation. *Cancer, 121*, 2757–2764. doi:10.1002/cncr.29414

Krok-Schoen, J.L., Kurta, M.L., Weier, R.C., Young, G.S., Carey, A.B., Tatum, C.M., & Paskett, E.D. (2015). Clinic type and patient characteristics affecting time to resolution after an abnormal cancer-screening exam. *Cancer Epidemiology, Biomarkers and Prevention, 24*, 162–168. doi:10.1158/1055-9965.EPI-14-0692

Lorhan, S., Cleghorn, L., Fitch, M., Pang, K., McAndrew, A., Applin-Poole, J., … Wright, M. (2013). Moving the agenda forward for cancer patient navigation: Understanding volunteer and peer navigation approaches. *Journal of Cancer Education, 28,* 84–91. doi:10.1007/s13187-012-0424-2

Madore, S., Kilbourn, K., Valverde, P., Borrayo, E., & Raich, P. (2014). Feasibility of a psychosocial and patient navigation intervention to improve access to treatment among underserved breast cancer patients. *Supportive Care in Cancer, 22,* 2085–2093. doi:10.1007/s00520-014-2176-5

Malone, P., Bruno, L., Hayden, B., & Carlson, J. (2014). Development and evolution of an oncology nurse navigation program: From formation to fruition. *Journal of Oncology Navigation and Survivorship, 5*(5), 19–24.

Marchand, P. (2010). Schering Lectureship 2008: The clinical nurse specialist as nurse navigator: Ordinary role presents extraordinary experience. *Canadian Oncology Nursing Journal, 20,* 80–83. doi:10.5737/1181912x2028083

Markossian, T.W., & Calhoun, E.A. (2011). Are breast cancer navigation programs cost-effective? Evidence from the Chicago Cancer Navigation Project. *Health Policy, 99,* 52–59. doi:10.1016/j.healthpol.2010.07.008

Markossian, T.W., Darnell, J.S., & Calhoun, E.A. (2012). Follow-up and timeliness after an abnormal cancer screening among underserved, urban women in a patient navigation program. *Cancer Epidemiology, Biomarkers and Prevention, 21,* 1691–1700. doi:10.1158/1055-9965.EPI-12-0535

Mays, D., Sharff, M.E., DeMarco, T.A., Williams, B., Beck, B., Sheppard, V.B., … Tercyak, K.P. (2012). Outcomes of a systems-level intervention offering breast cancer risk assessments to low-income underserved women. *Familial Cancer, 11,* 493–502. doi:10.1007/s10689-012-9541-7

McAllister, K.A., & Schmitt, M.L. (2015). Impact of a nurse navigator on genomic testing and timely treatment decision making in patients with breast cancer. *Clinical Journal of Oncology Nursing, 19,* 510–512. doi:10.1188/15.CJON.510-512

McClung, E.C., Davis, S.W., Jeffrey, S.S., Kuo, M.-C., Lee, M.M., & Teng, N.N.H. (2013). Impact of navigation on knowledge and attitudes about clinical trials among Chinese patients undergoing treatment for breast and gynecologic cancers. *Journal of Immigrant and Minority Health, 17,* 976–979. doi:10.1007/s10903-013-9901-x

McVay, S., Toney, T., & Kautz, D. (2014). The effect of different types of navigators on patient outcomes. *Journal of Oncology Navigation and Survivorship, 5*(2), 17–24.

Meade, C.D., Wells, K.J., Arevalo, M., Calcano, E.R., Rivera, M., Sarmiento, Y., … Roetzheim, R.G. (2014). Lay navigator model for impacting cancer health disparities. *Journal of Cancer Education, 29,* 449–457. doi:10.1007/s13187-014-0640-z

Mitchell, J.B., Bir, A., Hoover, S., & Subramanian, S. (2012). *Evaluation of the cancer prevention and treatment demonstration for ethnic and racial minorities: Final report to Congress.* Retrieved from https://innovation.cms.gov/Files/reports/CPTD-Final.pdf

National Accreditation Program for Breast Centers. (2014). *NAPBC standards manual* (2014 ed.). Retrieved from https://www.facs.org/~/media/files/quality%20programs/napbc/2014%20napbc%20standards%20manual.ashx

National Cancer Institute. (n.d.). Grid-Enabled Measures Database. Retrieved from https://www.gem-beta.org/Public/MeasureList.aspx?cat=2

National Cancer Institute. (2015, February 17). Patient Navigation Research Program (PNRP). Retrieved from http://www.cancer.gov/about-nci/organization/crchd/disparities-research/pnrp

National Comprehensive Cancer Network. (2017). *NCCN Clinical Practice Guidelines in Oncology (NCCN Guidelines®): Palliative care* [v.2.2017]. Retrieved from http://www.nccn.org/professionals/physician_gls/pdf/palliative.pdf

National Consortium of Breast Centers. (2016). *Breast patient navigator certification.* Retrieved from http://www2.bpnc.org/wp-content/uploads/2013/06/Navigator-processes-and-procedures-V2.pdf

Oluwole, S.F., Ali, A.O., Adu, A., Blane, B.P., Barlow, B., Oropeza, R., & Freeman, H.P. (2003). Impact of a cancer screening program on breast cancer stage at diagnosis in a medically underserved urban community. *Journal of the American College of Surgeons, 196,* 180–188. doi:10.1016/S1072-7515(02)01765-9

Oncology Nursing Certification Corporation. (n.d.). Certified breast care nurse (CBCN®). Retrieved at http://www.oncc.org/certifications/certified-breast-care-nurse-cbcn

Oncology Nursing Society. (2010). Oncology Nursing Society, the Association of Oncology Social Work, and the National Association of Social Workers joint position on the role of oncology nursing and oncology social work in patient navigation. Retrieved from https://www.ons.org/advocacy-policy/positions/education/patient-navigation

Paskett, E.D., Harrop, J.P., & Wells, K.J. (2011). Patient navigation: An update on the state of the science. *CA: A Cancer Journal for Clinicians, 61,* 237–249. doi:10.3322/caac.20111

Paskett, E.D., Katz, M.L., Post, D.M., Pennell, M.L., Young, G.S., Seiber, E.E., … Murray, D.M. (2012). The Ohio Patient Navigation Research Program: Does the American Cancer Society Patient Navigation Model improve time to resolution in patients with abnormal screening tests? *Cancer Epidemiology, Biomarkers and Prevention, 21,* 1620–1628. doi:10.1158/1055-9965.EPI-12-0523

Patient Navigator Outreach and Chronic Disease Prevention Act of 2005, Pub. L. No. 109-18. Retrieved from https://www.congress.gov/109/plaws/publ18/PLAW-109publ18.pdf

Patierno, S.R., LaVerda, N.L., Alexander, L.M., Levine, P.H., Young, H.A., & Hoffman, H.J. (2010). Longitudinal network patient navigation: Development of a city-wide integrative model to reduce breast cancer disparities in Washington, D.C. *Oncology Issues, 25*(2), 28–35.

Pedersen, A.E., Hack, T.F., McClement, S.E., & Taylor-Brown, J. (2014). An exploration of the patient navigator role: Perspectives of younger women with breast cancer. *Oncology Nursing Forum, 41,* 77–88. doi:10.1188/14.ONF.77-88

Perry, N. (1992, April). A recycled mom. *South Carolina Nursing Matters,* pp. 5–8.

Phillips, C.E., Rothstein, J.D., Beaver, K., Sherman, B.J., Freund, K.M., & Battaglia, T.A. (2011). Patient navigation to increase mammography screening among inner city women. *Journal of General Internal Medicine, 26,* 123–129. doi:10.1007/s11606-010-1527-2

Pieters, H.C., Heilemann, M.V., Grant, M., & Maly, R.C. (2011). Older women's reflections on accessing care across their breast cancer trajectory: Navigating beyond the triple barriers. *Oncology Nursing Forum, 38,* 175–184. doi:10.1188/11.ONF.175-184

Pratt-Chapman, M. (2015). Cancer survivorship: The role of the nurse navigator. *Journal of Oncology Navigation and Survivorship, 6*(6), 14–18.

Pratt-Chapman, M., & Willis, A. (2013). Community cancer center administration and support for navigation services. *Seminars in Oncology Nursing, 29,* 141–148. doi:10.1016/j.soncn.2013.02.009

Pratt-Chapman, M., Willis, A., & Masselink, L. (2015). Core competencies for oncology patient navigators. *Journal of Oncology Navigation and Survivorship, 6*(2), 16–21.

Rahm, A.K., Sukhanova, A., Ellis, J., & Mouchawar, J. (2007). Increasing utilization of cancer genetic counseling services using a patient navigator model. *Journal of Genetic Counseling, 16,* 171–177. doi:10.1007/s10897-006-9051-6

Raich, P.C., Whitley, E.M., Thorland, W., Valverde, P., & Fairclough, D. (2012). Patient navigation improves cancer diagnostic resolution: An individually randomized clinical trial in an underserved population. *Cancer Epidemiology, Biomarkers and Prevention, 21,* 1629–1638. doi:10.1158/1055-9965.EPI-12-0513

Raj, A., Ko, N., Battaglia, T.A., Chabner, B.A., & Moy, B. (2012). Patient navigation for underserved patients diagnosed with breast cancer. *Oncologist, 17,* 1027–1031. doi:10.1634/theoncologist.2012-0191

Ramachandran, A., Freund, K.M., Bak, S.M., Heeren, T.C., Chen, C.A., & Battaglia, T.A. (2015). Multiple barriers delay care among women with abnormal cancer screening despite patient navigation. *Journal of Women's Health, 24,* 30–36. doi:10.1089/jwh.2014.4869

Ramirez, A., Perez-Stable, E., Penedo, F., Talavera, G., Carrillo, J.E., Fernández, M., … Gallion, K. (2014). Reducing time-to-treatment in underserved Latinas with breast cancer: The Six Cities Study. *Cancer, 120,* 752–760. doi:10.1002/cncr.28450

Robinson-White, S., Conroy, B., Slavish, K.H., & Rosenzweig, M. (2010). Patient navigation in breast cancer: A systematic review. *Cancer Nursing, 33,* 127–140. doi:10.1097/NCC.0b013e3181c40401

Rousseau, S.J., Humiston, S.G., Yosha, A., Winters, P.C., Loader, S., Luong, V., … Fiscella, K. (2014). Patient navigation moderates emotion and information demands of cancer treatment: A qualitative analysis. *Supportive Care in Cancer, 22,* 3143–3151. doi:10.1007/s00520-014-2295-z

Sein, E. (2011). Building breast centers of excellence through patient navigation and care coordination. In S.M. Mahon (Ed.), *Site-specific cancer series: Breast cancer* (2nd ed., pp. 213–229). Pittsburgh, PA: Oncology Nursing Society.

Shockney, L.D. (2010a). Evolution of patient navigation. *Clinical Journal of Oncology Nursing, 14,* 405–407. doi:10.1188/10.CJON.405-407

Shockney, L.D. (2010b). The nurse navigator's role in preventing medical legal issues associated with breast cancer diagnosis and treatment: Part 2. Retrieved from https://www.aonnonline.org/the-nurse-navigator-s-role-in-preventing-medical-legal-issues-associated-with-breast-cancer-diagnosis-and-treatment-part-2

Shockney, L.D. (2011). *Becoming a breast cancer nurse navigator.* Burlington, MA: Jones & Bartlett Learning.

Shockney, L.D. (2015). The evolution of patient navigation and survivorship care. *Breast Journal, 21,* 104–110. doi:10.1111/tbj.12353

Shockney, L.D., Haylock, P.J., & Cantril, C. (2013). Development of a breast navigation program. *Seminars in Oncology Nursing, 29,* 97–104. doi:10.1016/j.soncn.2013.02.006

Sprandio, J.D. (2010). Oncology patient-centered medical home and accountable cancer care. *Community Oncology, 7,* 565–572. Retrieved from https://www.communityoncology.org/UserFiles/pdfs/co-js-medical-home.pdf

St. Germain, D., Dimond, E., Olesen, K. Ellison, C., Nacpil, L., Gansauer, L., ... Gonzalez, M. (2014). The NCCCP Patient Navigation Project: Using patient navigators to enhance clinical trial education and promote accrual. *Oncology Issues, 29*(3), 44–53.

Strusowski, T., Sein, E., Johnston, D., Gentry, S., Bellomo, C., Brown, E., ... Messier, N. (2017). Standardized evidence-based oncology navigation metrics for all models: A powerful tool in assessing the value and impact of navigation programs. *Journal of Oncology Navigation and Survivorship, 8,* 220–243.

Tejeda, S., Darnell, J.S., Cho, Y.I., Stolley, M.R., Markossian, T.W., & Calhoun, E.A. (2013). Patient barriers to follow-up care for breast and cervical cancer abnormalities. *Journal of Women's Health, 22,* 507–517. doi:10.1089/jwh.2012.3590

Thomas, M.A., & Peters, E.A. (2014). Setting-specific navigation. In K.D. Blaseg, P. Daugherty, & K.A. Gamblin (Eds.), *Oncology nurse navigation: Delivering patient-centered care across the continuum* (pp. 175–206). Pittsburgh, PA: Oncology Nursing Society.

Trevillion, K., Singh-Carlson, S., Wong, F., & Sherriff, C. (2015). An evaluation report of the nurse navigator services for the breast cancer support program. *Canadian Oncology Nursing Journal, 25,* 409–421. doi:10.5737/23688076254409414

Wagner, E.H., Ludman, E.J., Bowles, E.J.A., Penfold, R., Reid, R.J., Rutter, C.M., ... McCorkle, R. (2014). Nurse navigators in early cancer care: A randomized, controlled trial. *Journal of Clinical Oncology, 32,* 12–18. doi:10.1200/JCO.2013.51.7359

Weber, J.J., Mascarenhas, D.C., Bellin, L.S., Raab, R.E., & Wong, J.H. (2012). Patient navigation and the quality of breast cancer care: An analysis of the Breast Cancer Care Quality Indicators. *Annals of Surgical Oncology, 19,* 3251–3256. doi:10.1245/s10434-012-2527-8

Wells, K.J., Battaglia, T.A., Dudley, D.J., Garcia, R., Greene, A., Calhoun, E., ... Raich, P.C. (2008). Patient navigation; State of the art or is it science? *Cancer, 113,* 1999–2010. doi:10.1002/cncr.23815

Whitley, E., Valverde, P., Wells, K., Williams, L., Teschner, T., & Shih, Y.-C.T. (2011). Establishing common cost measures to evaluate the economic value of patient navigation programs. *Cancer, 117*(Suppl. S15), 3616–3623. doi:10.1002/cncr.26268

Willis, A., Reed, E., Pratt-Chapman, M., Kapp, H., Hatcher, E., Vaitones, V., ... Washington, C. (2013). Development of a framework for patient navigation: Delineating roles across navigator types. *Journal of Oncology Navigation and Survivorship, 4*(6), 20–26.

Wong, R.S.L., Vikram, B., Govern, F.S., Petereit, D.G., Maguire, P.D., Clarkson, M.R., ... Coleman, C.N. (2014). National Cancer Institute's Cancer Disparities Research Partnership program: Experience and lessons learned. *Frontiers in Oncology, 4,* 303. doi:10.3389/fonc.2014.00303

CHAPTER 11

Survivorship Care

Deborah K. Mayer, PhD, ANP-BC, AOCN®, FAAN, and
Anna Kate Owens, MSN, RN, FNP

Introduction

More than three million women are living in the United States who have had a breast cancer diagnosis (National Cancer Institute, 2016). Most women (89.7%) are alive at least five years after diagnosis, but those diagnosed with earlier stages of breast cancer have a greater chance of being alive (98.6%) at that time point. An estimated 2,600 new breast cancers occur in men, accounting for less than 1% of all breast cancers. On average, men are between 60 and 70 years old at the time of diagnosis. For more specific information about male breast cancer, see National Cancer Institute (2017). Progress in early detection and treatment is reflected in five-year survival statistics that have improved from 75.2% in 1975 to 89.7% in 2013. Many of these women will be cured, whereas others may be living with a local recurrence, new breast cancer, or distant metastases (Howlader et al., 2017; National Cancer Institute, 2016).

Survivorship Care

Definition

Survivorship focuses on the health and life of individuals from the time of their cancer diagnosis throughout the balance of their life (National Cancer Institute Office of Cancer Survivorship, 2014). It covers the physical, psychosocial, and economic issues of cancer, beyond the diagnosis and treatment phases. Survivorship includes issues related to the ability to get health care and follow-up treatment, late effects of treatment, second cancers, and quality of life (see Chapter 9 for more detailed information on symptom management).

Disparities

Disparities exist in breast cancer care. Women of minority racial and ethnic groups, older women, and rural- and urban-dwelling women may not have access to or receive the recommended survivorship care (Paskett, 2015a). Older women may not receive the same benefits as younger women because of ageism and lack of clinical trial data in older women (Hurria & Muss, 2015). Decisions about their treatment should be based on their functional status, not chronologic age. Minority women have worse breast cancer outcomes, including lower receipt of appropriate treatment (Reeder-Hayes, Wheeler, & Mayer, 2015; Wheeler, Reeder-Hayes, & Carey, 2013). Monitoring adherence to endocrine therapy and for follow-up will be important during the survivorship phase of care to ensure patients receive the standard of care.

Multiple Chronic Conditions

Breast cancer is diagnosed most frequently in women aged 55–64 years (25%), yet 41.8% is diagnosed in women aged 65 years or older. Older women may have more comorbidities, which need to be considered and actively managed during cancer treatment (National Cancer Institute, 2016).

Guidelines for Survivorship Care

The frequency of survivorship care depends on patients' diagnosis and stage, treatment, and time since diagnosis. The American Society of Clinical Oncology and the American Cancer Society (ASCO/ACS) collaborated on the frequency and type of survivorship care recommended for patients with breast cancer (Runowicz et al., 2016). ASCO/ACS recommendations include the following:
• Visits every 3–6 months for the first 3 years after primary therapy, then every 6–12 months for years 4 and 5, and then annually thereafter
• Assessment and updating of cancer family history on regular basis
• Referral for genetic counseling if hereditary risk factors have developed since diagnosis. Risk factors include a strong family history of breast, colon, or endometrial cancers, triple-negative breast cancer in women aged 60 years or younger, or bilateral breast cancer (see Chapter 2).

Adherence to Oral Therapies

Assessing and encouraging adherence to ongoing oral therapies is an important guideline for survivorship care. Adherence to endocrine therapy declines over time (Huang, Chen, Lin, & Chang, 2016). Both early discontinuation and nonadherence to endocrine therapy are independent predictors of mortality (Hershman et al., 2011). Factors negatively influencing adherence include experiencing side effects and being followed by generalists instead of oncologists (Cahir, Guinan, Dombrowski, Sharp, & Bennett, 2015). Healthcare providers should assess barriers and beliefs regarding adherence and encourage strategies to facilitate adherence (Huang et al., 2016). The Oncology Nursing Society (n.d.) has an oral adherence toolkit that may be useful in addressing these issues.

Physical Examination

When conducting a physical examination, the healthcare provider should complete an assessment of areas at risk for recurrence, as well as long-term or late effects. This includes an assessment of the regional axillary, clavicular, and cervical lymphatics; breast and chest wall; the skin, cardiovascular, pulmonary, gastrointestinal, and musculoskeletal systems, including bone and back pain, range of motion in the affected arm, and evidence of lymphedema; and neurologic and psychological effects of the cancer or its treatment.

Surveillance

Surveillance for breast cancer recurrence is a necessary component of survivorship care. Recurrences peak by the second year after diagnosis and decline throughout the first 10 years; rates are higher for women with four or more involved lymph nodes or in the first three years in women with triple-negative breast cancer (Colleoni et al., 2016). Although the rates decline over time, breast cancer recurrences can occur much later. The annual hazard of recurrence was 2.2% from 10–15 years, 1.5% for years 15–20, and 0.7% for years 20–25 (Colleoni et al., 2016). Research is ongoing to identify predictive biomarkers or multigene signatures that may help to identify women at higher risk for later recurrence (Sestak & Cuzick, 2015).

Testing

Women should receive an annual mammogram—bilateral if both breasts are still present and unilateral if a mastectomy has been performed. This should be initiated at least six months after completion of radiation therapy and then repeated annually (Khatcheressian et al., 2013). If reconstruction occurred following mastectomy, imaging of the reconstructed breast is not indicated.

Women should not be routinely referred for a screening magnetic resonance imaging (MRI) of the breast unless the patient meets high-risk criteria. ACS guidelines recommend performing an MRI if the woman has a *BRCA* mutation, a first-degree relative who is a *BRCA* carrier, or a lifetime risk of approximately 20%–25% or greater based on predictive models (Saslow et al., 2007). These models and risk calculators include but are not limited to the BRCAPRO, CancerMath.net, and Breast Cancer Risk Assessment Tool and can be found at www.surgonc.org/resources/models -nomograms/breast-cancer-risk-models (Merajver & Milliron, 2003). In certain situations when a woman's breast cancer was not visible on diagnostic mammography, MRI may be recommended by her providers; however, this occurs infrequently and should be evaluated on a case-by-case basis. At this time, tomosynthesis (three-dimensional mammography) should only be ordered to evaluate dense breasts when recommended by the provider (Tagliafico et al., 2016).

Although the U.S. Preventive Services Task Force (2016) recommends screening mammography until age 74, the decision for when to stop cancer screening in someone with a history of breast cancer should be based on the woman's health status and life expectancy (Soung, 2015). Highly functioning women at age 75 and older who would be considered good candidates for surgery may still choose to have an annual mammogram. At any point after this, however, changing to routine clinical breast examination is appropriate.

Routine laboratory tests or imaging is not recommended. Avoid using positron-emission tomography (PET) or positron-emission tomography–computed tomography (PET-CT) scanning as part of routine follow-up care to monitor for a cancer recurrence in asymptomatic patients who have finished initial treatment with curative intent. Without high-level evidence that such imaging will change the outcome, false positives generated by screening asymptomatic individuals can lead to unnecessary and invasive procedures, overtreatment, unnecessary radiation exposure, and incorrect diagnoses, as well as unwarranted anxiety (ASCO, 2013).

Recurrence Identification

Patient Education

Women should be educated about common signs and symptoms of recurrence. Common sites of recurrence include the breast, chest wall, lymph nodes, bones, or visceral organs. Signs and symptoms vary for each of these sites. Locoregional recurrences include recurrences in the same (ipsilateral) breast or axilla or infraclavicular/supraclavicular lymph nodes. These recurrences are influenced by clinical features of the cancer and the effectiveness of local (surgery and radiation) and systemic therapies. Lumps, bumps, and rashes may be noted by the woman or clinician on examination. Distant recurrences include sites away from the affected breast and regional lymph nodes and are not curable in most situations. The most common sites include bone, lung, liver, lymph nodes, brain, and soft tissue but also can include the gastrointestinal tract, ovaries, peritoneum, and other less common locations. Although bone is the most common metastatic site, it is usually diagnosed in more than one distant site at the time of first recurrence. About three-fourths of recurrences are in distant sites. Persistent pain, fatigue, shortness of breath, nausea, loss of appetite, and headaches may be reported. Given that the fear of recurrence is common, healthcare providers should inform women to report anything they are worried about that might be related to the cancer coming back, including any new or persistent symptoms.

Imaging

Appropriate imaging should be ordered to evaluate signs or symptoms of recurrences.
- Musculoskeletal pain: Plain films may be used initially, as they are cost-effective and are relatively low risk to the patient. A nuclear medicine bone scan or ^{18}F-fluorodeoxyglucose–PET-CT scan is more sensitive, however, and is useful if a patient complains of persistent pain in more than one area.
- Visceral symptoms: CT scans are frequently used to evaluate chest and abdominal symptoms. PET-CT scans also are gaining in popularity as more evidence to validate their use in breast cancer emerges (Hildebrandt et al., 2016).
- Neurologic symptoms and headaches: Gadolinium-enhanced MRI is preferred over head CT for the detection of central nervous system recurrences. In cases where MRI is not possible, CT is used but has less sensitivity (Barajas & Cha, 2012). Lumbar puncture is also occasionally used in patients with suspected central nervous system metastases.

Screening for Second Primary Cancers

Survivorship care includes screening for other cancers as recommended for the general public. New cancers in the opposite breast (contralateral) may occur and should be screened for with an annual mammogram. Colon cancer screening should be performed as recommended for the average-risk population. According to ACS (n.d.), this includes any of the following in someone aged 50 years or older: flexible sigmoidoscopy every 5 years; colonoscopy every 10 years; double-contrast barium enema every 5 years; CT colonography (virtual colonoscopy) every 5 years; guaiac-based fecal occult blood test every year; fecal immunochemical test every year; or stool DNA test every 3 years.

Annual gynecologic assessment for endometrial cancer should be performed if the woman is on one of the selective estrogen receptor modulator therapies, such as tamoxifen, raloxifene, or toremifene, and has a uterus. Otherwise, women should undergo human papillomavirus and Pap testing as recommended. Hypertension, gallbladder diseases, and thyroid disease also increase a woman's odds of developing endometrial cancer (Torres et al., 2015).

In regard to skin cancer screening, insufficient evidence exists at this time for whole body screening in the general population. However, breast cancer survivors also may have a history of skin cancer and, if so, should be screened regularly.

The incidence of thyroid cancer is higher in women with breast cancer, and the incidence of breast cancer is higher in women with a history of thyroid cancer (Kuo, Chabot, & Lee, 2016; Nielsen et al., 2016). Although no specific recommendations exist for screening for thyroid cancer, clinicians should keep this risk in mind when performing a history and physical examination.

Assessment and Management of Long-Term and Late Effects

Body Image and Appearance Concerns

Breast cancer treatments can cause disfiguration (scarring, skin tanning) and weight changes that may affect a woman's body image, causing physical and psychologic distress and changes in sexual functioning and intimacy (Paterson, Lengacher, Donovan, Kip, & Tofthagen, 2016). These concerns may be increased in younger women. Clinicians should offer and discuss adaptive devices or surgery (e.g., prostheses, reconstruction). They may also consider referring patients to the Look Good Feel Better program (http://lookgoodfeelbetter.org).

When considering the use of adaptive devices or undergoing surgery, healthcare providers should assess the patient's physical functioning. Fatigue is a consideration, with causative factors including anemia, thyroid, and cardiac dysfunction. Clinicians should treat or refer for treatment of factors contributing to fatigue, including pain, sleep disturbances, and depression. Patients should be encouraged to engage in regular physical activity to reduce fatigue (Meneses-Echávez, González-Jiménez, & Ramírez-Vélez, 2015). Cognitive behavioral therapy is an additional consideration, as needed.

Clinicians should assess cancer survivors for pain and neuropathy on a regular basis. This includes consideration of the patient's current pain scale, pain history, and workup for causative factors. When treating symptoms, the underlying mechanisms should be treated if possible. Treatment could be pharmacologic or nonpharmacologic. As needed, healthcare providers should refer patients to appropriate specialists (e.g., pain specialist).

Lymphedema

Lymphedema can affect anywhere from 3%–60% of breast cancer survivors (Paskett, 2015b). Swelling, pain, reduced function, and increased risk for infection can affect quality of life. Shoulder mobility should be assessed as well. Patients should undergo prevention and risk reduction education, including maintaining a healthy weight, as being overweight or obese increases risk (Das et al., 2015). Patients can be referred to a lymphedema therapist, such as a certified lymphedema therapist, physical therapist, or occupational therapist, for treatment (see Chapter 9). Therapists should be certified by the Lymphology Association of North America and can be found at www.clt-lana.org/search/therapists. Treatments can be found through the National Lymphedema Network at www.lymphnet.org/find-treatment.

Bone and Musculoskeletal Health

Women with breast cancer are at increased risk for developing osteoporosis and fractures. Bones are sensitive to estrogen, and many breast cancer treatments block estrogenic effects. Healthy postmenopausal women are expected to have a 2%–3% bone loss for the first one to two years after menopause and then about 1% per year thereafter (Milat & Vincent, 2015). With the exception of tamoxifen, which is not associated with bone loss, chemotherapy and aromatase inhibitors are associated with increased loss of bone density (approximately 8% and 3% loss, respectively) compared to normal menopause at one year (Milat & Vincent, 2015). See Figure 11-1 for a summary of evaluation and management of bone health in women with breast cancer.

- Encourage adequate calcium and vitamin D intake: calcium 1,200 mg per day and vitamin D greater than 50 nmol/L per day in divided doses.
- Encourage recommended levels of physical activity.
- Recommend yoga, evaluation by physical therapy, or rehabilitation for unrelieved symptoms (Irwin et al., 2015).
- Perform baseline bone density scan (dual-energy x-ray absorptiometry [DEXA]) for postmenopausal women at initiation of endocrine therapy; repeat bone density scan (DEXA) every two years if the patient is on an aromatase inhibitor (anastrozole, exemestane, letrozole) or taking tamoxifen and a gonadotropin-releasing hormone agonist (goserelin) or has chemotherapy-induced menopause.
- Consider treatment with bisphosphonates or denosumab to maintain or improve bone density, but a dental examination should be performed prior to initiation, as osteonecrosis of the jaw is a low-risk but serious side effect.

Cardiotoxicity

Cardiotoxicity is associated with anthracyclines, trastuzumab, and other HER2-directed therapies, and left-sided radiation cardiotoxicity includes left ventricular dysfunction and ischemic heart disease (Xie et al., 2015). Toxicity is greater with combinations than single-agent treatment and increases over time (see Figure 11-2). Women with breast cancer are at greater risk of dying from cardiovascular disease (CVD) than women without breast cancer; those who received chemotherapy are at greater risk for cardiovascular mortality beginning seven years after diagnosis (Bradshaw et al., 2016). Autonomic dysfunction represents a loss of normal autonomic control of the cardiovascular system associated with both sympathetic nervous system overdrive and reduced efficacy of the parasympathetic nervous system. Autonomic dysfunction is a strong predictor of future coronary heart

Figure 11-1. Summary of Evaluation and Management of Bone Health in Women With Breast Cancer

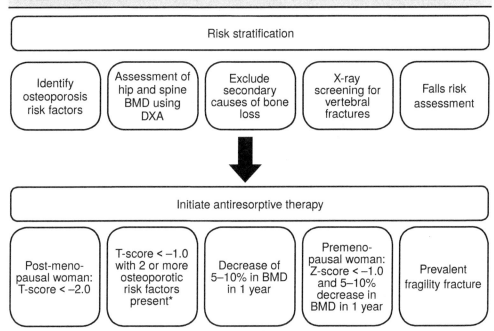

Management involves (1) risk stratification with identification of osteoporotic risk factors, assessment of bone mineral density (BMD) using dual x-ray absorptiometry (DXA), exclusion of secondary causes of bone loss and falls risk assessment; (2) lifestyle approaches including optimization of calcium intake, adequate vitamin D, exercise, avoidance of excess alcohol and cessation of smoking; and (3) initiation of antiresorptive therapy where indicated.

* Osteoporotic risk factors for initiation of antiresorptive therapy with aromatase inhibitor treatment include: age > 65 years, body mass index < 20, T-score < –1.5, family history of hip fracture, personal history of fragility fracture after age 50, current/previous smoking and oral glucocorticoid use > 6 months.

Note. From "Management of Bone Disease in Women After Breast Cancer," by F. Milat and A.J. Vincent, 2015, *Climacteric, 18*(Suppl. 2), p. 50. Copyright 2015 by Taylor and Francis. Reprinted with permission.

disease, vascular disease, and sudden cardiac death (Lakoski, Jones, Krone, Stein, & Scott, 2015; Vigo et al., 2015). Nurses should monitor lipid levels and provide cardiovascular monitoring and management, as indicated. They also should assess left ventricular function in patients with a history of anthracyclines or HER2-targeted therapies who have symptoms of heart failure (e.g., unusual fatigue, fluid overload). Patients should be encouraged to engage in regular physical activity to prevent heart disease and reduce cardiovascular morbidity and mortality (Kirkham & Davis, 2015). Survivors should receive education on healthy lifestyle modifications and potential treatment-related cardiac risk factors. Signs and symptoms of cardiac issues include shortness of breath, fatigue, and chest pain. Women may also have atypical symptoms of CVD, including nausea and regional pain related to angina that does not present as classic anginal heart pain. Use of angiotensin-converting enzyme inhibitors, statins, or beta-blockers to prevent cardiotoxicity is still experimental (Valachis & Nilsson, 2015). They are, however, used in the management of cardiovascular disorders once diagnosed.

Figure 11-2. Potential Mechanisms Associated With Autonomic Dysfunction and Increased Cardiovascular Disease Risk in Breast Cancer Patients

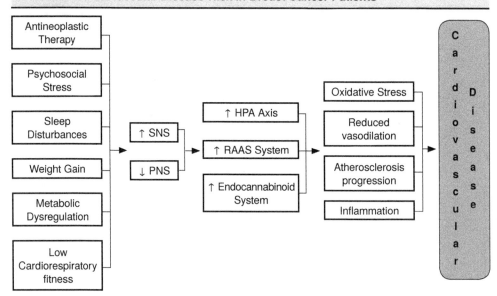

Breast cancer diagnosis is associated with therapy-induced cardiovascular injury and lifestyle perturbations leading to increased activation of the SNS (sympathetic nervous system) and decreased activation of the PNS (parasympathetic nervous system). In turn, this autonomic imbalance triggers the HPA (hypothalamic-pituitary-adrenal axis), RAAS (renin-angiotensin-aldosterone system), and the endocannabinoid system, leading to oxidative stress, reduced vasodilation, inflammation, and atherosclerosis progression that promotes CVD.

Note. From "Autonomic Dysfunction in Early Breast Cancer: Incidence, Clinical Importance, and Underlying Mechanisms," by S.G. Lakoski, L.W. Jones, R.J. Krone, P.K. Stein, and J.M. Scott, 2015, *American Heart Journal, 170,* p. 235. Copyright 2015 by Elsevier. Reprinted with permission.

Cognitive Impairment

Cognitive impairment is a decline in function in one or multiple cognitive domains, including attention and concentration, executive function, information processing speed, language, visuospatial skill, psychomotor ability, and learning and memory (Jansen, Von Ah, Allen, Merriman, & Myers, 2017). These anatomic and functional changes may be seen before treatment or after hormone therapy or chemotherapy, or more often with both treatments, leading to a decline in cognitive reserve (Buchanan et al., 2015; Frank, Vance, Triebel, & Meneses, 2015; Patel et al., 2015; Zwart, Terra, Linn, & Schagen, 2015). An increase in inflammatory cytokines has been noted and is theorized to play a role (Henneghan, 2016).

Healthcare providers should ask patients about issues related to and assess for cognitive difficulties. Self-reported cognitive issues were reported by 60% of patients after treatment, but only 37% discussed their concerns with a healthcare provider, and even fewer (15%) were referred for treatment (Buchanan et al., 2015). Patients' perceived cognitive abilities may help identify problems with verbal memory and executive functioning (Von Ah & Tallman, 2015). Depression and other contributing factors need to be ruled out before these changes can be attributed to treatment (Seliktar, Polek, Brooks, & Hardie, 2015).

Problems affecting cognition, such as poor sleep, should be treated. If signs of cognitive impairment exist, patients should be referred for neurocognitive assessment and rehabilitation, cognitive training, or rehabilitation as needed (Ercoli et al., 2015; Poppelreuter, Weis, & Bartsch, 2009; Roscoe et al., 2015; Vance et al., 2017; Von Ah et al., 2012). Nurses should recommend increased physical activity, as it can increase working memory and overall cardiopulmonary fitness (Chaddock-Heyman et al., 2015; Mackenzie et al., 2016). Other modifiable factors to increase cognitive function include improved sleep and improved stress management.

Coping and Emotional Functioning

Survivorship care includes assessment of patients' coping and emotional functioning. Psychological adjustment varies, but depression, anxiety, and fear of recurrence are common (Stanton & Bower, 2015; Stanton et al., 2015). Interventions, especially cognitive behavioral therapy, mindfulness, and supportive–expressive therapy, can assist with adaptation and reduce these mood disturbances (Carlson et al., 2015; Jassim, Whitford, Hickey, & Carter, 2015). Nurses should assess for social support, as it can also help ameliorate symptoms (Garner et al., 2015), and refer patients for psychosocial care and support as needed. Assessment can be performed using a distress screener or specific screening tools. Distress levels are highest during and for the first three months after treatment but begin declining for most women by six months after treatment (Lester, Crosthwaite, et al., 2015).

Depression screening can be performed using a standardized tool such as the PHQ-9 (www.phqscreeners.com), with referral as appropriate.

Anxiety can occur in different patterns but usually decreases over the first year during the transition from treatment (Saboonchi, Petersson, Wennman-Larsen, Alexanderson, & Vaez, 2015). Patients can experience fear of recurrence; this changes over time, with increases prior to mammograms or checkups and declines after receiving a negative result (McGinty, Small, Laronga, & Jacobsen, 2016). Patients also may experience greater fears of pain, suffering, and death (Thewes, Lebel, Leclair, & Butow, 2016). Patients may use distraction and avoidance as coping strategies and may need help in developing additional coping strategies. Social cognitive processing—talking about stressful events in a supportive environment—has been helpful in reducing this fear (Cohee et al., 2017).

A small percentage of women will experience symptoms of post-traumatic stress during diagnosis and treatment, but fewer actually meet the *Diagnostic and Statistical Manual of Mental Disorders, Fifth Edition* criteria for post-traumatic stress disorder (Voigt et al., 2017). These symptoms include involuntary recurrent memories, dreams, or flashbacks or reexperience of the stressor (intrusion); efforts to avoid memories, thoughts, feelings, or reminders associated with the stressor (avoidance); emotional numbing; and hyperarousal, including difficulty concentrating, outbursts of anger, hypervigilance, and difficulty falling or staying asleep (Voigt et al., 2017). These symptoms may decline over time, but for some, this does not happen and referral for management should be made.

Post-traumatic growth also can occur after the diagnosis of breast cancer. This is a positive psychological change, including hope and optimism, that occurs over time as a result of dealing with a life challenge and contributes to greater psychosocial well-being (Kolokotroni, Anagnostopoulos, & Tsikkinis, 2014; Parikh et al., 2015).

Sexual Health

Sexual health should be assessed as part of routine follow-up care. Oncology nurses should educate patients about the impact of treatment on sexual organs and on sexual functioning, such as decreased libido. Vaginal symptoms may include dryness, pain, dyspareunia, and itching related to urogenital atrophy (Lester, Pahouja, Andersen, & Lustberg, 2015; Mazzarello et al., 2015). Nurses should assess for signs or symptoms of sexual dysfunction using standardized sexual assessment such as PLISSIT or BETTER (Dow & Sheldon, 2015; see Chapter 9). Pharmacologic interventions include vaginal moisturizers and lubricants, topical lidocaine for dyspareunia, and low-dose topical estrogens in those without history of hormone-sensitive tumors. For patients with premature menopause symptoms, hot flashes, or vaginal symptoms, pharmacologic interventions include venlafaxine, citalopram, gabapentin, and clonidine, which are typically effective and can be combined for symptoms refractory to a single class of drug (Stuenkel et al., 2015). Nonpharmacologic interventions may include acupuncture, meditation, music therapy, and yoga (Chiu, Shyu, Chang, & Tsai, 2016; Greenlee et al., 2017).

Health Promotion

Information needs continue for years after diagnosis and treatment and are related to unmet needs regarding ongoing physical and emotional needs and distress (Brédart, Kop, Fiszer, Sigal-Zafrani, & Dolbeault, 2015; Cheng, Wong, & Koh, 2016; Hodgkinson et al., 2007; Knobf, 2015). When needs are not addressed by their health professionals, women turn to other sources such as support groups (Vivar & McQueen, 2005). Women may find diagnosis and treatment to be stressful and feel abandoned when treatment ends (Williams & Jeanetta, 2015). Symptoms and existential concerns include lack of energy, neuropathic pain, numbness or tingling in hands and feet, pain, phantom breast sensations, menopausal symptoms, sleep disruption, increased weight and appetite, gastrointestinal complaints, and psychological issues such as fear of recurrence and depression (Marshall et al., 2016; Pereira et al., 2015). Most cancer survivors have at least one comorbid condition that may affect quality of life, physical function, energy level, and pain (Fu et al., 2015). Hypertension, arthritis, and diabetes with breast cancer lead to poorer quality of life and obesity (Christian et al., 2015; Fu et al., 2015).

Health professionals can recommend measures to improve a patient's health during the years after diagnosis and treatment, including reaching and maintaining a healthy weight, promoting physical activity, and encouraging smoking cessation. Additionally, nurses should refer patients to preventive services appropriate for their age group. See www.womenshealth.gov/nwhw/by-age.

Weight Loss

Weight gain and body composition shifting (sarcopenia or increasing adipose tissue and declining muscle mass) are common during treatment. This continues during the first few years after the end of treatment, especially after chemotherapy (Gross et al., 2015). Healthy lifestyle behaviors may improve after cancer for some women, but others may require encouragement to follow dietary and physical activity guidelines (DeNysschen et al., 2015).

Nurses should counsel survivors on nutrition and recommend a healthy diet with an emphasis on plant foods, including increased consumption of whole foods such as fruits, vegetables, whole grains, legumes, fish, and poultry, and limited consumption of refined grains, refined carbohydrate foods, sugar-sweetened beverages, processed meat, and red meat. Patients should choose portions that promote a healthy weight. Alcohol consumption should be limited (one drink a day or less for women) (Kushi et al., 2012). Dietary supplement use, including vitamins and minerals, should be based on existing deficiencies with the exception of calcium and vitamin D.

Patients should manage obesity by achieving and maintaining a healthy weight (body mass index between 18–24.9 kg/m²; calculate at www.nhlbi.nih.gov/health /educational/lose_wt/BMI/bmicalc.htm). Even a 5%–10% weight loss can be beneficial. Obesity is a risk factor for many cancers, including breast, colon and rectum, and endometrial, among others. It also may increase the risk of recurrence and decrease overall survival (Rock et al., 2012). Nurses should refer patients to a registered dietitian or recommend commercial or self-help weight loss programs such as Weight Watchers (Marrero et al., 2016; Tsai, Morton, Mangione, & Keeler, 2005).

Physical Activity

Encouraging patients to engage in physical activity is another recommendation for improving overall health. Recommendations include avoiding inactivity, returning to normal daily activities after treatment ends, engaging in moderate exercise for at least 150 minutes per week, and performing strength training exercises at least two days per week (Rock et al., 2012). Strong evidence suggests that physical activity (aerobic and resistance exercise) can improve cardiopulmonary fitness, muscular strength, bone health, mood, sleep, and overall quality of life (Dieli-Conwright & Orozco, 2015; Giallauria et al., 2015; Irwin et al., 2005, 2015). When available, refer patients to existing exercise-based cancer rehabilitation programs at the completion of surgery, radiation, or chemotherapy, such as the Livestrong programs available through local YMCA branches (see www.livestrongattheymca.org).

Smoking Cessation

The smoking rates of breast cancer survivors are low (Mayer & Carlson, 2011), but if a woman is a current smoker, encourage smoking cessation and refer for support in that process (e.g., http://smokefree.gov).

Integrative Therapies

A majority of women use integrative therapies during and after breast cancer treatment (Greenlee et al., 2017). The evidence supports that integrative therapy use can decrease anxiety, mood disorders, stress, and fatigue and improve quality of life. The most commonly used therapies include meditation, yoga, relaxation with imagery, and massage. Yoga can also be helpful in women on aromatase inhibitors who have musculoskeletal symptoms (Peppone et al., 2015).

Survivorship Care Delivery Models and Practice Implications

Many different models exist for delivering survivorship care but all have implications for communication and coordination of care among team members. Care coordination relies on communication between the survivor, family, and providers. The survivorship care plan is a tool that includes a diagnosis and treatment summary along with a plan for follow-up care. Women should receive this document from their cancer care provider at the end of initial treatment and share it with their primary care provider of record. Primary care providers want information about surveillance plans and potential cancer- or treatment-related problems in a clear, short document to feel more confident in providing care to women with a history of breast cancer (Mayer, Gerstel, Leak, & Smith, 2012; O'Brien, Grunfeld, Sussman, Porter, & Mobilio, 2015).

In the oncology-led care model, follow-up care is delivered among surgery, radiation, and medical oncology specialties, depending on the treatment delivered. Medical oncology providers often feel responsible for follow-up care (Neuman et al., 2016).

Breast cancer programs are another approach, in which survivorship care is embedded into existing breast programs. The timing and location of the follow-up care should be determined with sensitivity to these women and others being seen in the breast program (e.g., have the follow-up clinic be separate from the active treatment clinic). Established time points should identify when women will be discharged and transition and to receive follow-up from their primary care provider, with visits to the oncologist occurring on an as-needed basis only.

Cancer survivorship programs are another care delivery model. Some facilities may have specific clinics to see women who have completed treatment.

In the primary care provider–led care model, the primary care provider understands and provides follow-up care, including clinical breast examination, mammograms, adherence to endocrine therapy, and management of ongoing or new symptoms (Railton et al., 2015). Primary care providers may not be comfortable in providing care without additional training and guidance about the use of surveillance guidelines and the management of endocrine therapy (Dawes et al., 2015).

The last model is that of shared care delivered by both oncology and primary care. This model requires communication to coordinate care to ensure that both cancer follow-up care and general health care are provided to avoid over- or undertesting.

Resources

- For survivors and families—Breast Cancer Survivorship Guidelines: http://onlinelibrary.wiley.com/doi/10.3322/caac.21322/pdf
- For healthcare providers
  - Cancer Survivorship E-Learning Series for Primary Care Providers (Module 9—Spotlight Breast Cancer Survivorship: Clinical Follow-Up Care Guidelines for Primary Care Providers): http://gwcehp.learnercommunity.com/elearning-series
  - National Cancer Institute Breast Cancer PDQ®: www.cancer.gov/types/breast/hp
  - National Comprehensive Cancer Network®: www.nccn.org

Summary

An ever-growing pool of breast cancer survivors will need ongoing care over a lifetime. Oncology nurses should be aware of emerging evidence-based guidelines for survivorship care to promote prevention and early detection of recurrence and second primary malignancies. Survivorship care is no longer an option. Multiple models for survivorship care exist, and oncology nurses play a key role in coordinating care between the oncology team and primary care team.

References

American Cancer Society. (n.d.). Colorectal cancer: Early detection, diagnosis, and staging. Retrieved from https://www.cancer.org/content/cancer/en/cancer/colon-rectal-cancer/detection-diagnosis -staging.html

American Society of Clinical Oncology. (2013). ASCO's 2013 top five list in oncology. Retrieved from http://www.asco.org/practice-guidelines/cancer-care-initiatives/value-cancer-care/choosing-wisely

Barajas, R.F., Jr., & Cha, S. (2012). Imaging diagnosis of brain metastasis. In L.D. Lunsford (Ed.), *Progress in Neurological Surgery: Vol. 25: Current and future management of brain metastasis* (pp. 55–73). doi:10 .1159/000331174

Bradshaw, P.T., Stevens, J., Khankari, N., Teitelbaum, S.L., Neugut, A.I., & Gammon, M.D. (2016). Cardiovascular disease mortality among breast cancer survivors. *Epidemiology, 27,* 6–13. doi:10.1097/EDE .0000000000000394

Brédart, A., Kop, J.-L., Fiszer, C., Sigal-Zafrani, B., & Dolbeault, S. (2015). Breast cancer survivors' perceived medical communication competence and satisfaction with care at the end of treatment. *Psycho-Oncology, 24,* 1670–1678. doi:10.1002/pon.3836

Buchanan, N.D., Dasari, S., Rodriguez, J.L., Smith, J.L., Hodgson, M.E., Weinberg, C.R., & Sandler, D.P. (2015). Post-treatment neurocognition and psychosocial care among breast cancer survivors. *American Journal of Preventive Medicine, 49*(6, Suppl. 5), S498–S508. doi:10.1016/j.amepre.2015.08.013

Cahir, C., Guinan, E., Dombrowski, S.U., Sharp, L., & Bennett, K. (2015). Identifying the determinants of adjuvant hormonal therapy medication taking behaviour in women with stages I–III breast cancer: A systematic review and meta-analysis. *Patient Education and Counseling, 98,* 1524–1539. doi:10.1016/j.pec .2015.05.013

Carlson, L.E., Beattie, T.L., Giese-Davis, J., Faris, P., Tamagawa, R., Fick, L.J., ... Speca, M. (2015). Mindfulness-based cancer recovery and supportive-expressive therapy maintain telomere length relative to controls in distressed breast cancer survivors. *Cancer, 121,* 476–484. doi:10.1002/cncr.29063

Chaddock-Heyman, L., Mackenzie, M.J., Zuniga, K., Cooke, G.E., Awick, E., Roberts, S., ... Kramer, A.F. (2015). Higher cardiorespiratory fitness levels are associated with greater hippocampal volume in breast cancer survivors. *Frontiers in Human Neuroscience, 9,* 465. doi:10.3389/fnhum.2015.00465

Cheng, K.K., Wong, W.H., & Koh, C. (2016). Unmet needs mediate the relationship between symptoms and quality of life in breast cancer survivors. *Supportive Care in Cancer, 24,* 2025–2033. doi:10.1007 /s00520-015-2994-0

Chiu, H.-Y., Shyu, Y.-K., Chang, P.-C., & Tsai, P.-S. (2016). Effects of acupuncture on menopause-related symptoms in breast cancer survivors: A meta-analysis of randomized controlled trials. *Cancer Nursing, 39,* 228–237. doi:10.1097/NCC.0000000000000278

Christian, A., Hudson, S.V., Miller, S.M., Bator, A., Ohman-Strickland, P.A., Somer, R.A., & Ferrante, J. (2015). Perceptions of primary care among breast cancer survivors: The effects of weight status. *Health Services Research and Managerial Epidemiology, 2,* 10. doi:10.1177/2333392815587487

Cohee, A.A., Adams, R.N., Johns, S.A., Von Ah, D., Zoppi, K., Fife, B., ... Champion, V.L. (2017). Long-term fear of recurrence in young breast cancer survivors and partners. *Psycho-Oncology, 26,* 22–28. doi:10.1002/pon.4008

Colleoni, M., Sun, Z., Price, K.N., Karlsson, P., Forbes, J.F., Thürlimann, B., ... Goldhirsch, A. (2016). Annual hazard rates of recurrence for breast cancer during 24 years of follow-up: Results from the International Breast Cancer Study Group Trials I to V. *Journal of Clinical Oncology, 34,* 927–935. doi:10 .1200/JCO.2015.62.3504

Das, N., Baumgartner, R.N., Riley, E.C., Pinkston, C.M., Yang, D., & Baumgartner, K.B. (2015). Treatment-related risk factors for arm lymphedema among long-term breast cancer survivors. *Journal of Cancer Survivorship, 9,* 422–430. doi:10.1007/s11764-014-0416-9

Dawes, A.J., Hemmelgarn, M., Nguyen, D.K., Sacks, G.D., Clayton, S.M., Cope, J.R., ... Maggard-Gibbons, M. (2015). Are primary care providers prepared to care for survivors of breast cancer in the safety net? *Cancer, 121,* 1249–1256. doi:10.1002/cncr.29201

DeNysschen, C., Brown, J.K., Baker, M., Wilding, G., Tetewsky, S., Cho, M.H., & Dodd, M.J. (2015). Healthy lifestyle behaviors of breast cancer survivors. *Clinical Nursing Research, 24,* 504–525. doi:10 .1177/1054773814553298

Dieli-Conwright, C.M., & Orozco, B.Z. (2015). Exercise after breast cancer treatment: Current perspectives. *Breast Cancer, 7,* 353–362. doi:10.2147/BCTT.S82039

Dow, J., & Sheldon, L.K. (2015). Breast cancer survivors and sexuality: A review of the literature concerning sexual functioning, assessment tools, and evidence-based interventions. *Clinical Journal of Oncology Nursing, 19,* 456–461. doi:10.1188/15.CJON.456-461

Ercoli, L.M., Petersen, L., Hunter, A.M., Castellon, S.A., Kwan, L., Kahn-Mills, B.A., … Ganz, P.A. (2015). Cognitive rehabilitation group intervention for breast cancer survivors: Results of a randomized clinical trial. *Psycho-Oncology, 24,* 1360–1367. doi:10.1002/pon.3769

Frank, J.S., Vance, D.E., Triebel, K.L., & Meneses, K.M. (2015). Cognitive deficits in breast cancer survivors after chemotherapy and hormonal therapy. *Journal of Neuroscience, 47,* 302–312. doi:10.1097/JNN .0000000000000171

Fu, M.R., Axelrod, D., Guth, A.A., Cleland, C.M., Ryan, C.E., Weaver, K.R., … Melkus, G.D. (2015). Comorbidities and quality of life among breast cancer survivors: A prospective study. *Journal of Personalized Medicine, 5,* 229–242. doi:10.3390/jpm5030229

Garner, M.J., McGregor, B.A., Murphy, K.M., Koenig, A.L., Dolan, E.D., & Albano, D. (2015). Optimism and depression: A new look at social support as a mediator among women at risk for breast cancer. *Psycho-Oncology, 24,* 1708–1713. doi:10.1002/pon.3782

Giallauria, F., Maresca, L., Vitelli, A., de Magistris, M.S., Chiodini, P., Mattiello, A., … Vigorito, C. (2015). Exercise training improves heart rate recovery in women with breast cancer. *SpringerPlus, 4,* 388. doi:10 .1186/s40064-015-1179-0

Greenlee, H., DuPont-Reyes, M.J., Balneaves, L.G., Carlson, L.E., Cohen, M.R., Deng, G., … Tripathy, D. (2017). Clinical practice guidelines on the evidence-based use of integrative therapies during and after breast cancer treatment. *CA: A Cancer Journal for Clinicians, 67,* 194–232. doi:10.3322/caac.21397

Gross, A.L., May, B.J., Axilbund, J.E., Armstrong, D.K., Roden, R.B., & Visvanathan, K. (2015). Weight change in breast cancer survivors compared to cancer-free women: A prospective study in women at familial risk of breast cancer. *Cancer Epidemiology, Biomarkers and Prevention, 24,* 1262–1269. doi:10.1158 /1055-9965.EPI-15-0212

Henneghan, A. (2016). Modifiable factors and cognitive dysfunction in breast cancer survivors: A mixed-method systematic review. *Supportive Care in Cancer, 24,* 481–497. doi:10.1007/s00520-015-2927-y

Hershman, D.L., Shao, T., Kushi, L.H., Buono, D., Tsai, W.Y., Fehrenbacher, L., … Neugut, A.I. (2011). Early discontinuation and non-adherence to adjuvant hormonal therapy are associated with increased mortality in women with breast cancer. *Breast Cancer Research and Treatment, 126,* 529–537. doi:10.1007 /s10549-010-1132-4

Hildebrandt, M.G., Gerke, O., Baun, C., Falch, K., Hansen, J.A., Farahani, Z.A., … Høilund-Carlsen, P.F. (2016). [^{18}F]fluorodeoxyglucose (FDG)-positron emission tomography (PET)/computed tomography (CT) in suspected recurrent breast cancer: A prospective comparative study of dual-time-point FDG-PET/CT, contrast-enhanced CT, and bone scintigraphy. *Journal of Clinical Oncology, 34,* 1889–1897. doi:10.1200/JCO.2015.63.5185

Hodgkinson, K., Butow, P., Hunt, G.E., Pendlebury, S., Hobbs, K.M., & Wain, G. (2007). Breast cancer survivors' supportive care needs 2–10 years after diagnosis. *Supportive Care in Cancer, 15,* 515–523. doi:10 .1007/s00520-006-0170-2

Howlader, N., Noone, A.M., Krapcho, M., Miller, D., Bishop, K., Kosary, C.L., … Cronin, K.A. (Eds.). (2017). *SEER cancer statistics review, 1975–2014.* Retrieved from https://seer.cancer.gov/csr/1975_2014

Huang, W.-C., Chen, C.-Y., Lin, S.-J., & Chang, C.-S. (2016). Medication adherence to oral anticancer drugs: Systematic review. *Expert Review of Anticancer Therapy, 16,* 423–432. doi:10.1586/14737140.2016.1159515

Hurria, A., & Muss, H. (2015). Special issues in older women with breast cancer. In P.A. Ganz (Ed.), *Advances in Experimental Medicine and Biology: Vol. 862. Improving outcomes for breast cancer survivors* (pp. 23–37). doi:10.1007/978-3-319-16366-6_3

Irwin, M.L., Cartmel, B., Gross, C.P., Ercolano, E., Li, F., Yao, X., … Ligibel, J. (2015). Randomized exercise trial of aromatase inhibitor-induced arthralgia in breast cancer survivors. *Journal of Clinical Oncology, 33,* 1104–1111. doi:10.1200/JCO.2014.57.1547

Irwin, M.L., McTiernan, A., Baumgartner, R.N., Baumgartner, K.B., Bernstein, L., Gilliland, F.D., & Ballard-Barbash, R. (2005). Changes in body fat and weight after a breast cancer diagnosis: Influence of demographic, prognostic, and lifestyle factors. *Journal of Clinical Oncology, 23,* 774–782. doi:10.1200 /JCO.2005.04.036

Jansen, C.E., Von Ah, D., Allen, D.H., Merriman, J.D., & Myers, J.S. (2017, April 3). ONS PEP resource: Cognitive impairment. Retrieved from https://www.ons.org/practice-resources/pep/cognitive-impairment

Jassim, G.A., Whitford, D.L., Hickey, A., & Carter, B. (2015). Psychological interventions for women with non-metastatic breast cancer. *Cochrane Database of Systematic Reviews, 2015*(5). doi:10.1002/14651858.CD008729.pub2

Khatcheressian, J.L., Hurley, P., Bantug, E., Esserman, L.J., Grunfeld, E., Halberg, F., ... Davidson, N.E. (2013). Breast cancer follow-up and management after primary treatment: American Society of Clinical Oncology clinical practice guideline update. *Journal of Clinical Oncology, 31*, 961–965. doi:10.1200/JCO.2012.45.9859

Kirkham, A.A., & Davis, M.K. (2015). Exercise prevention of cardiovascular disease in breast cancer survivors. *Journal of Oncology, 2015*, 917606. doi:10.1155/2015/917606

Knobf, M.T. (2015). The transition experience to breast cancer survivorship. *Seminars in Oncology Nursing, 31*, 178–182. doi:10.1016/j.soncn.2015.02.006

Kolokotroni, P., Anagnostopoulos, F., & Tsikkinis, A. (2014). Psychosocial factors related to posttraumatic growth in breast cancer survivors: A review. *Women and Health, 54*, 569–592. doi:10.1080/03630242.2014.899543

Kuo, J.H., Chabot, J.A., & Lee, J.A. (2016). Breast cancer in thyroid cancer survivors: An analysis of the Surveillance, Epidemiology, and End Results-9 database. *Surgery, 159*, 23–30. doi:10.1016/j.surg.2015.10.009

Kushi, L.H., Doyle, C., McCullough, M., Rock, C.L., Demark-Wahnefried, W., Bandera, E.V., ... Gansler, T. (2012). American Cancer Society Guidelines on nutrition and physical activity for cancer prevention: Reducing the risk of cancer with healthy food choices and physical activity. *CA: A Cancer Journal for Clinicians, 62*, 30–67. doi:10.3322/caac.20140

Lakoski, S.G., Jones, L.W., Krone, R.J., Stein, P.K., & Scott, J.M. (2015). Autonomic dysfunction in early breast cancer: Incidence, clinical importance, and underlying mechanisms. *American Heart Journal, 170*, 231–241. doi:10.1016/j.ahj.2015.05.014

Lester, J., Crosthwaite, K., Stout, R., Jones, R.N., Holloman, C., Shapiro, C., & Andersen, B.L. (2015). Women with breast cancer: Self-reported distress in early survivorship [Online exclusive]. *Oncology Nursing Forum, 42*, E17–E23. doi:10.1188/15.ONF.E17-E23

Lester, J., Pahouja, G., Andersen, B., & Lustberg, M. (2015). Atrophic vaginitis in breast cancer survivors: A difficult survivorship issue. *Journal of Personalized Medicine, 5*, 50–66. doi:10.3390/jpm5020050

Mackenzie, M.J., Zuniga, K.E., Raine, L.B., Awick, E.A., Hillman, C.H., Kramer, A.F., & McAuley, E. (2016). Associations between physical fitness indices and working memory in breast cancer survivors and age-matched controls. *Journal of Women's Health, 25*, 99–108. doi:10.1089/jwh.2015.5246

Marrero, D.G., Palmer, K.N.B., Phillips, E.O., Miller-Kovach, K., Foster, G.D., & Saha, C.K. (2016). Comparison of commercial and self-initiated weight loss programs in people with prediabetes: A randomized control trial. *American Journal of Public Health, 106*, 949–956. doi:10.2105/AJPH.2015.303035

Marshall, S.A., Yang, C.C., Ping, Q., Zhao, M., Avis, N.E., & Ip, E.H. (2016). Symptom clusters in women with breast cancer: An analysis of data from social media and a research study. *Quality of Life Research, 25*, 547–557. doi:10.1007/s11136-015-1156-7

Mayer, D.K., & Carlson, J. (2011). Smoking patterns in cancer survivors. *Nicotine and Tobacco Research, 13*, 34–40. doi:10.1093/ntr/ntq199

Mayer, D.K., Gerstel, A., Leak, A.N., & Smith, S.K. (2012). Patient and provider preferences for survivorship care plans. *Journal of Oncology Practice, 8*, e80–e86. doi:10.1200/JOP.2011.000401

Mazzarello, S., Hutton, B., Ibrahim, M.F.K., Jacobs, C., Shorr, R., Smith, S., ... Clemons, M. (2015). Management of urogenital atrophy in breast cancer patients: A systematic review of available evidence from randomized trials. *Breast Cancer Research and Treatment, 152*, 1–8. doi:10.1007/s10549-015-3434-z

McGinty, H.L., Small, B.J., Laronga, C., & Jacobsen, P.B. (2016). Predictors and patterns of fear of cancer recurrence in breast cancer survivors. *Health Psychology, 35*, 1–9. doi:10.1037/hea0000238

Meneses-Echávez, J.F., González-Jiménez, E., & Ramírez-Vélez, R. (2015). Effects of supervised exercise on cancer-related fatigue in breast cancer survivors: A systematic review and meta-analysis. *BMC Cancer, 15*, 77. doi:10.1186/s12885-015-1069-4

Merajver, S.D., & Milliron, K. (2003). Breast cancer risk assessment: A guide for clinicians using the NCCN Breast Cancer Risk Reduction Guidelines. *Journal of the National Comprehensive Cancer Network, 1*, 297–301. Retrieved from http://www.jnccn.org/content/1/2/297.long

Milat, F., & Vincent, A.J. (2015). Management of bone disease in women after breast cancer. *Climacteric, 18*(Suppl. 2), 47–55. doi:10.3109/13697137.2015.1100383

National Cancer Institute. (2016). Cancer stat facts: Female breast cancer. Retrieved from http://seer.cancer.gov/statfacts/html/breast.html

National Cancer Institute. (2017). Male breast cancer treatment (PDQ®) [Health professional version]. Retrieved from https://www.cancer.gov/types/breast/hp/male-breast-treatment-pdq

National Cancer Institute Office of Cancer Survivorship. (2014). Definitions. Retrieved from https://cancercontrol.cancer.gov/ocs/statistics/definitions.html

Neuman, H.B., Steffens, N.M., Jacobson, N., Tevaarwerk, A., Anderson, B., Wilke, L.G., & Greenberg, C.C. (2016). Oncologists' perspectives of their roles and responsibilities during multi-disciplinary breast cancer follow-up. *Annals of Surgical Oncology, 23,* 708–714. doi:10.1245/s10434-015-4904-6

Nielsen, S.M., White, M.G., Hong, S., Aschebrook-Kilfoy, B., Kaplan, E.L., Angelos, P., ... Grogan, R.H. (2016). The breast–thyroid cancer link: A systematic review and meta-analysis. *Cancer Epidemiology, Biomarkers and Prevention, 25,* 231–238. doi:10.1158/1055-9965.EPI-15-0833

O'Brien, M.A., Grunfeld, E., Sussman, J., Porter, G., & Mobilio, M.H. (2015). Views of family physicians about survivorship care plans to provide breast cancer follow-up care: Exploration of results from a randomized controlled trial. *Current Oncology, 22,* 252–259. doi:10.3747/co.22.2368

Oncology Nursing Society. (n.d.). ONS oral adherence toolkit. Retrieved from https://www.ons.org/practice-resources/toolkits/oral-adherence

Parikh, D., De Ieso, P., Garvey, G., Thachil, T., Ramamoorthi, R., Penniment, M., & Jayaraj, R. (2015). Post-traumatic stress disorder and post-traumatic growth in breast cancer patients—A systematic review. *Asian Pacific Journal of Cancer Prevention, 16,* 641–646. doi:10.7314/APJCP.2015.16.2.641

Paskett, E.D. (2015a). Breast cancer among special populations: Disparities in care across the cancer control continuum. In P.A. Ganz (Ed.), *Advances in Experimental Medicine and Biology: Vol. 862. Improving outcomes for breast cancer survivors* (pp. 39–52). doi:10.1007/978-3-319-16366-6_4

Paskett, E.D. (2015b). Symptoms: Lymphedema. In P.A. Ganz (Ed.), *Advances in Experimental Medicine and Biology: Vol. 862. Improving outcomes for breast cancer survivors* (pp. 101–113). doi:10.1007/978-3-319-16366-6_8

Patel, S.K., Wong, A.L., Wong, F.L., Breen, E.C., Hurria, A., Smith, M., ... Bhatia, S. (2015). Inflammatory biomarkers, comorbidity, and neurocognition in women with newly diagnosed breast cancer. *Journal of the National Cancer Institute, 107*(8), djv131. doi:10.1093/jnci/djv131

Paterson, C.L., Lengacher, C.A., Donovan, K.A., Kip, K.E., & Tofthagen, C.S. (2016). Body image in younger breast cancer survivors: A systematic review. *Cancer Nursing, 39,* E39–E58. doi:10.1097/NCC .0000000000000251

Peppone, L.J., Janelsins, M.C., Kamen, C., Mohile, S.G., Sprod, L.K., Gewandter, J.S., ... Mustian, K.M. (2015). The effect of YOCAS©® yoga for musculoskeletal symptoms among breast cancer survivors on hormonal therapy. *Breast Cancer Research and Treatment, 150,* 597–604. doi:10.1007/s10549-015-3351-1

Pereira, S., Fontes, F., Sonin, T., Dias, T., Fragoso, M., Castro-Lopes, J.M., & Lunet, N. (2015). Neurological complications of breast cancer: A prospective cohort study. *Breast, 24,* 582–587. doi:10.1016/j.breast.2015.05.006

Poppelreuter, M., Weis, J., & Bartsch, H.H. (2009). Effects of specific neuropsychological training programs for breast cancer patients after adjuvant chemotherapy. *Journal of Psychosocial Oncology, 27,* 274–296. doi:10.1080/07347330902776044

Railton, C., Lupichuk, S., McCormick, J., Zhong, L., Ko, J.J., Walley, B., ... Giese-Davis, J. (2015). Discharge to primary care for survivorship follow-up: How are patients with early-stage breast cancer faring? *Journal of the National Comprehensive Cancer Network, 13,* 762–771. Retrieved from http://www.jnccn .org/content/13/6/762.long

Reeder-Hayes, K.E., Wheeler, S.B., & Mayer, D.K. (2015). Health disparities across the breast cancer continuum. *Seminars in Oncology Nursing, 31,* 170–177. doi:10.1016/j.soncn.2015.02.005

Rock, C.L., Doyle, C., Demark-Wahnefried, W., Meyerhardt, J., Courneya, K.S., Schwartz, A.L., ... Gansler, T. (2012). Nutrition and physical activity guidelines for cancer survivors. *CA: A Cancer Journal for Clinicians, 62,* 242–274. doi:10.3322/caac.21142

Roscoe, J.A., Garland, S.N., Heckler, C.E., Perlis, M.L., Peoples, A.R., Shayne, M., ... Morrow, G.R. (2015). Randomized placebo-controlled trial of cognitive behavioral therapy and armodafinil for insomnia after cancer treatment. *Journal of Clinical Oncology, 33,* 165–171. doi:10.1200/JCO.2014.57.6769

Runowicz, C.D., Leach, C.R., Henry, N.L., Henry, K.S., Mackey, H.T., Cowens-Alvarado, R.L., ... Ganz, P.A. (2016). American Cancer Society/American Society of Clinical Oncology breast cancer survivorship care guideline. *CA: A Cancer Journal for Clinicians, 66,* 43–73. doi:10.3322/caac.21319

Saboonchi, F., Petersson, L.-M., Wennman-Larsen, A., Alexanderson, K., & Vaez, M. (2015). Trajectories of anxiety among women with breast cancer: A proxy for adjustment from acute to transitional survivorship. *Journal of Psychosocial Oncology, 33,* 603–619. doi:10.1080/07347332.2015.1082165

Saslow, D., Boetes, C., Burke, W., Harms, S., Leach, M.O., Lehman, C.D., ... Russell, C.A. (2007). American Cancer Society guidelines for breast screening with MRI as an adjunct to mammography. *CA: A Cancer Journal for Clinicians, 57,* 75–89. doi:10.3322/canjclin.57.2.75

Seliktar, N., Polek, C., Brooks, A., & Hardie, T. (2015). Cognition in breast cancer survivors: Hormones versus depression. *Psycho-Oncology, 24,* 402–407. doi:10.1002/pon.3602

Sestak, I., & Cuzick, J. (2015). Markers for the identification of late breast cancer recurrence. *Breast Cancer Research, 17,* 10. doi:10.1186/s13058-015-0516-0

Soung, M.C. (2015). Screening for cancer: When to stop? A practical guide and review of the evidence. *Medical Clinics of North America, 99,* 249–262. doi:10.1016/j.mcna.2014.11.002

Stanton, A.L., & Bower, J.E. (2015). Psychological adjustment in breast cancer survivors. In P.A. Ganz (Ed.), *Advances in Experimental Medicine and Biology: Vol. 862. Improving outcomes for breast cancer survivors* (pp. 231–242). doi:10.1007/978-3-319-16366-6_15

Stanton, A.L., Wiley, J.F., Krull, J.L., Crespi, C.M., Hammen, C., Allen, J.J.B., ... Weihs, K.L. (2015). Depressive episodes, symptoms, and trajectories in women recently diagnosed with breast cancer. *Breast Cancer Research and Treatment, 154,* 105–115. doi:10.1007/s10549-015-3563-4

Stuenkel, C.A., Davis, S.R., Gompel, A., Lumsden, M.A., Murad, M.H., Pinkerton, J.V., & Santen, R.J. (2015). Treatment of symptoms of the menopause: An Endocrine Society clinical practice guideline. *Journal of Clinical Endocrinology and Metabolism, 100,* 3975–4011. doi:10.1210/jc.2015-2236

Tagliafico, A., Calabrese, M., Mariscotti, G., Durando, M., Tosto, S., Monetti, F., ... Houssami, N. (2016). Adjunct screening with tomosynthesis or ultrasound in women with mammography-negative dense breasts: Interim report of a prospective comparative trial. *Journal of Clinical Oncology, 34,* 1882–1888. doi:10.1200/JCO.2015.63.4147

Thewes, B., Lebel, S., Leclair, C.S., & Butow, P. (2016). A qualitative exploration of fear of cancer recurrence (FCR) amongst Australian and Canadian breast cancer survivors. *Supportive Care in Cancer, 24,* 2269–2276. doi:10.1007/s00520-015-3025-x

Torres, D., Myers, J.A., Eshraghi, L.W., Riley, E.C., Soliman, P.T., & Milam, M.R. (2015). Risk factors for the development of uterine cancer in breast cancer survivors: An army of women study. *Annals of Surgical Oncology, 22,* 1974–1979. doi:10.1245/s10434-014-4193-5

Tsai, A.C., Morton, S.C., Mangione, C.M., & Keeler, E.B. (2005). A meta-analysis of interventions to improve care for chronic illnesses. *American Journal of Managed Care, 11,* 478–488.

U.S. Preventive Services Task Force. (2016, January). Final recommendation statement: Breast cancer: Screening. Retrieved from https://www.uspreventiveservicestaskforce.org/Page/Document/RecommendationStatementFinal/breast-cancer-screening1

Valachis, A., & Nilsson, C. (2015). Cardiac risk in the treatment of breast cancer: Assessment and management. *Breast Cancer, 7,* 21–35. doi:10.2147/BCTT.S47227

Vance, D.E., Frank, J.S., Bail, J., Triebel, K.L., Niccolai, L.M., Gerstenecker, A., & Meneses, K. (2017). Interventions for cognitive deficits in breast cancer survivors treated with chemotherapy [Online exclusive]. *Cancer Nursing, 40,* E11–E27. doi:10.1097/NCC.0000000000000349

Vigo, C., Gatzemeier, W., Sala, R., Malacarne, M., Santoro, A., Pagani, M., & Lucini, D. (2015). Evidence of altered autonomic cardiac regulation in breast cancer survivors. *Journal of Cancer Survivorship, 9,* 699–706. doi:10.1007/s11764-015-0445-z

Vivar, C.G., & McQueen, A. (2005). Informational and emotional needs of long-term survivors of breast cancer. *Journal of Advanced Nursing, 51,* 520–528. doi:10.1111/j.1365-2648.2005.03524.x

Voigt, V., Neufeld, F., Kaste, J., Bühner, M., Sckopke, P., Wuerstlein, R., ... Hermelink, K. (2017). Clinically assessed posttraumatic stress in patients with breast cancer during the first year after diagnosis in the prospective, longitudinal, controlled COGNICARES study. *Psycho-Oncology, 26,* 74–80. doi:10.1002/pon.4102

Von Ah, D., Carpenter, J.S., Saykin, A., Monahan, P., Wu, J., Yu, M., ... Unverzagt, F. (2012). Advanced cognitive training for breast cancer survivors: A randomized controlled trial. *Breast Cancer Research and Treatment, 135,* 799–809. doi:10.1007/s10549-012-2210-6

Von Ah, D., & Tallman, E.F. (2015). Perceived cognitive function in breast cancer survivors: Evaluating relationships with objective cognitive performance and other symptoms using the Functional Assessment of Cancer Therapy-Cognitive Function instrument. *Journal of Pain and Symptom Management, 49,* 697–706. doi:10.1016/j.jpainsymman.2014.08.012

Wheeler, S.B., Reeder-Hayes, K.E., & Carey, L.A. (2013). Disparities in breast cancer treatment and outcomes: Biological, social, and health system determinants and opportunities for research. *Oncologist, 18,* 986–993. doi:10.1634/theoncologist.2013-0243

Williams, F., & Jeanetta, S.C. (2015). Lived experiences of breast cancer survivors after diagnosis, treatment and beyond: Qualitative study. *Health Expectations, 19,* 631–642. doi:10.1111/hex.12372

Xie, Y., Collins, W.J., Audeh, M.W., Shiao, S.L., Gottlieb, R.A., Goodman, M.T., ... Mehta, P.K. (2015). Breast cancer survivorship and cardiovascular disease: Emerging approaches in cardio-oncology. *Current Treatment Options in Cardiovascular Medicine, 17,* 60. doi:10.1007/s11936-015-0421-y

Zwart, W., Terra, H., Linn, S.C., & Schagen, S.B. (2015). Cognitive effects of endocrine therapy for breast cancer: Keep calm and carry on? *Nature Reviews Clinical Oncology, 12,* 597–606. doi:10.1038/nrclinonc .2015.124

Index

The letter f after a page number indicates that relevant content appears in a figure; the letter t, in a table.

A

absolute risk, 18
Academy of Oncology Nurse and Patient Navigators (AONN), 251, 252
accelerated partial breast irradiation (APBI), 136–137, 137f
accreditation agencies for breast navigation, 228
accreditation measures for comprehensive breast centers, 6–10
  interprofessional breast conferences as, 7–9
  leadership as, 7
  management guidelines as, 9–10
  National Accreditation Program for Breast Centers as, 6–7, 8t–9t
  standards of care as, 7
accreditation review, 14–15
adaptive devices in survivorship care, 265
adenomas, 83
adenosis, nonsclerosing, 83
adherence
  breast navigation and, 247
  to endocrine therapy, 186–187, 187t, 262
  to oral therapies, 262
adjuvant therapy, 156, 157f
administration
  of comprehensive breast center, 4t
  in risk assessment, 43

ado-trastuzumab emtansine, 164–165, 169t
Advisory Board Company Oncology Roundtable, 228
advocacy in breast navigation, 234t
age as risk factor, 20
alcohol consumption as risk factor, 23
alkylating agents
  cardiotoxicity of, 169t
  cutaneous toxicities of, 170t
allogeneic reconstructive procedures, 120–121
alloplastic reconstructive procedures, 120–121
alopecia, chemotherapy-induced, 170–171
ambulatory care, 227
amenorrhea, 202f
amorphous calcifications, 56, 56f
anastrozole, 184
anatomic landmarks, 81
anatomy of breast, 81, 82f
ancillary services, navigation of, 236, 236t
angiolymphatic invasion, 88
anthracyclines
  cardiotoxicity of, 169t
  cutaneous toxicities of, 170t
anticoagulation, 109
antimetabolites
  cardiotoxicity of, 169t
  cutaneous toxicities of, 170t
anti-Müllerian hormone (AMH), 203

antitumor antibiotics
  cardiotoxicity of, 169t
  cutaneous toxicities of, 170t
anxiety, survivorship care for, 269
appearance concerns, survivorship care for, 265
architectural distortion, 58
areola tattoo, 121, 122f
arm volume, objective assessment of, 194–195, 194f, 195f
aromatase inhibitors (AIs), 180t, 183–185
  anastrozole as, 184
  exemestane as, 184
  letrozole as, 184–185
  for prevention, 37
asymmetries, 58, 59f–60f
ataxia telangiectasia, 29t
ATM gene, 29t
attitudes as barrier to care, 243t
atypia, proliferative lesions with, 84
atypical ductal hyperplasia, 84
autologous reconstructive procedures, 119–120
autosomal hereditary breast cancer syndrome, 28, 28t–32t
axilla, evaluation of, 109–110
axillary node dissection, 93–94, 110, 111
  brachial plexopathy due to, 200
  total mastectomy with, 113–114

D